Challenging Cases in Pediatric Diagnosis

CASES FROM *PEDIATRICS IN REVIEW* INDEX OF SUSPICION AND VISUAL DIAGNOSIS

EDITOR
DEEPAK KAMAT, MD, PhD, FAAP

American Academy of Pediatrics
DEDICATED TO THE HEALTH OF ALL CHILDREN®

American Academy of Pediatrics Publishing Staff

Mark Grimes, *Director, Department of Publishing*

Mary Lou White, *Director, Department of Marketing and Sales*

Peter Lynch, *Manager, Digital Strategy and Product Development*

Shannan Martin, *Publishing and Production Services Specialist*

Amanda Helmholz, *Editorial Specialist*

Peg Mulcahy, *Manager, Art Direction and Production*

Linda Smessaert, *Brand Manager, Clinical and Professional Publications*

Published by the American Academy of Pediatrics
141 Northwest Point Blvd
Elk Grove Village, IL 60007-1019
Telephone: 847/434-4000
Facsimile: 847/434-8000
www.aap.org

First edition published 2016.

Printed in the United States of America

9-374 1 2 3 4 5 6 7 8 9 10

MA0749

ISBN: 978-1-61002-016-9

eBook: 978-1-61002-017-6

Library of Congress Control Number: 2015956184

Contents

PART 14. OBSTETRICS AND GYNECOLOGY

PART 15. OPHTHALMOLOGY

PART 16. ORTHOPEDICS

PART 17. SURGERY

PART 18. UROLOGY

Preface

It is with great honor and immense pleasure I present to you *Challenging Cases in Pediatric Diagnosis.* I am indebted to Lawrence Nazarian, MD, FAAP, former editor in chief of *Pediatrics in Review,* for appointing me editor for the Index of Suspicion section of *Pediatrics in Review.* He is an outstanding mentor and great role model.

In this book, we present 90 cases from Index of Suspicion and 10 cases from Visual Diagnosis that have been published since the year 2000. My sincere thanks to Joseph Zenel, MD, FAAP, editor in chief, and Hugh Allen, MD, deputy editor, *Pediatrics in Review,* for helping me select the 10 cases from Visual Diagnosis that have been included. Since the year 2000 through 2014, 574 cases have been published in Index of Suspicion and 70 cases, in Visual Diagnosis. The Index of Suspicion cases that I selected were ones that I believed to be true diagnostic challenges, in that they covered either rare conditions or unusual clinical manifestations of common conditions. We have presented cases as they were originally published in *Pediatrics in Review.* Because some of the cases were published as early as 2000, wherever we felt that the information regarding evaluation or management of a particular case or condition may have been outdated, we sought expert input to update the information; the expert comments are published immediately following the case.

During the 6 years in which I have served as editor for the Index of Suspicion, I have had the pleasure of interacting with large numbers of medical students, residents, fellows, practicing pediatricians, faculty in academic institutions at all levels in their careers, and nurse practitioners from all over the world. The quality of writing and scientific content of cases submitted has been very variable, and it has been a gratifying experience mentoring the "inexperienced" writers and creating a wonderful educational product.

As Dr Nazarian said in his introduction to *Challenges in Pediatric Diagnosis* (the book that inspired this one), we, the physicians, learn best from our experiences and interactions with our patients. I hope this book will be useful to both the learners and trainers at all levels of clinical practice and training to provide the best possible care to our patients.

My sincere thanks to Mr Peter Lynch, manager, digital strategy and product development, American Academy of Pediatrics, for helping me put together the book. I wish to thank Dr Joseph Zenel, editor in chief, *Pediatrics in Review;* Ms Luann Zanzola, managing editor, *Pediatrics in Review;* and Ms Sara Strand, editorial associate, *Pediatrics in Review,* for their support and encouragement. I could not have done this without the support of my wife, Dr Ambika Mathur, and my children, Amol and Aarti, for putting up with me as I worked late nights and weekends, editing to meet the deadlines for finalizing the cases for publication. I would like to extend my sincere thanks to all the authors for submitting their interesting and challenging cases so that we can all learn from their experiences.

And, finally, I would like express my sincere gratitude to all our patients and their families for teaching us so that we can be better at what we do: take care of children.

Part 1

Autoimmune

CHAPTER 1

Growth Failure and Diarrhea in a 6-Week-Old

Presentation

A 6-week-old term boy is admitted to the hospital for a 3-week history of growth failure and diarrhea. At age 36 days, he had been admitted for vomiting and diarrhea, at which time abdominal ultrasonography was negative for pyloric stenosis and other abnormalities. An upper gastrointestinal (GI) series showed GI reflux to the thoracic inlet, but findings were otherwise normal. Blood, stool, and urine culture results were negative. He continued on exclusive breastfeeding, gained weight, and was discharged with the diagnosis of GI reflux and an antireflux medication. Now, he is readmitted for increased diarrhea, decreased interest in feedings, and weight loss.

Physical examination reveals a small, wasted infant who is alert and has a weight of 3.3 kg (<3rd percentile), length of 53 cm (10th percentile), and head circumference of 39 cm (50th percentile). No dysmorphic features are evident, but facial and temporal wasting and a large, soft, flat fontanelle are present. His abdomen is scaphoid without organomegaly, and his extremities show decreased subcutaneous fat and loose skin. He has no abnormal pulmonary or cardiovascular findings. Despite suspension of oral feedings, the baby continues to pass more than 6 loose, watery stools daily. Repeated viral and bacterial stool cultures are negative. Additional evaluation reveals the diagnosis.

- **What is your differential diagnosis at this point?**
- **Are there any elements of history or physical examination that would help you?**
- **What additional diagnostic studies would you like performed?**

Discussion

This infant presented with the common complaint of diarrhea. However, his presentation became complicated by weight loss and continuation of the diarrhea. The evaluation began by ruling out the most likely causes, including infections. His stool was analyzed for pH, reducing substances, fecal fats, elastase, trypsin, and alpha$_1$-antitrypsin to assess for malabsorption. Immunoglobulins were measured, and human immunodeficiency virus testing was performed. Urine organic acid and plasma amino acid values were normal.

He was given an elemental formula, but his diarrhea persisted, and he was taken off of feedings to distinguish between osmotic and secretory diarrhea. The diarrhea and weight loss continued. Esophagogastroduodenoscopy and flexible sigmoidoscopy with biopsies were performed. Biopsies showed marked chronic active enteritis with severe villous blunting and lymphocytic infiltrate. In this age group, such findings are consistent with autoimmune processes or severe allergy. Antienterocyte antibodies were found in his blood, and autoimmune enteropathy was diagnosed.

Making the Diagnosis

The term *protracted* (or intractable) diarrhea of infancy was described in 1968 as diarrhea lasting longer than 2 weeks in an infant younger than 3 months who does not have infection (>3 negative stool cultures). At this time in history, affected patients experienced a high mortality rate, and the cause remained unknown in many cases.

With the advancement of parenteral nutrition and improved diagnostic tools, it has become possible to diagnose more causes of protracted diarrhea. The term is used now to describe infants who have prolonged diarrhea unresponsive to conventional therapy, and the differential diagnosis includes a heterogeneous group of disorders. When presented with an infant experiencing prolonged diarrhea, the physician must take into account diet, exposures, birth history, and growth. Infectious causes and immunodeficiencies must be ruled out.

Prolonged diarrhea can be divided into secretory and osmotic types. Osmotic diarrhea occurs when digestion or absorption is impaired, resulting in unabsorbed nutrients remaining in the lumen of the gut. Osmotic diarrhea tends to be associated with a lower pH and produces positive reducing substances on stool studies. The diarrhea stops when enteral feedings stop. Osmotic disorders include congenital lactase deficiency, sucrase-isomaltase deficiency, lipase deficiency, and glucose-galactose malabsorption. Secretory diarrhea is characterized by large volumes of watery stool resulting from secretion by enterocytes of more electrolytes and water into the intestinal lumen. Electrolyte testing of the stool reveals normal osmolality, with stool sodium concentration greater than 70 mEq/L (70 mmol/L). The stools persist despite removal of food.

Esophagogastroduodenoscopy and flexible sigmoidoscopy with biopsies should be performed in cases of protracted diarrhea. Microscopic examination of tissue is necessary to determine whether villous atrophy and inflammatory cells are present. Conditions that have normal villus architecture include transport defects such as congenital chloride and congenital sodium diarrhea, congenital carbohydrate malabsorptive disorders, congenital bile acid malabsorption, and deficiencies of micronutrients such as zinc.

Several disorders can manifest villous atrophy and can be categorized further by the presence or absence of inflammatory cells. Microvillus inclusion disease and tufting enteropathy are examples of structural enteropathies (disorders having villous atrophy but no inflammatory cells). Electron microscopy is needed for definitive diagnosis of the 2 entities. Causes of protracted diarrhea of infancy associated with villous atrophy and inflammatory cells on histologic examination are considered inflammatory or immune mediated. The differential diagnosis includes infectious or postinfectious enteropathy, allergic enteropathy, and, less commonly, autoimmune enteropathy.

The Condition

Autoimmune enteropathy is a rare condition; only a few hundred cases have been reported. Affected patients undergo extensive evaluation in the pursuit of a diagnosis. In the initial evaluation, allergic enteropathy is high among the differential diagnoses because it is a much more common process. However, infants with autoimmune enteropathy continue to have diarrhea despite food withdrawal and cannot tolerate even elemental formulas. This feature should make the physician pursue another diagnosis.

Autoimmune enteropathy is a heterogeneous disorder that is characterized by protracted diarrhea in infancy that continues despite withdrawal of feedings as well as the presence of circulating autoantibodies to enterocytes. Affected patients have normal immunoglobulin concentrations and white blood cell counts, but the presence of other circulating autoantibodies and other autoimmune disorders is not uncommon. Biopsies taken from the bowel demonstrate total villous atrophy and marked infiltration with T lymphocytes in the lamina propria. Immunohistochemistry shows increases in $CD3^+$ lymphocytes.

Definitive diagnosis requires testing for autoantibodies to enterocytes by indirect immunofluorescence. As with most tests for rare conditions, only a few centers perform the test. The antibodies are not found in other bowel diseases, such as celiac disease, Crohn disease, or ulcerative colitis. Their role in autoimmune enteropathy is unclear.

Autoimmune enteropathy can be categorized further into 3 types. Type 1, the IPEX syndrome (**i**mmune dysregulation, **p**olyendocrinopathy, **e**nteropathy, **X**-linked), is the most well-defined cause of autoimmune enteropathy and results from a defect in the *FOXP3* gene. It occurs in males and is associated with early diabetes mellitus and eczema. Type 2 occurs in males but is not associated with *FOXP3* mutations or extraintestinal manifestations. Type 3 occurs in females and is often associated with extraintestinal autoimmune manifestations.

Once the diagnosis is made, management consists of nutrition support and immunosuppression. In most cases, affected infants require parenteral nutrition even before the diagnosis is made, a need that continues until enteral intake is adequate. Dietary tolerance is achieved through immunosuppression with systemic steroids. Unfortunately, steroid dependency is the norm, and resistance is common. Other immunosuppressive drugs have been tried in hopes of weaning these infants from steroids. This approach continues to be a source of investigation.

Lessons for the Physician

When presented with an infant who has protracted diarrhea, the most important first step is assessment of nutrition status. Enteral nutrition is preferable, but not uncommonly, hyperalimentation is required and should be initiated even in the absence of a diagnosis. Other important information during the evaluation includes prenatal history, exposures, and dietary history. Infectious causes should be ruled out with viral stool culture and at least 3 negative bacterial stool cultures. Immunodeficiencies must also be excluded. Studies of the composition of the stool are warranted and can help in deciding if dietary changes can be of benefit. If the diarrhea is unresponsive to dietary changes, referral to a gastroenterologist should be made for endoscopy with biopsy and additional management.

Rebecca Scherr, MD, Emory University School of Medicine, Children's Healthcare of Atlanta, GA

COMMENTARY BY DR MOHAMMAD EL-BABA, PEDIATRIC GASTROENTEROLOGIST, CHILDREN'S HOSPITAL OF MICHIGAN

Autoimmune enteropathy (AE), first described in 1982 by Walker-Smith et al, is a rare disorder that typically manifests in the first few weeks of life, although adult-onset cases have been reported. Estimated incidence in children is less than 1/100,000 infants and much of the existing literature is from case reports or small series.

The diagnosis of AE in young infants should be made on the basis of clinical picture and histopathologic findings of the small intestine. Diagnostic criteria include protracted secretory diarrhea that fails to respond to exclusion diets; intestinal villous atrophy and inflammatory infiltration with hyperplastic crypts, with or without other associated autoimmune disease; and absence of severe immunodeficiency. The presence of antienterocyte antibodies is supportive of the diagnosis, but not specific, as they may be found in other inflammatory conditions such as inflammatory bowel diseases and allergic enetritis.

Management of patients with AE can be challenging. Many patients develop malnutrition and require parenteral nutrition and chronic immunosuppressive therapy with corticosteroids, azathioprine, 6-mercaptopurine, cyclosporine, tacrolimus, or mycophenolate. The successful use of biologic therapy such as infliximab and rituximab has recently been reported in patients who were refractory to corticosteroid therapy.

The prognosis is dependent on the extent and severity of gastrointestinal involvement and on the presence of other autoimmune disorders. Patients with AE are at higher risk of infections due to malnutrition, immunosuppressive therapy, and central lines.

Our knowledge of AE remains limited and more research is required to elucidate the pathophysiology and optimal management of the disease.

CHAPTER 2

Fever, Diarrhea, and Rash in a 9-Month-Old Boy

Presentation

A previously healthy 9-month-old boy is brought to the emergency department having 3 days of fever and diarrhea and a rash that appeared today.

Physical examination reveals an alert infant whose vital signs are normal except for a temperature of 101.6°F (38.7°C). A palpable purpuric rash is visible over his face, ears, arms, and legs, but the trunk is spared. The remainder of the examination is unremarkable. Urinalysis is negative for blood or protein. A complete evaluation for sepsis, including lumbar puncture, yields normal findings. Intravenous antibiotics are started.

Over the following days, the fever subsides and the rash starts to clear. Blood and cerebrospinal culture results are sterile, antibiotics are stopped, and the infant is discharged. Two days later he is readmitted because of a flare-up of the rash and the development of tender edema of the right lower extremity with no signs of arthritis. His temperature is 100.2°F (37.9°C), and he looks well. The results of a technetium bone scan are normal. Serologic testing for seasonal viruses gives negative results. Levels of complement and immunoglobulins are normal. A skin biopsy reveals the diagnosis.

- **What is your differential diagnosis at this point?**
- **Are there any elements of history or physical examination that would help you?**
- **What additional diagnostic studies would you like performed?**

Discussion

The skin biopsy revealed leukocytoclastic vasculitis (LCV), prompting the diagnosis of acute hemorrhagic edema of infancy (AHEI). *Leukocytoclastic vasculitis* is a histopathologic term used to denote a small-vessel vasculitis, in which the infiltration of polymorphonuclear white blood cells forms "nuclear dust" (leukocytoclasis).

The Condition

Acute hemorrhagic edema of infancy, or Finkelstein disease, was reported initially by Snow in 1913 and is an acute benign form of LCV occurring in children younger than 2 years. This benign disorder is characterized by the abrupt onset of fever, peripheral edema, and large tender palpable purpuric plaques, typically involving the face, ears, and extremities. Internal organs are usually spared, although renal (hematuria, mild proteinuria) and gastrointestinal (bloody stools) involvement have been reported. Complete recovery usually occurs within 2 to 3 weeks, leaving no sequelae.

Histopathology

The characteristic findings of LCV in skin biopsies are infiltration of blood vessels and perivascular areas by polymorphonuclear white blood cells and eosinophils, with formation of nuclear dust, extravasation of red blood cells, and fibrinoid necrosis of the vessel walls. Immunofluorescence studies have revealed deposition of fibrinogen, complement C_3, IgA, IgM, and IgE. IgA deposits are found only in approximately one-third of the patients, in contrast to Henoch-Schönlein purpura (HSP), in which most of the deposits are composed of IgA.

Pathogenesis

The pathogenesis of AHEI is unknown. The LCV found on skin biopsy is probably mediated by immune complexes. Factors believed to be associated with the condition are bacterial or viral infections (including cytomegalovirus), vaccination, and drug therapy, mostly involving antibiotics.

Differential Diagnosis

The association of fever with a purpuric rash in an infant or child is alarming and requires prompt evaluation. Although a septicemic disease must be ruled out, other conditions should be considered.

Purpura occurs following extravasation of red blood cells into the dermis. Purpura (≥3 mm) or petechiae (≤2 mm) are divided into 2 major groups: palpable and nonpalpable. The causes of nonpalpable purpura include trauma, clotting disorders (thrombocytopenia, abnormal platelet function), capillary fragility, and the formation of thrombi (disseminated intravascular coagulation, purpura fulminans).

Palpable purpuras are subdivided further into those having embolic and vasculitic causes. Embolic lesions are usually irregular in outline, indicative of a cutaneous infarct that corresponds in size to the area of the skin receiving blood supply from an arteriole. Most infectious emboli are due to gram-negative cocci such as *Neisseria meningitidis* (meningococcemia) and *Neisseria gonorrhoeae* (disseminated gonococcal infection), but other bacteria have been implicated (Enterobacteriaceae and staphylococci). In these cases, organisms can sometimes be recovered from the lesions. An additional cause is rickettsiae (Rocky Mountain spotted fever). Rarely, infection with *Pseudomonas aeruginosa* causes a condition termed *ecthyma gangrenosum,* the lesions of which begin as edematous erythematous papules or plaques and then develop central purpura and necrosis.

Leukocytoclastic vasculitis is the most common vasculitic disorder. The lesions are circular because the red blood cells diffuse from postcapillary venules evenly as a result of inflammation. The most common LCV is HSP. Although some authors identify AHEI as a variant of HSP, most agree that it is a distinct disorder. Acute hemorrhagic edema of infancy occurs in younger children; edema is more prominent, fever is more common, and internal organ involvement and long-term complications are rare. The distribution of the rash also differs. In AHEI, there are large palpable purpuric lesions, sometimes with central clearing (targetlike) on the face, ears, and upper and lower extremities. The lesions of HSP are smaller and polymorphic and usually involve the extensor surfaces of the legs and the buttocks.

Besides HSP and AHEI, other vasculitic conditions include polyarteritis nodosa, serum sickness, and Sweet syndrome.

Nonvasculitic conditions that can be confused with AHEI are hypersensitivity phenomena such as urticarial vasculitis, angioedema, and erythema multiforme, the lesions of which are targetlike papules with an erythematous outer border, an inner pale ring, and a dusky purple center. The rash is symmetric and involves primarily the extensor surfaces of the upper extremities. Lesions are sparse on the face, trunk, and legs. Biopsy findings comprise perivascular and interstitial mononuclear infiltrates.

Lessons for the Physician

The occurrence of a purpuric rash associated with fever should always alert the physician to the possibility of a life-threatening disease such as meningococcemia. Evaluation for sepsis and prompt antibiotic treatment should not be deferred. However, when an infant or young child has the typical presentation of acute hemorrhagic edema of infancy, that condition should be considered. A skin biopsy should be obtained to confirm the diagnosis of this benign disorder, which is self-limited and requires no specific treatment.

Galia Barkai, MD, and Levana Sinai, MD, Kaplan Medical Center, Rehovot, Israel

CHAPTER 3

Recurrent Fevers in a 10-Year-Old Girl

Presentation

A 10-year-old Hispanic girl presents with a history of recurrent fevers (temperature up to 104.0°F [40.0°C]) over the past 4 years. She has had 4 to 5 episodes of fever, each lasting 1 to 2 weeks. The episodes are accompanied by chills, malaise, periorbital swelling, rash, myalgias, arthralgias, and diffuse abdominal pain. She denies weight loss, night sweats, and oral or genital ulcers. Medical and family histories are noncontributory.

Physical examination reveals a well-nourished girl who has a temperature of 102.2°F (39.0°C), heart rate of 130 beats/min, respiratory rate of 20 breaths/min, and blood pressure of 101/64 mm Hg. Erythematous, nonpruritic, polymorphous, blanching maculopapular lesions of 0.5 to 3 cm in size are apparent on her trunk and upper extremities. The rest of her physical findings are normal.

Her hemoglobin level is 10.7 g/dL (107 g/L), white blood cell count is 13.24 × 10^3/mcL (13.24 × 10^9/L) (54% neutrophils, 2% bands, 30% lymphocytes, 14% monocytes), and platelet count is 424 × 10^3/mcL (424 × 10^9/L). Her C-reactive protein value is 15.1 mg/dL (143.8 nmol/L), and erythrocyte sedimentation rate is 82 mm/h. Results of her liver function tests, pancreatic enzymes panel, urine protein to creatinine ratio, and serum complement assessments are normal. The antinuclear antibody, antibody to double-stranded DNA, antinuclear cytoplasmic antibody, and direct Coombs tests show negative results. Quantitative serum immunoglobulin concentrations, including serum IgD, are normal. A computed tomography scan of the abdomen and pelvis is read as normal. Additional laboratory evaluation establishes the diagnosis.

- **What is your differential diagnosis at this point?**
- **Are there any elements of history or physical examination that would help you?**
- **What additional diagnostic studies would you like performed?**

Discussion

Genetic testing for the tumor necrosis factor (TNF) receptor abnormality (*TNFRSF1A* gene mutation) was positive, and the diagnosis of TNF receptor–associated periodic fever syndrome (TRAPS) was established.

Differential Diagnosis

Periodic fever syndromes are characterized by distinct febrile episodes that occur in a predictable frequency, often with associated symptoms and signs.

Infectious causes are the most common source of periodic fevers, generally in the form of recurrent viral upper respiratory tract infections. If there is exposure to brucellosis or borreliosis, these infectious diseases should be considered. Brucellosis (undulant fever) is contracted by ingestion of contaminated or unpasteurized milk products. Affected patients present with weight loss, abdominal pain, lymphadenopathy, hepatosplenomegaly, chronic monoarthritis, and skin manifestations ranging from erythema nodosum to ulcerative lesions.

Infection with *Borrelia recurrentis,* which causes relapsing fever, is transmitted by ticks or lice. Onset in these cases is sudden, and symptoms include photophobia, headache, myalgia, arthralgia, an erythematous macular rash, meningeal signs, and cranial neuropathy.

Rheumatic and inflammatory disorders that can present with recurrent febrile episodes include Crohn disease, sarcoidosis, systemic inflammatory arthritis, and Behçet disease. Cyclic neutropenia manifests as febrile episodes of 3 to 10 days' duration with associated absolute neutrophil counts of less than 200/mcL (0.20×10^9/L). Fevers in cyclic neutropenia may occur independent of concomitant infection, although the propensity for infection is high. Periodic fever with aphthous stomatitis, pharyngitis, and adenitis syndrome is a benign condition, with episodes generally occurring every month and onset before age 5 years.

Hereditary recurrent fever syndromes are a class of autoinflammatory syndromes that manifest with periodic fever and characteristic clinical findings. Familial Mediterranean fever is an autosomal recessive illness characterized by bouts of fever, serositis, synovitis, and rash and can result in systemic amyloidosis. Familial Mediterranean fever attacks last 1 to 3 days. Abdominal symptoms range from mild discomfort to severe pain. The characteristic exanthem consists of erysipeloid, erythematous lesions on the dorsal surface of the lower extremities. Hyper-IgD with periodic fever syndrome is an autosomal recessive disease resulting from abnormalities in mevalonate kinase enzyme activity. Attacks occur every 1 to 3 months, are heralded by high fevers with chills and abdominal symptoms, and can be precipitated by environmental stressors such as immunizations or viral illnesses. Clinical manifestations last 3 to 7 days and include a nonmigratory maculopapular rash, headache, splenomegaly, and cervical adenopathy. Oral and vaginal ulcers may be present during an acute attack.

The Condition

Tumor necrosis factor receptor–associated periodic fever syndrome, also known as familial Hibernian fever, is an autosomal dominant autoinflammatory disease with incomplete penetrance. More than 50 mutations in the *TNFR1* gene have been identified. The TNF receptor is widely expressed on cell surfaces, mediating a number of proinflammatory effects. Mutations in the receptor result in repeated signaling and prolongation of the inflammatory response. Originally described in patients of Irish and Scottish descent, the syndrome occurs in people from a broad range of ethnic backgrounds. It is the second most common periodic fever disorder, with a median age of onset at 3 to 5 years.

Clinical manifestations are similar to those of familial Mediterranean fever, with fevers often accompanied by abdominal pain, arthralgia, cutaneous vasculitis, and migratory myalgias. The dreaded complication of amyloidosis occurs in 8% to 10% of patients. Episodes generally last 1 to 4 weeks and, as in hyper-IgD with periodic fever syndrome, may be precipitated by illness or environmental stressors. A distinctive feature of TRAPS is ocular inflammation, which manifests as a nonpurulent conjunctivitis or periorbital edema. Serum concentrations of complements, inflammatory markers, and amyloid protein are elevated. Genetic testing for mutations of the TNF receptor gene is diagnostic.

Amyloidosis is the most severe complication of TRAPS, with the prognosis directly related to the development of amyloidosis. This complication generally manifests later in life. Risk factors include mutations involving the cysteine residues of *TNFRSF1A* and a positive family history. Other genetic and environmental factors may also modulate susceptibility to amyloidogenesis. Amyloidosis results from a sequence of changes in protein folding that leads to the deposition of insoluble amyloid fibrils in the extracellular spaces of organs and tissues. Amyloidosis in patients who have TRAPS generally presents as nephrosis. Renal disease ranges from proteinuria to renal failure and is usually irreversible. Cardiac amyloidosis can present with congestive failure and fatal arrhythmias. Although hepatic involvement is common, liver function abnormalities are minimal and generally occur late in the disease. Neurologic, gastrointestinal, respiratory, cutaneous, and endocrine involvement may also occur.

Treatment and Prognosis

Preventing recurrent attacks and reducing the risk for developing amyloidosis are the goals of therapy. Treatment is guided by severity of disease. Commonly used drugs include prednisone and etanercept. Etanercept is a pharmacological agent that is composed of human soluble TNF receptor and the Fc component of IgG1 and is produced by recombinant DNA technology. It binds TNF and thus downregulates the proinflammatory effects mediated by TNF. Etanercept has reduced the acute-phase response and corticosteroid requirement in patients who have TRAPS and amyloidosis. Its use has been recommended for patients born with mutations that are highly associated with renal amyloid disease. Another agent recently being used is anakinra, a recombinant human IL-1 receptor antagonist.

Average survival in familial amyloid disease is 7 to 15 years, with major causes of death generally attributed to arrhythmias and progressive cardiac and renal failure. The use of hemodialysis, transplantation, and etanercept has improved the prognosis for patients having renal amyloidosis.

Follow-up

This patient has had additional self-limited bouts of fever, abdominal pain, and exanthems but has not developed signs of amyloidosis. Currently, she is receiving corticosteroids only when she develops fever and abdominal pain. Etanercept therapy has not been used because of the relative infrequency of her attacks and her lack of a mutation associated with increased risk of amyloidosis.

Lessons for the Physician

Although fever is common in children, periodic fever can present a diagnostic challenge to physicians. The autoinflammatory hereditary fever syndromes should be considered in patients who experience recurrent fevers and associated manifestations, such as abdominal pain, pleuritis, synovitis, rash, and elevated concentrations of inflammatory markers. Early diagnosis is important because prompt initiation of therapy may prevent complications and reduce morbidity. Tumor necrosis factor receptor–associated periodic fever syndrome is an important condition to entertain in the differential diagnosis of periodic fever, and close monitoring for the development of amyloidosis is essential in affected patients.

Nicole Rizkalla, MD, and Edward Hu, MD, Children's Hospital of Los Angeles, CA

COMMENTARY BY DR MATTHEW ADAMS, PEDIATRIC RHEUMATOLOGIST, CHILDREN'S HOSPITAL OF MICHIGAN

Up to 90 known mutations in the *TNFRSF1A* on 12p13 can cause tumor necrosis factor receptor–associated periodic syndrome. Many involve cysteine residues and are thought to be involved in protein folding. Colchicine doesn't prevent amyloidosis in tumor necrosis factor receptor–associated periodic syndrome as it does in familial Mediterranean fever.

CHAPTER 4

Increasing Fatigue, Dyspnea on Exertion, and a 3.6-kg Weight Loss in a 14-Year-Old Boy

Presentation

A 14-year-old boy is sent to the emergency department by his pediatrician because of a 2-month history of increasing fatigue, dyspnea on exertion, and a 3.6-kg weight loss. A chest radiograph performed yesterday shows bilateral patchy infiltrates. He denies fever, vomiting, diarrhea, changes in appetite, or feeling light-headed. The boy recently visited Puerto Rico for 10 days and works in a dog kennel on weekends. He has had no significant past illnesses and does not take any medications on a regular basis.

On physical examination, his temperature is 97.6°F (36.4°C), heart rate is 102 beats/min, respiratory rate is 20 breaths/min, and blood pressure is 114/68 mm Hg. There are diminished breath sounds bilaterally throughout his lung fields, but he has no respiratory distress. His oxygen saturation is 92% on room air.

The boy's white blood cell count is 6.8 × 10^3/mcL (6.8 × 10^9/L), hemoglobin value is 16.1 g/dL (161 g/L), hematocrit is 45.6% (0.456), and platelet count is 283 × 10^3/mcL (283 × 10^9/L). Electrolyte concentrations, liver function tests, and protein and albumin concentrations are within reference range. Blood glucose concentration is 92 mg/dL (5.1 mmol/L), calcium is 12.4 mg/dL (3.1 mmol/L), and ionized calcium is 5.6 mg/dL (1.4 mmol/L). His erythrocyte sedimentation rate is 3 mm/h. A computed tomography scan of his chest reveals bilateral ground-glass opacities with prominent mediastinal and hilar lymph nodes bilaterally. He is admitted to the hospital for intravenous hydration, treatment of his hypercalcemia and oxygen requirement, and additional evaluation of his pulmonary disease.

- **What is your differential diagnosis at this point?**
- **Are there any elements of history or physical examination that would help you?**
- **What additional diagnostic studies would you like performed?**

Discussion

An extensive infectious evaluation revealed no evidence of bacterial infection, *Mycoplasma* or *Legionella* infection, or viral infection, including Epstein-Barr virus, cytomegalovirus, and human immunodeficiency virus. An endocrinologic evaluation failed to identify a cause for his hypercalcemia. No evidence of malignancy was found.

The boy's pulmonary function tests (PFTs) showed a restrictive pattern, including a forced expiratory volume in 1 second (FEV_1) and forced vital capacity (FVC) at 58% of predicted value. The FEV_1:FVC ratio was 100%, correlating with his restrictive pattern. His angiotensin-converting enzyme level was elevated at 196 IU/L (reference range, 18–90 IU/L), and a bronchial biopsy obtained during bronchoscopy showed multiple noncaseating coalescing granulomas suggestive of sarcoidosis. He was started on oral prednisone (1 mg/kg/d). He required a short stay in the intensive care unit to control his hypercalcemia (ionized calcium level rose to 7.9 mg/dL [2 mmol/L]) and oxygen requirement.

Repeat PFTs showed significant improvement less than 1 week after the initiation of corticosteroids. The FVC and FEV_1 improved to 72% and 68% of predicted values, respectively, and the FEV_1:FVC ratio was 94% of its predicted value. He was discharged from the hospital on hospital day 11 and instructed to follow up with a pediatric pulmonologist and pediatric rheumatologist. He will continue daily steroids while having his PFTs monitored serially. The goal is to taper his maintenance steroid dosing to an every-other-day regimen. Pulse high-dose steroids along with methotrexate was considered, but it was decided to pursue the more classic treatment of corticosteroids dosed conventionally.

The Condition

Sarcoidosis is a generalized inflammatory process that most often affects the lungs but can involve almost any body system, including the skin, eyes, kidneys, lymphatics, and heart. In one series, 75% of patients had multisystem involvement. In infants, sarcoidosis typically presents with skin involvement (including erythema nodosum) and joint and eye disease. In older children and adolescents, sarcoidosis tends to affect the pulmonary system, lymphatics, and eyes (uveitis) more frequently.

Clinical features of sarcoidosis vary and depend on the specific organ systems involved. This patient displayed the classic findings of a restrictive pattern on PFTs, although he had no eye findings typical of uveitis or rash characteristic of cutaneous sarcoidosis.

Sarcoidosis can be staged by the following criteria: stage I is defined as the presence of hilar lymphadenopathy on radiographs without parenchymal infiltrates, stage II includes pulmonary infiltrates, and stage III is defined as infiltrates without lymphadenopathy.

The pathogenesis of sarcoidosis remains obscure, primarily because of the variety of manifestations it can produce. Both environmental and genetic factors have been linked to the condition. Infectious agents, chemicals, drugs, autoimmune factors, and genetic factors have all been explored as potential causes of the disease. The current belief is that sarcoidosis represents the exposure of a genetically susceptible individual to a specific environmental agent that triggers an exaggerated cellular immune response. Sarcoidosis most commonly affects young adults and in the United States occurs more frequently in African Americans.

Pathologic Findings

Sarcoidosis is characterized by a focused, overwhelming inflammatory response to an unknown antigen. The noncaseating granuloma is the classic pathologic finding. The pathogenesis of the granuloma includes accumulation of mononuclear inflammatory cells in the target organ, following which macrophages aggregate and differentiate into epithelioid and multinucleated cells. Activated lymphocytes and macrophages within the granuloma release mediators, including IL-1, IL-2, interferon, and other cytokines that promote and maintain the granulomatous lesion. During active disease, lymphocytes in the granulomas are predominantly helper T (CD4) lymphocytes.

Three processes have been identified in the initiation of sarcoidosis: exposure to antigen, cellular immunity directed against the antigen mediated through antigen-presenting cells and antigen-specific T lymphocytes, and the appearance of immune cells that produce a nonspecific immune response. This extensive inflammation often results in fibrosis, as with pulmonary sarcoidosis.

Differential Diagnosis

Sarcoidosis is a diagnosis of exclusion. Because no specific test confirms the diagnosis, other causes of granulomatous disease must be ruled out. Tuberculosis, chronic beryllium disease, hypersensitivity pneumonitis, pulmonary alveolar proteinosis, Wegener granulomatosis, and other conditions must be considered when evaluating a patient who has granulomatous disease with diffuse pulmonary involvement.

Clues to the diagnosis of sarcoidosis include an elevated angiotensin-converting enzyme level, hypercalcemia (33% of patients), uveitis, elevated erythrocyte sedimentation rate, hyperproteinemia, eosinophilia, and a diffuse pulmonary process.

Treatment

The mainstay of treatment is oral corticosteroids, with the dose and duration of treatment tailored to the individual because absolute guidelines regarding steroid use are not available. Initial dosing is 1 mg/kg/d and may be tapered according to clinical response. Duration of therapy is based on an individual patient's response to therapy. Corticosteroid therapy has been associated with improvements in dyspnea, PFTs, and the appearance of the chest radiograph, as well as suppression of granuloma formation. However, evidence that corticosteroids can prevent long-term pulmonary fibrosis does not exist, and adverse effects often limit their usefulness.

Second-line therapy is with immunosuppressants and cytotoxic agents, including methotrexate, hydroxychloroquine, azathioprine, and antitumor necrosis factor drugs (etanercept and infliximab). Of these agents, methotrexate is the best studied and has been found to reduce the need for corticosteroid therapy as well as to delay the decline in PFT parameters, such as the FEV_1 and diffusing capacity of carbon monoxide. One limitation of methotrexate is hepatotoxicity, which is minimized when folic acid supplementation is provided.

Other therapies are useful in treating specific symptoms of sarcoidosis: nonsteroidal anti-inflammatory drugs for erythema nodosum, joint involvement, and fevers; topical corticosteroids for mild cases of erythema nodosum; ophthalmic corticosteroids for prevention of permanent damage in suspected cases of uveitis; hydroxychloroquine for cutaneous sarcoidosis unresponsive to steroids and for hypercalcemia; and implantable defibrillators for cardiac sequelae. In general, therapy for a patient who has sarcoidosis requires a multidisciplinary approach, which can involve primary care physicians, pulmonologists, rheumatologists, dermatologists, ophthalmologists, cardiologists, and neurologists.

Prognosis

More than 60% of patients with sarcoidosis have a good prognosis; they do not require therapy and their disease remits spontaneously. Poor prognostic indicators include advanced staging by chest radiographs, cardiac or neurologic disease, and pulmonary hypertension. Of these, the initial stage is the most important prognostic factor: 95% of patients who have stage I disease are asymptomatic at 5 years compared with 25% of patients who have stage III disease. In general, asymptomatic patients undergo spontaneous resolution of their disease, while symptomatic patients tend toward multisystem involvement and chronic disease, with irreversible sequelae in up to 20% of cases.

Sarcoidosis in children and adolescents usually carries a better prognosis than in adults. However, children who have early-onset sarcoidosis with eye, joint, or skin involvement carry a guarded prognosis; most experience a chronic course and multiple irreversible sequelae. Determining the prognosis for a patient who has sarcoidosis must involve screening for multiorgan disease, using scales such as the ACCESS Organ Assessment Instrument as well as determining the effect of pulmonary, systemic, and cutaneous symptoms on the patient's perceived quality of life.

Lessons for the Physician

Sarcoidosis remains an unusual disease in children and adolescents but must be considered when evaluating a patient who has a diffuse pulmonary process that cannot be explained by other causes. Sarcoidosis can present with involvement of almost any organ system but most commonly involves the lungs, lymphatics, eyes, and skin in children. Consultation with a pediatric pulmonologist, rheumatologist, and ophthalmologist should be considered when the diagnosis is a possibility.

Michael Wolf, MD, and Sibel Algon, MD, Bristol Myers Squibb Children's Hospital/UMDNJ-Robert Wood Johnson University Hospital, New Brunswick, NJ

CHAPTER 5

Right-Sided Lower Back and Lower Quadrant Abdominal Pain and Intermittent Hematuria

Presentation

A 14-year-old boy has experienced right-sided lower back and lower quadrant abdominal pain and intermittent hematuria for 3 months. The pain is colicky, poorly localized, and does not radiate to the groin. He has a history of weight loss and decreased appetite but no dysuria, increased urinary frequency, or fever. There is no history of taking medications, exposure to tuberculosis, prior surgery, trauma to the abdomen, urinary tract infection, or foreign travel. Family history is negative for collagen vascular diseases, kidney stones, and malignancy.

Findings on physical examination are unremarkable except for tenderness at the right costovertebral angle. An abdominal radiograph shows normal findings. Abdominal ultrasonography reveals right-sided hydronephrosis with pyelocalyceal dilatation. Urinalysis shows abundant red blood cells but no protein, casts, or crystals. Complete blood cell count, electrolyte and comprehensive blood chemistry levels, liver function tests, thyroid functions, and lipid profiles are within reference range. The erythrocyte sedimentation rate (Westergren) is 98 mm/h. A tuberculin test is negative. Cultures for bacteria and mycobacteria grow nothing. Antinuclear antibody, anti–double-stranded DNA antibody, rheumatoid factor, antineutrophil cytoplasmic antibodies (both cytoplasmic and perinuclear), antimitochondrial antibody, thyroglobulin antibody, antiperoxidase antibody, anti-Ro antibody, and anti-Jo antibody are absent. An additional diagnostic procedure is performed.

- **What is your differential diagnosis at this point?**
- **Are there any elements of history or physical examination that would help you?**
- **What additional diagnostic studies would you like performed?**

Discussion

A computed tomography scan of the abdomen demonstrated an extensive, ill-defined soft-tissue density in the right perirenal space, anterior to the right psoas muscle, and marked right-sided hydronephrosis with pyelocalyceal dilatation. This finding is consistent with unilateral localized retroperitoneal fibrosis (RPF).

The Condition

Retroperitoneal fibrosis is an uncommon clinical entity that is being recognized with increasing frequency. It is characterized by fibrosis or chronic inflammation of the normal tissue of the retroperitoneum. The fibrotic process may spread contiguously to involve multiple structures and usually causes ureteral obstruction with subsequent development of renal insufficiency.

The available evidence suggests strongly that idiopathic RPF represents an immunologic hypersensitivity disorder. A number of conditions are reported to be associated with RPF, including scleroderma, systemic lupus erythematosus, polyarteritis nodosa, ankylosing spondylitis, sclerosing cholangitis, thyroiditis, primary biliary cirrhosis, inflammatory bowel diseases, amyloidosis, histiocytosis, tuberculosis, radiation therapy, prior surgery, trauma, retroperitoneal hemorrhage, urinary extravasations, and medications such as methysergide, β-blockers, and pergolide.

Pathologic Findings

Macroscopically, RPF appears as a gray-white fibrous plaque, usually arising between the level of the lower aorta and the common iliac arteries in the retroperitoneal space. Microscopically, a mixture of lymphocytes, eosinophils, polymorphonuclear white blood cells, and other inflammatory cells is seen at an early stage. As the disease progresses, the process can become acellular, manifesting only diffuse fibrosis.

Clinical Features

The signs and symptoms of RPF are nonspecific and are related to entrapment and compression of retroperitoneal structures. The most common symptom is poorly localized back pain. Other clinical features include anorexia, fatigue, weight loss, mild fever, and malaise. The diagnosis usually is made late after the development of hydronephrosis. There has been one case report of renal vein obstruction and gross hematuria due to RPF.

Differential Diagnosis

Unilateral hydronephrosis caused by clinically significant obstruction at the ureteropelvic junction is encountered commonly in children and adolescents. Ureteropelvic junction obstruction is caused by either intrinsic or extrinsic factors. Intrinsic factors include absence or reduction of smooth muscle at the ureteropelvic junction, ureteral valves, ureteral polyps, or ureteral leiomyoma. Extrinsic causes include aberrant blood vessels, inflammatory processes leading to fibrous bands, postsurgical stricture, or entrapment due to RPF. Rarer causes of ureteral obstruction include calculi, ureterocele, extrinsic compression secondary to neoplasia (neuroblastoma, lymphoma, or other pelvic tumor), and inflammatory conditions (such as Crohn disease) or chronic granulomatous diseases (such as tuberculosis). Dilatation of the ureter may be associated with vesicoureteral reflux disease without any obstruction being present.

The differential diagnosis of lower back pain in older children and adolescents includes bad posture, lumbar kyphosis, diskitis, tuberculous spondylitis, vertebral osteomyelitis, paraspinal abscess, and bone tumors. Lower back pain can result from vertebral collapse and compression caused by leukemia, eosinophilic granuloma, or osteoporosis due to chronic steroid use. Common bone disorders that can present with back pain are aneurysmal bone cyst, osteoid osteoma, Ewing sarcoma, neuroblastoma, lymphoma, leukemia, hemangioma, fibrous dysplasia, and giant cell tumor. Rarer causes of back pain in older children include herniated intervertebral disk, spondylolisthesis, spondylolysis, and ankylosing spondylitis.

Radiologic Diagnosis

Previously, RPF was diagnosed by intravenous urography, which demonstrated the triad of medial deviation of the ureters, extrinsic compression, and hydronephrosis. However, these patterns are nonspecific. Ureteral tumors, inflammatory processes, and adenopathy can mimic RPF. On ultrasonography, RPF appears as a retroperitoneal, hypoechoic, ill-defined mass. Computed tomography and magnetic resonance imaging are the modalities of choice for evaluating the extent of the process. On unenhanced computed tomography, RPF appears as a plaque, isodense with muscle, which encases the aorta and inferior vena cava without causing displacement and usually spreads laterally to incorporate the ureters. After administration of intravenous contrast medium, the plaque shows variable degrees of enhancement, depending on the stage of the fibrotic process. The advantage of magnetic resonance imaging is its ability to provide better anatomic details of the RPF.

Treatment

The primary goal of therapy is to relieve the urinary obstruction. Surgical ureterolysis is the treatment of choice. Because studies indicate that idiopathic RPF is an immunologic condition involving the actions of T cells, agents such as corticosteroids, tamoxifen, cyclosporine, and azathioprine are used for additional treatment. Some reports state that tamoxifen therapy in the acute stages of RPF not only helps retard the growth of fibrous tissue but also dissolves the fibrous growth already present. There is a high likelihood of the fibrosis recurring if surgical intervention is not coupled with immunosuppressive therapy, which is effective when administered in the early stages of the disease. The combination of immunosuppressive medication and surgical management results in an excellent outcome.

The long-term prognosis for patients who have idiopathic RPF depends on the structures affected by the fibrous growth, with renal failure being the most serious complication. Questions persist about the optimal duration of therapy as well as the effectiveness of treatment and persistence of improvement because of the small number of cases studied. No data are available on the effects of long-term treatment of this condition.

In this case, an idiopathic, localized form of RPF was diagnosed after all known associated disorders were excluded. Exploratory laparotomy with lysis of the right ureter was performed. A double J–stent was placed, and the right ureter was repaired. The diagnosis of RPF was confirmed histologically. The patient also received corticosteroid therapy in the perioperative period and for 3 additional months. The boy remains asymptomatic 12 months after surgery.

Lessons for the Physician

After excluding the more common causes of extrinsic or intrinsic ureteral obstruction, the physician should consider retroperitoneal fibrosis as a cause of unilateral hydronephrosis.

Bibhuti B. Das, MD, Lincoln Medical Center, Bronx, NY

Sunati Sahoo, MD, New York Presbyterian Hospital/Weill Cornell Center, New York, NY

CHAPTER 6

High Temperature, Vomiting, Facial Pain, and Congestion in a 16-Year-Old Girl

Presentation

A 16-year-old Hispanic girl is seen because of temperatures up to 102.0°F (38.9°C), vomiting, facial pain, and congestion. Her pediatrician had diagnosed sinusitis and prescribed amoxicillin. At first, she showed improvement, but 1 week later, she developed a painful rash on her lower extremities with bilateral foot swelling. She denies upper respiratory and gastrointestinal (GI) tract symptoms. She is admitted to the hospital for persistent pain and swelling of her legs, with concern for cellulitis.

She has mild asthma, has a cat at home, and traveled to Mexico 3 months ago. No findings of note are reported in her family history.

On physical examination, the girl has normal vital signs, a mildly injected throat, and extensive dark, nodular, 1- to 2-cm lesions covering the anterior aspects of both thighs and pretibial regions. The lesions are erythematous, warm, and painful to palpation. Both feet are markedly swollen but have normal pulses and sensation. All other findings are normal.

Laboratory results are white blood cell count of 10.4×10^3/mcL (10.4×10^9/L) with 67% neutrophils and 26% lymphocytes, hemoglobin of 13.4 g/dL (134.0 g/L), platelet count of 442.0×10^3/mcL (442.0×10^9/L), C-reactive protein of 15.3 mg/dL (153 mg/L) (reference range, 0–0.5 mg/dL [0–5 mg/L]), erythrocyte sedimentation rate (ESR) of 85 mm/h (reference range, 4–25 mm/h), creatine kinase of 31 U/L (0.52 mckat/L) (reference range, 10–80 U/L [0.17–1.3 mckat/L]), aspartate aminotransferase of 56 U/L (0.94 mckat/L), alanine aminotransferase of 93 U/L (1.6 mckat/L), antistreptolysin of 30 IU/mL (reference range, <200 IU/mL), coccidioidomycosis titer of less than 1:2, negative antinuclear antibody titer, and normal findings on urinalysis. Blood culture and tuberculin test results are negative. Radiographs of the lower extremities show soft-tissue swelling.

Cefazolin and subsequently clindamycin are prescribed because of concern for cellulitis but are discontinued when the diagnosis is made. An additional test reveals the likely cause of her condition.

- **What is your differential diagnosis at this point?**
- **Are there any elements of history or physical examination that would help you?**
- **What additional diagnostic studies would you like performed?**

Discussion

The additional test was a stool culture, which grew non-*typhi* group D *Salmonella* species. The clinical findings suggested erythema nodosum (EN), in this case presenting as an extraintestinal manifestation of salmonellosis. At the time of this adolescent's evaluation, no GI symptoms were present. Because *Salmonella* was isolated only from the stool, antibiotics were not administered. Asymptomatic *Salmonella* infection is rare, and detection in the stool of a healthy individual may reflect a carrier state. Although an extensive infectious and noninfectious evaluation was performed for this patient, only *Salmonella* was isolated. Thus, *Salmonella* appears to be the likely causative organism responsible for the EN in this case.

Erythema nodosum has long been associated with GI infection, particularly with *Yersinia*. Erythema nodosum only rarely has been reported as a presentation of *Salmonella* infection, but in one series, *Salmonella* was the primary organism isolated from stool samples in patients who had EN. To date, more than 40 cases have been reported in the literature.

Differential Diagnosis

Largely a clinical diagnosis, EN can resemble other dermatologic conditions manifesting as panniculitis (inflammation of subcutaneous fat). Panniculitis can be caused by infection, cold, and corticosteroids. Other, less common entities include nodular panniculitis (erythema induratum) and cytophagic histiocytic panniculitis. Subcutaneous infections such as those caused by *Staphylococcus* can resemble EN and should be considered.

Nodular pretibial lymphangitis caused by *Francisella, Mycobacterium, Nocardia, Sporothrix,* and *Leishmania* species can resemble EN. Systemic illnesses that have dermatologic presentations and can mimic EN include lupus erythematosus profundus, alpha$_1$-antitrypsin deficiency, and pancreatic disease. Rare dermatologic diseases should be considered if the EN cannot be diagnosed clearly, on the basis of history and physical findings, or if symptoms persist beyond what is expected.

These symptoms include necrobiosis lipoidica and subcutaneous granuloma annulare. In these conditions, dermatologic consultation and deep incisional skin biopsy may be required.

The Condition

Erythema nodosum is a self-limited hypersensitivity panniculitis associated with several noninfectious and infectious agents. Antigens trigger a type 4 delayed hypersensitivity reaction, resulting in septal inflammation of subcutaneous fat. The overall incidence has been estimated to be 1 to 5 per 100,000 persons, with the peak incidence seen between 20 and 30 years of age and a male to female ratio of 1 to 6. Although not common, cases in young children and adolescents do occur, with both sexes affected equally.

Erythema nodosum causes painful, erythematous, palpable nodules over the extensor surfaces of the lower extremities, upper extremities, and trunk. Pretibial involvement is typical. As the nodules evolve, they undergo color changes similar to those of a resolving bruise. Nodules subside over a period of 2 to 8 weeks in adults, with new lesions appearing as late as 6 weeks after onset. The duration of EN may be shorter in children because the underlying illness is usually not chronic. In general, EN heals completely without ulceration or scarring.

A prodrome of fever, malaise, weight loss, and arthralgia is common 1 to 3 weeks prior to the appearance of nodules. In contrast to adults, arthralgias are less likely in children. The ESR is frequently elevated but may be normal in up to 40% of cases. In children, an elevated ESR correlates significantly with the number of skin lesions.

Finding EN on examination of an ill child should prompt investigation into an underlying systemic illness. Most often, no identifiable cause is found (up to 72% in one series). In conditions for which a cause is identified, streptococcal pharyngitis remains the most common.

Other infectious causes of EN include pertussis, gonorrhea, meningococcal infection, brucellosis, *Yersinia* infection, salmonellosis, shigellosis, *Campylobacter* infection, secondary syphilis, lymphogranuloma venereum, viral hepatitis, Epstein-Barr virus infection, blastomycosis, histoplasmosis, coccidioidomycosis, mycobacteria infection (including tuberculosis and leprosy), *Mycoplasma* infection, *Chlamydophila* infection, *Bartonella* infection, BCG vaccination, and immune reconstitution associated with treatment of human immunodeficiency virus.

Inflammatory bowel disease is the most common noninfectious trigger, but celiac disease, Behçet disease, sarcoidosis, leukemia, lymphoma, pregnancy, and medications are also possibilities. Sulfonamides, penicillins, estrogens (particularly oral contraceptive pills), bromides, and iodides are the most frequent medications implicated in causing EN.

Basic evaluation should include a complete blood cell count with differential, liver function tests, basic metabolic panel, antistreptolysin-O titer, stool culture, and placement of a tuberculin test. Chest radiography should be performed to rule out pneumonia and hilar adenopathy, which may indicate tuberculosis or sarcoidosis.

Some individuals develop chronic EN, EN migrans, or subacute nodular migratory panniculitis. These variants of classic EN may require long-term management.

Therapy and Prognosis

Erythema nodosum is a self-limited panniculitis that heals completely in 1 to 2 months without residual dermatologic or neurologic sequelae. This adolescent's pain and erythema resolved over 2 months. Treatment is primarily supportive and includes bed rest. Pain is the most significant symptom and, in most cases, can be managed with nonsteroidal anti-inflammatory drugs. More aggressive pain management may be needed for recurrent or prolonged cases. Oral potassium iodide has been used in small trials to treat various forms of panniculitis. Although some benefit has been shown, this agent has not been studied objectively in children, nor is its mechanism understood completely. In difficult or prolonged cases of EN for which malignancy and infection have been excluded, glucocorticoids have been used.

Management should also focus on treatment of any underlying disease. Therapies that treat the underlying condition may hasten resolution of the EN.

Lessons for the Physician

- Because erythema nodosum (EN) is a dermatologic manifestation of systemic disease, its discovery on physical examination should generate a thorough search for a cause. Results of history, physical examination, and basic laboratory testing can guide the physician.
- Many cases of EN are idiopathic, but infection, autoimmune disease, malignancy, pregnancy, and medications may be responsible and should be ruled out. Gastrointestinal causes of EN should be investigated even in individuals who have no gastrointestinal symptoms, as was the case in this patient.

David Michalik, DO, Miller Children's Hospital, Long Beach, CA

CHAPTER 7

Fever, Neck Swelling, and Weight Loss in a 17-Year-Old Boy

Presentation

A 17-year-old boy is referred for evaluation of fever, malaise, left-sided neck swelling, headache, and a 4.0-kg weight loss. Symptoms began 2 weeks ago. He has had multiple medical evaluations, including an urgent care visit during which a rapid streptococcal antigen test result was negative and a subsequent emergency department visit during which he was treated for cervical lymphadenitis with oral clindamycin. He denies rash, sore throat, conjunctivitis, shortness of breath, cough, joint swelling, or pain. He denies exposure to kittens and has no risk factors for tuberculosis.

Vital signs are as follows: temperature, 101.5°F (38.6°C); heart rate, 104 beats/min; respiratory rate, 18 breaths/min; and blood pressure, 116/54 mm Hg. He appears tired but is not in acute distress. There is left-sided neck swelling in the posterior cervical triangle with no overlying erythema or warmth. The area of swelling is tender but not fluctuant. Neck range of motion is limited because of pain. The oropharynx is normal. He has no other lymphadenopathy or hepatosplenomegaly, and the remainder of his physical examination findings are normal.

Laboratory evaluation reveals the following values: a white blood cell count of 3,000/mcL (3.0×10^9/L) with 46% neutrophils (absolute neutrophil count, 1,400), 37% lymphocytes, and 15% monocytes; hemoglobin, 14.4 g/dL (144 g/L); and hematocrit, 40% (0.40). Further laboratory test results are unremarkable, including normal erythrocyte sedimentation rate, C-reactive protein level, comprehensive metabolic panel, lactate dehydrogenase level, uric acid level, and urinalysis, as well as negative monospot test. Screening for numerous infections, including human immunodeficiency virus, Epstein-Barr virus, cytomegalovirus, gonorrhea, *Chlamydia, Bartonella,* and tuberculosis, yields negative results. Computed tomography reveals the left-sided lymphadenopathy without a drainable abscess (Figures 7.1 and 7.2). Surgical biopsy confirms the diagnosis.

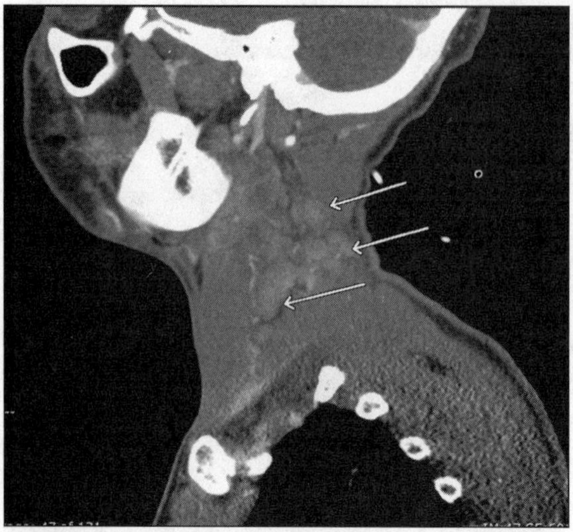

Figure 7.1. The coronal cut of head and neck computed tomography scan shows enlarged lymph nodes of left jugular chain, some of them with necrotic centers.

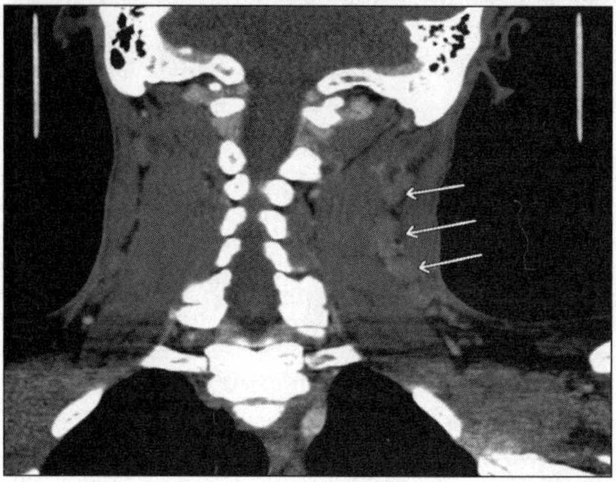

Figure 7.2. The sagittal cut of neck computed tomography scan shows enlarged lymph nodes on the left side of the neck.

- **What is your differential diagnosis at this point?**
- **Are there any elements of history or physical examination that would help you?**
- **What additional diagnostic studies would you like performed?**

Discussion

After failing to respond to intravenous antibiotics, the patient underwent an excisional biopsy of the cervical lymph nodes. The histopathologic analysis established the diagnosis of Kikuchi-Fujimoto disease (KFD). Treatment thereafter consisted of symptomatic management, including antipyretics and pain control. He initially responded well to intravenous ketorolac for pain and was transitioned to oral naproxen at discharge. He was also treated with ranitidine for gastric prophylaxis while taking nonsteroidal anti-inflammatory drugs. He was discharged home while still febrile with instructions to follow-up with his primary care physician. He recovered from his illness within 4 months of discharge.

The Condition

Kikuchi-Fujimoto disease is a self-limited and benign condition characterized by regional cervical lymphadenitis. The cause is unknown, although infectious and autoimmune triggers have been postulated. The clinical manifestations of KFD are usually acute or subacute and evolve during a period of 2 to 3 weeks. The hallmark features include fever and lymphadenopathy, particularly of the cervical chain. The lymph nodes in the posterior cervical triangle are most commonly involved, but generalized lymphadenopathy has been reported. The lymphadenopathy can be painful and is usually unilateral, and the lymph nodes can vary in size. The nodes typically range from 0.5 to 4 cm, but much larger nodes have been reported. Patients may present with other symptoms, such as malaise, headache, nausea, vomiting, sore throat, arthritis, and arthralgia. Weight loss, night sweats, and nonspecific rashes are reported in less than 10% of patients.

No specific laboratory tests contribute to the diagnosis. In fact, the results of a wide range of laboratory evaluation are usually normal. Abnormal laboratory findings may include leukopenia and a mildly elevated erythrocyte sedimentation rate. Other rare, but possible, abnormal results include anemia, elevated liver enzymes, positive antinuclear antibody test results, increased lactate dehydrogenase, positive viral serologic test results, thrombocytopenia, and leukocytosis. The histopathologic findings are distinctive and include patchy, irregular paracortical areas of coagulative necrosis without a polymorphonuclear white blood cell infiltration (Figure 7.3).

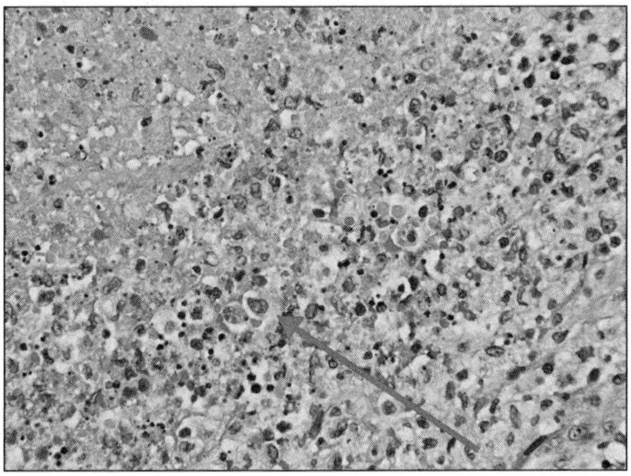

Figure 7.3. Lymph node histopathologic analysis reveals numerous histiocytes and plasmacytoid cells surrounding areas of necrosis.

Kikuchi-Fujimoto disease typically lasts 1 to 4 months and resolves spontaneously. There is no specific treatment aside from supportive care and symptomatic management. Corticosteroids have been used for patients with more severe or persistent disease. Physicians should know that there is an association between KFD and systemic lupus erythematosus (SLE) because some patients may have SLE preceding, occurring concomitantly, or postdating the diagnosis of KFD.

Differential Diagnosis

The differential diagnosis for lymphadenopathy or lymphadenitis includes infectious and noninfectious conditions. Because KFD is diagnosed only by the characteristic histopathologic findings of the lymph node, other conditions that cause lymphadenopathy and fever are typically explored before confirming the diagnosis of KFD. Infections with viruses such as Epstein-Barr virus, cytomegalovirus, and herpes simplex virus and bacterial infections such as *Staphylococcus aureus,* group A *Streptococcus, Bartonella henselae,* nontuberculous mycobacterium, and *Mycobacterium tuberculosis* can all cause lymphadenitis and fever. Noninfectious conditions that closely mimic KFD include lymphoma, SLE-associated lymphadenopathy, Castleman disease, and Kawasaki syndrome. In fact, it is often difficult to histologically distinguish KFD, lymphoma, and SLE. Therefore, expert review of the histopathologic findings by someone experienced with these conditions is essential.

Lessons for the Physician

- Kikuchi-Fujimoto disease should always be considered in the differential of patients with prolonged fever and lymphadenopathy, particularly of the posterior cervical chain.
- An excisional biopsy of the lymph node is essential for the diagnosis.
- Treatment is symptomatic only (analgesics, antipyretics, and rarely corticosteroids).
- Kikuchi-Fujimoto disease resolves spontaneously.

Stephanie Todd, MD, Children's National Health System, Washington, DC

Part 2

Behavioral

CHAPTER 8

Daily Paroxysmal Episodes in a 1-Year-Old Girl

Presentation

A 1-year-old girl who has developed normally has experienced as many as 40 paroxysmal episodes daily since age 6 months. Each episode occurs while she is lying prone or is on her knees. She crouches down, pelvis pressed on the floor; lifts herself onto her extended arms; looks up; arches her back; and throws her head back. Her legs shake, and she goes stiff. Her face appears strained and frightened. She sometimes dribbles, looks vacant, and stares as if "in a trance." Her eyes appear glazed but move erratically. She suddenly becomes floppy and goes to sleep. During an episode, she immediately comes round when spoken to.

Sometimes, as if anticipating an "attack," she runs to her mother, appearing frightened; grips her mother's clothes intermittently; looks vacant; and then becomes floppy and sleeps for a few minutes. These episodes occur primarily when she is tired or bored and never when she is playing or distracted.

On hospital admission, the girl's mother prefers observation in a cubicle, convinced that nothing will happen if she is distracted by other children. The girl's physical findings are normal, and no psychosocial issues are identified in the family.

Serum chemistry and metabolic studies yield normal results. Computed tomography of the head and electroencephalography (EEG) yield normal results, despite the occurrence of an episode during the EEG. There is no response to carbamazepine or valproate therapy.

- **What is your differential diagnosis at this point?**
- **Are there any elements of history or physical examination that would help you?**
- **What additional diagnostic studies would you like performed?**

Discussion

The girl's parents were asked to videotape the episodes at home. The tapes showed that the manifestations were always stereotypical and reproducible and provided clear evidence of voluntary control and distractibility. All the episodes were remarkably similar to what has been reported previously as self-stimulatory behavior, called by some "infantile masturbation." The diagnosis was explained to the parents, who accepted it with great relief.

The Disorder

Although self-stimulation of the genitalia in a young boy is recognized easily, this specific behavior is rare in young girls, making it more difficult to determine what is happening, with resulting unnecessary investigations and treatment.

This activity occurs at any age, the youngest child reported being 2 months of age. It has been detected in a male fetus by ultrasonography. A minor perineal focus of irritation, such as dermatitis, urinary tract infection, pinworms, or constipation, may precede the manifestations. Stressful events, such as weaning, birth of a sibling, or separation from the parents, may also be precipitating factors. Self-stimulatory behaviors tend to occur during boredom, loneliness, anxiety, or excitement.

In young girls, tightening the thighs, rocking pelvic movements or other rhythmic activities, and application of mechanical pressure to the suprapubic area are characteristic, as are grunting, facial flushing, irregular breathing, and sweating. These activities may be misinterpreted as representing abdominal pain or urinary symptoms. A vacant and glassy stare, associated with rigidity, grunting, or rocking movements, may suggest seizures. These episodes may last from a minute to several hours, consciousness is not altered, and the child usually stops when told. The physical findings are usually normal or there may be mild perineal irritation. Causes of local irritation in the perineum should be sought, and the possibility of child sexual abuse must be considered.

Diagnosis

Taking a detailed history is essential, and personal observation of the episodes helps confirm the diagnosis. Videotaping the episodes at home is also very helpful and aids in the management of this condition.

Continuous ambulatory EEG recording with video monitoring is readily available in many medical centers and unequivocally distinguishes seizure activity from non-seizure activity.

Natural History and Management

Spontaneous resolution is the norm and occurs in approximately 78% of the children within 2 years. Improvement may be delayed in younger patients, those who begin to stimulate earlier, and those who stimulate more frequently.

It is more helpful and certainly more acceptable to most families when physicians use the term *autostimulation* or *habit* rather than *masturbation* when discussing this entity. Management consists of explaining to the parents the harmless and painless nature of the autostimulatory activity and attempting to avoid inappropriate responses, such as punishment, that might have a reinforcing effect.

Lessons for the Physician

Self-stimulation is a normal and common behavior in young children and may mimic common medical conditions. Failure to recognize this activity for what it is may lead to considerable parental anxiety, unnecessary investigations, and inappropriate and potentially harmful therapy. Physicians should be familiar with this benign condition and always include it in the differential diagnosis of the common conditions it may mimic. The diagnostic value of videotaping unusual activity or spells should be appreciated by physicians.

Hassib Narchi, MD, Sandwell General Hospital, Lyndon, West Bromwich, United Kingdom

CHAPTER 9

Pain, Swelling, and Redness of Left Leg in a 17-Year-Old Girl

Presentation

A 17-year-old Caucasian girl is admitted to the hospital because of pain, swelling, and redness of her left leg for 6 months, with occasional low-grade fevers.

Previously, cellulitis had been diagnosed and antistaphylococcal antibiotics prescribed on more than one occasion, with temporary improvement. Cultures of the cellulitis had yielded *Staphylococcus aureus* sensitive to all antistaphylococcal antibiotics. Complete blood cell count, erythrocyte sedimentation rate, liver and renal function tests, calcium, phosphorous, antinuclear antibody, rheumatoid factor, and blood cultures resulted in normal or negative findings. Radiographs of the pelvis, hip, femur, knee, tibia, fibula, ankle, and lumbosacral spine, as well as a venogram and bone scan, were interpreted as normal. Arthrocentesis yielded normal results. Additionally, she had been admitted repeatedly for strict bed rest, elevation of the extremity, and intravenous antibiotics, with no sustained resolution of swelling, redness, or pain.

She had been traveling to various islands of the western Pacific as a member of a soccer team prior to the onset of her symptoms.

Physical findings today are normal with the exception of redness, pain, and warmth over the left calf and anterior portion of the left leg, with pitting edema involving the calf, pretibial region, ankle, foot, and knee area, although results of the knee examination are normal. Pulses and strength are normal.

- **What is your differential diagnosis at this point?**
- **Are there any elements of history or physical examination that would help you?**
- **What additional diagnostic studies would you like performed?**

Discussion

This patient had experienced numerous episodes of disease in her left leg that involved variable degrees of swelling, erythema, warmth, and pain. Her clinical picture suggested both inflammation of unknown cause and secondary infection. To complicate the picture, she demonstrated features of chondromalacia of the left patella, which physicians thought might be related to the lower extremity disease, perhaps through infection. The differential diagnosis included cellulitis, septic arthritis, osteomyelitis, thrombophlebitis, collagen vascular disease, necrotizing fasciitis, pyomyositis, compartment syndrome, immunodeficiency, venomous insect bite or snakebite, and lymphedema.

By the time of admission to this hospital, an extensive evaluation had been completed, eliminating many of the diagnoses on the list, including septic arthritis (negative arthrocentesis), chronic osteomyelitis (negative radiograph, bone scan, and blood culture), thrombophlebitis (negative venogram), and collagen vascular disease (negative rheumatoid factor and antinuclear antibody and normal erythrocyte sedimentation rate).

With necrotizing fasciitis, progression should be more acute. Signs and symptoms of pyomyositis should progress and by 6 months would require surgical management for resolution. With compartment syndrome, there should be a history of pain on exercising. Immunodeficiency is unlikely given the onset of symptoms at age 17 years and absence of risk factors for human immunodeficiency virus. There was no history of snakebite or insect bite.

One other important diagnostic consideration is lymphedema. This finding can occur in lymphedema praecox (Meige disease), which is a primary lymphedema with onset in adolescence and is usually a diagnosis of exclusion. In addition, several secondary causes of lymphedema include tumors, postradiation fibrosis, retroperitoneal fibrosis, infection (including filariasis), and postinflammatory scarring from trauma, surgery, or burns. Lymphoscintigraphy can be used to differentiate primary from secondary lymphedema.

In this patient, filariasis was an intriguing possibility given her travel history. Filariasis is a roundworm infestation that can lead to massive lymphedema of the legs and genitalia. Diagnosis is made by reviewing blood smears for microfilariae or by antigen immunoassay. In this case, blood smears were negative.

The Condition

This patient's diagnostic dilemma was solved dramatically one day on rounds when she was discovered to be applying a constrictive tourniquet around her leg just above the knee. When she was confronted, she became withdrawn and denied she was doing anything. With one-to-one nursing supervision to ensure no further placement of the tourniquet, the redness and swelling resolved rapidly. A psychiatrist was consulted, and factitious illness was diagnosed.

This unusual presentation is a striking example of how physicians can be deceived by patients who have factitious disorders and can be compelled into performing extensive and invasive diagnostic procedures. In retrospect, one diagnostic clue could have been a zone of demarcation between the normal and edematous areas caused by the tourniquet. Careful reexamination after the true cause had been revealed did show that finding, which had not been evident on previous examinations.

Psychosomatic illnesses have a wide spectrum of presentations and are common in adolescents. Frequently, they are manifestations of underlying psychological disease, but they can also be seen in healthy adolescents during stressful situations. Examples include adjustment disorders, somatization disorders, conversion disorders, hypochondriasis, malingering, and factitious disorder.

According to the American Psychiatric Association *Diagnostic and Statistical Manual of Mental Disorders*, Fifth Edition, adjustment disorders relate to a difficult adjustment to a situation that is out of proportion to the circumstances. In these disorders, stress can lead to physical symptoms. Examples include tension headaches, palpitations, neurodermatitis, and tremor.

In somatization disorders such as conversion disorder and hypochondriasis, a variety of symptoms can present vaguely and imprecisely over a period of several years. There must be a significant impairment in functioning or a history of no explanation of symptoms after an appropriate assessment. The patient often goes to many different physicians and frequently has underlying anxiety and depression.

Conversion disorder is characterized by neurologic or other somatic symptoms that do not fit biological explanations. The patient benefits from these symptoms by avoiding stressful conflict (primary gain) and evokes attention and sympathy for being stricken with often dramatic symptoms (secondary gain). Patients who have hypochondriasis experience an exaggerated preoccupation or belief that they have a serious disease.

There are 3 mental health disorders in which an individual intentionally produces symptoms: malingering, factitious illness, and factitious illness by proxy. In malingering, the patient voluntarily, deliberately, and purposefully produces his or her symptoms to achieve some goal, such as gaining insurance money, avoiding military service, obtaining drugs, or avoiding work.

In factitious illness, or Munchausen syndrome, the patient produces signs or symptoms to assume the sick role. Examples of clinical presentations include factitious fever, induced infections, and hypoglycemia caused by exogenous insulin injections. There was one reported case of a tourniquet placed around the wrist, which mimicked reflex sympathetic dystrophy. *Münchausen syndrome by proxy* is a term used when a caregiver induces signs or symptoms in a child.

Patients who have factitious illness often have a vague and inconsistent history. When questioned in detail, they frequently have an extensive knowledge of diseases and may have a medical background. Patients commonly become hostile about not being diagnosed correctly and demand and request medications and procedures that are medically unnecessary. The cause of factitious illness is unknown. The diagnosis requires a high degree of suspicion and is often difficult to prove. The patient frequently uses the symptoms to gain attention and recognition. Prolonged psychotherapy is recommended.

Lessons for the Physician

This case reminds physicians to always consider the possibility of factitious illness in patients who present with atypical clinical manifestations. Careful observation of the patient in the hospital, including video surveillance, may be necessary to confirm the diagnosis, although physicians contemplating video surveillance should consult the hospital attorney and risk management office to be sure they are acting legally. Once the diagnosis is considered, physicians should avoid harmful invasive procedures or treatment with potentially toxic medications.

James J. Burns, MD, Baystate Medical Center, Springfield, MA

Part 3

Cardiology

CHAPTER 10

5-Day-Old Girl With Labored Breathing and Fast-Beating Heart

Presentation

A 5-day-old girl is brought to the emergency department because of labored breathing. Her parents noticed that her heart was "beating very fast." There has been no fever, cyanosis, or diaphoresis. A good feeder initially, she now takes only small amounts of formula and appears to tire during feedings.

The neonate weighed 4.63 kg at birth. Her mother received complete prenatal care, and there were no complications, including gestational diabetes. There is no family history of congenital heart disease.

The neonate's temperature is 99.3°F (37.4°C), pulse is 180 beats/min, respiratory rate is 85 breaths/min, and blood pressure is 72/45 mm Hg. She is pink without mottling but in moderate respiratory distress. Her lungs sound clear. She has a hyperdynamic precordium, her carotid and extremity pulses are 3/4 in intensity, and a grade 2/6 crescendo-decrescendo murmur is heard at the left midsternal border. The S_1 and S_2 are loud. The liver edge can be palpated 2 cm below the midcostal margin. No skin lesions or birthmarks are present.

Evaluation for sepsis yields results that make infection unlikely. Laboratory findings include normal electrolyte levels; hemoglobin, 16.9 g/dL (10.48 mmol/L); thyroxine, 6.7 mcg/dL (20.1 nmol/L) (reference range, 6.0–15.9 mcg/dL [78.0–206.7 nmol/L]); and thyroid-stimulating hormone, 3.8 µIU/dL (reference range, 3–18 µIU/mL). A radiograph of the chest shows an enlarged cardiac silhouette. Echocardiography demonstrates dilatation of the right atrium and ventricle and tricuspid regurgitation.

A detailed examination of the neonate's head and neck suggests a diagnosis that is confirmed by imaging.

- **What is your differential diagnosis at this point?**
- **Are there any elements of history or physical examination that would help you?**
- **What additional diagnostic studies would you like performed?**

Discussion

Differential Diagnosis

Findings on cardiovascular examination (hyperdynamic precordium, increased pulses, and loud heart sounds) and enlarged cardiac silhouette on the chest radiograph suggested that this neonate was in high-output congestive heart failure.

The differential diagnosis of high-output heart failure includes anemia, fever, sepsis, hyperthyroidism, and arteriovenous malformation (AVM). High-output states are also termed *hyperdynamic states.* It is extremely important to recognize a high cardiac output state in an infant or child for several reasons. Many hyperdynamic states result from conditions that can be ameliorated by medication or other interventions; without therapy, the heart failure will progress. Also, the physician would not want to prescribe a vasodilating agent for a neonate or infant in high-output failure because this state is usually associated with decreased peripheral vascular resistance. Finally, identification of a high-output state can lead the diagnostician to look more thoroughly for a systemic disorder such as thyrotoxicosis or AVM.

In patients who are anemic, arteriolar dilatation is a direct consequence of tissue hypoxia. The hypoxia leads to the production of lactate, a vasodilatory metabolite. When the arterial vessels dilate, more blood is delivered to the venous circulation, and the heart attempts to compensate for the increased venous return by increasing its rate. The high-output state in anemic patients may be due, to a lesser degree, to decreased blood viscosity and a noncatecholamine inotropic agent that increases contractility. It is prudent to consider anemia when an infant presents with high-output heart failure in the first week of life. This neonate's hemoglobin level and hematocrit ruled out anemia.

The physiology of thyrotoxicosis includes increased cardiac output due to an increase in total body oxygen consumption and a decrease in peripheral vascular resistance. Studies in animal models suggest that thyrotoxicosis may lead to increased ATPase activity, increasing both the contraction and relaxation phases in the myocardium. Hyperthyroidism was another possible cause of high-output heart failure in this neonate but was ruled out by laboratory investigation.

In septic shock, lactic acid levels tend to rise early because of glycolysis in the peripheral tissues. Lactic acid release leads to vasodilation, decreased peripheral vascular resistance, hypoperfusion, and hypoxia. A patient in septic shock may present in an extreme hyperdynamic state, although cardiac output can also be normal in this condition. Physicians must treat infants who might be septic with antibiotics until convinced that infection is not present. An evaluation for sepsis in this neonate failed to show any signs of infection.

Diagnosis

The examination of every neonate or infant who has congestive heart failure must include complete palpation of the carotid pulses and auscultation of the head and neck. Auscultation and palpation of these regions in this neonate revealed an impressive grade 4/6 cranial bruit and a palpable thrill. Magnetic resonance imaging of the brain revealed mildly reduced brain substance and a direct arteriovenous fistula between the occipital artery and transverse sinus. In retrospect, many other physical findings in this neonate, particularly the nonspecific flow murmur, hepatomegaly, loud heart sounds, and bounding pulses, were consistent with the diagnosis of AVM. Although she had a different lesion, this neonate's clinical picture was typical of that seen in infants who have AVMs involving the vein of Galen, a defect well known for its association with congestive heart failure.

An AVM shunts blood from a high-pressure artery into a low-pressure vein without the modulating effects of an intervening capillary bed. Heart rate and stroke volume increase because of the low systemic vascular resistance.

There are many sites and causes of AVMs. These fistulas may be congenital or acquired. Congenital lesions may be single or multiple and are most often located in the cerebrum or liver. They are situated less frequently in the cerebellum, brainstem, spinal cord, lung, kidney, or other anatomic locations. The finding of hepatic or pulmonary arteriovenous communications should lead the diagnostician to consider the possibility of Osler-Weber-Rendu disease, also known as hereditary hemorrhagic telangiectasia. Other types of arteriovenous communications include capillary hemangiomas, such as nevus flammeus (port-wine stain) or nevus vasculosus (strawberry hemangioma). These vascular lesions are highly unlikely to have hemodynamic manifestations, however. In addition, percutaneous femoral artery catheterization is an iatrogenic cause of arteriovenous communication that the physician always must consider.

Management

The immediate management of this neonate consists of mechanical ventilation, if needed. Some physicians also recommend manual compression of the fistula, although the benefit of this maneuver has not been proven. Such compression leads to a decrease in the hyperdynamic circulation and slowing of the heart rate (Branham sign). The neonate in this case had a complete neurosurgical evaluation while hospitalized and later underwent successful coil embolization of the AVM after she had gained more weight. She will require careful, serial follow-up clinical and radiographic examinations because recanalization and recurrence of abnormal blood flow can occur in as many as 50% of patients treated solely by endovascular coil techniques.

Lessons for the Physician

The process of arriving at a definitive diagnosis in a neonate or infant who is in heart failure can be intimidating because of the sheer number of diagnostic possibilities and because the infant is likely to be acutely ill. This case underscores the importance of a thorough clinical examination, which in this instance successfully led the diagnostician to recognize high-output heart failure, and emphasizes the need to include auscultation of the cranium as part of the physical evaluation.

Beth Carter, MD, Children's Hospital of Orange County, Orange, CA

CHAPTER 11

Chest Pain in a Boy With Duchenne Muscular Dystrophy and Cardiomyopathy (Visual Diagnosis)

Presentation

A 17-year-old boy with Duchenne muscular dystrophy (DMD) due to a deletion of exons 18 to 37 in the *DMD* gene was diagnosed in our clinic as having cardiomyopathy at age 12 years. His current medications include deflazacort (30 mg/d), lisinopril (10 mg once daily for cardiomyopathy), and metoprolol succinate (50 mg twice daily for disordered automaticity). His cardiac function had been stable, with ejection fractions (EFs) ranging from 47% to 55%.

After 1 day of headache and vomiting, he presents to a local emergency department with acute onset of chest pain and shortness of breath. Electrocardiogram (ECG) reveals ST-segment elevation in the inferolateral leads and ST-segment depression in the midprecordial leads, which prompts further testing (Figure 11.1). His initial troponin I level is elevated. He is transferred to a tertiary care facility for further evaluation. At the time of admission, his chest pain is substantially improved without intervention, but his troponin I level is now 40.27 ng/mL (40.27 mcg/L) (reference range, <0.04 ng/mL [<0.04 mcg/L]). Further laboratory evaluation reveals a white blood cell count of 12,900/mcL (12.9×10^9/L) with 72% neutrophils and 20% lymphocytes, a C-reactive protein level of 299.8 mg/L (2855.3 nmol/L) (reference range, <12.0 mg/L [114.3 nmol/L]), and a lactate level of 7.2 mg/dL (0.8 mmol/L) (reference range, 4.5–19.8 mg/dL [0.5–2.2 mmol/L]). Cardiac magnetic resonance imaging (CMRI) with late-gadolinium enhancement (LGE) reveals extensive left ventricular lateral wall epicardial enhancement (Figure 11.2A) and an EF of 50%. Quantitative T2 mapping reveals an increased T2 signal (80 milliseconds compared with 48 milliseconds in the unaffected interventricular septum) in the same region consistent with acute inflammation and injury (Figure 11.3A).

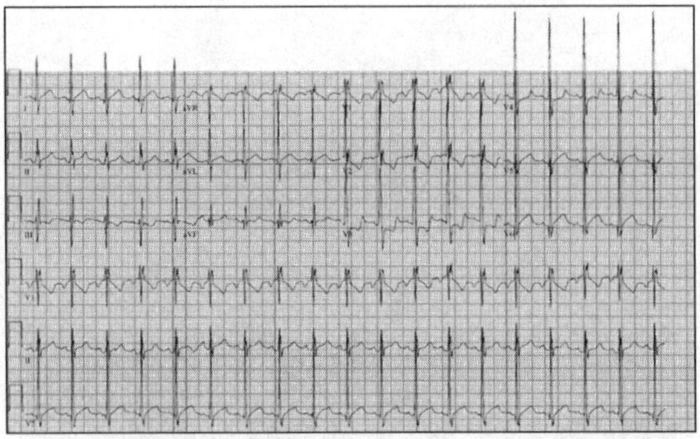

Figure 11.1. Electrocardiogram on admission to the tertiary care facility reveals sinus tachycardia (heart rate, 112 beats/min), incomplete right bundle branch block, possible left atrial enlargement, voltage criteria for left ventricular hypertrophy, minimal ST-segment elevation in the inferolateral leads, and marked ST-segment depression in the mid-precordial leads.

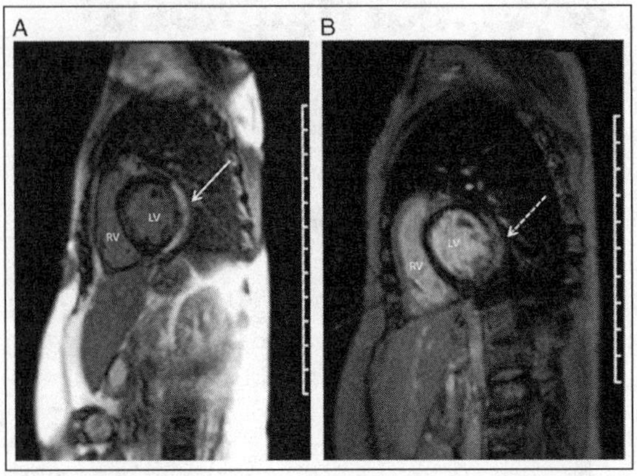

Figure 11.2. Sagittal cardiac magnetic resonance image of late-gadolinium enhancement reveals the right ventricle and left ventricle (LV) in short axis in the acute care setting at the time of diagnosis (A) and follow-up 3 months later (B). In the acute care setting, there was extensive LV lateral wall epicardial enhancement with late-gadolinium enhancement imaging (solid white arrow). At follow-up imaging, the LV lateral wall remained unchanged (dashed white arrow).

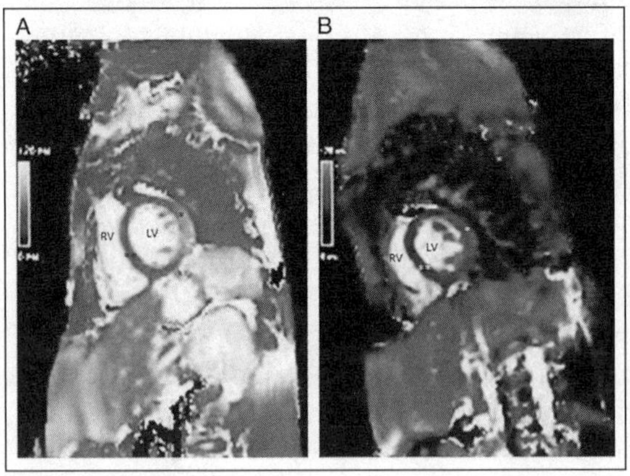

Figure 11.3. Colorized, sagittal, T2 cardiac magnetic resonance image reveals the right ventricle and left ventricle (LV) in short axis in the acute care setting at the time of diagnosis (A) and follow-up 3 months later (B). At the time of diagnosis, the T2 signal of the LV lateral free wall (black single asterisk) was 80 milliseconds. The T2 signal of the unaffected interventricular septum (black double asterisk) at that time was normal (48 milliseconds). At follow-up imaging 3 months later, the LV lateral free wall T2 signal (white single asterisk) was 53 milliseconds, and the unaffected interventricular septum T2 signal (white double asterisk) was 52 milliseconds.

- **What is your differential diagnosis at this point?**
- **Are there any elements of history or physical examination that would help you?**
- **What additional diagnostic studies would you like performed?**

Diagnosis

A diagnosis of acute myocarditis superimposed on left ventricular cardiomyopathy secondary to DMD was made. Chest pain can certainly be a presenting sign of myocarditis, although this is not necessary and may be absent. In this patient's case, the initial ECG is markedly abnormal with ST-segment changes. Although the most common ECG abnormality in myocarditis is diffuse T-wave inversion, the finding of ST-segment elevation, combined with the presenting symptoms, appropriately warrants further evaluation of a cardiac cause of his chest pain. The elevated C-reactive protein and troponin I levels should significantly raise the concern for myocarditis as a possible cause of his symptoms and abnormal laboratory test results. In this case, further evaluation was performed using CMRI, including T2 mapping, which revealed evidence of inflammation and confirmed a case of acute myocarditis superimposed on his underlying cardiomyopathy related to DMD.

Discussion

Chest pain, especially when coupled with shortness of breath, presents an extensive differential diagnosis that includes musculoskeletal, pulmonary, gastrointestinal, cardiac, and psychogenic causes. Musculoskeletal causes can include trauma, costochondritis, muscle strain, and rib or thoracic spine abnormalities. Respiratory causes may include severe cough related to viral or bacterial pneumonia, pleural effusions, and asthma.

Although patients with neuromuscular disorders may have multiple causes of chest pain, they still remain at risk for nonneuromuscular causes of chest pain. In patients with neuromuscular disorders who experience shortness of breath, one must consider respiratory muscle weakness and restrictive lung disease secondary to thoracic cage deformities and scoliosis. Some neuromuscular disorders can also cause chest pain secondary to esophageal spasms. Cardiac causes can include pericarditis, myocarditis, arrhythmias (including both supraventricular and ventricular arrhythmias), coronary artery abnormalities, and ischemic heart disease. Although many of these cardiac manifestations are rare, patients with neuromuscular disorders and cardiac manifestations are at the same risk for cardiac causes of chest pain as the general population. As such, they require thorough evaluation for potentially treatable causes of chest pain. In this case, appropriate screening led to evaluation of troponin I and, ultimately, CMRI, confirming the diagnosis of acute myocarditis.

Acute myocarditis is an inflammatory disease that affects the heart muscle. It is underrecognized in the general population because chest pain may resolve by the time the patient is evaluated. The true incidence of myocarditis is not known. Myocarditis is typically secondary to an antecedent viral infection or postviral immune-mediated response. The most common infectious causes include adenovirus, enterovirus (coxsackieviruses A and B), parvovirus B19, cytomegalovirus, herpesvirus, influenza A virus, and Epstein-Barr virus. Of interest, abnormal *DMD* has been identified as a susceptibility gene for myocardial viral infections, and dystrophin deficiency has been found to increase enteroviral-induced cardiomyopathy. There have been previous reports of boys with DMD diagnosed as acute myocarditis. However, these boys were younger than this patient and had normal left ventricular function before their diagnosis. In addition, rapid deterioration of left ventricular function in boys with DMD has been found after evidence of myocardial inflammation, defined by LGE on CMRI. In this study, two-thirds of the endomyocardial biopsy specimens obtained from the interventricular septum remote from the area of LGE had evidence of myocarditis, either active or healing.

In the current era, endomyocardial biopsy and the Dallas criteria are infrequently used for the diagnosis of acute myocarditis, and a current multi-institution study found that endomyocardial biopsy was performed in less than one-fifth of cases of pediatric myocarditis. Physicians now typically rely on the history, serologic evidence of a viral infection typical for myocarditis, echocardiogram, and CMRI, which is able to produce evidence of acute inflammation as evidenced by LGE of the involved myocardium. In the standard approach to endomyocardial biopsy, only the right ventricle myocardium is sampled. Combined with the patchy myocardial involvement in acute myocarditis, endomyocardial biopsy has a significant false-negative rate. Advantages of CMRI for the assessment of acute myocarditis include the noninvasive nature of the testing, the ability to study the myocardium of the left and right ventricles, and the ability to detect inflammation and edema using techniques such as LGE and T2 mapping. Late-gadolinium enhancement imaging is performed several minutes after the initial injection of gadolinium and allows visualization of injured myocardium and fibrosis, appearing as hyperintense areas, because the contrast is retained in these tissues longer than healthy myocardium. Quantitative T2 mapping is a technique used to assess for myocardial edema. It is similar to T2-weighted imaging, but it eliminates many of the limitations of T2-weighted sequences and allows for a quantitative, rather than qualitative, assessment of the myocardium.

In the DMD population, CMRI typically reveals subepicardial enhancement of the posterobasal regions of the left ventricle, which is thought to be secondary to fibrosis. Although our patient had the expected pattern of LGE consistent with that previously reported in patients with DMD, he also had evidence of increased T2 signal on quantitative T2 mapping consistent with edema from acute injury and inflammation. Quantitative T2 mapping reliably identifies the extent of myocardial involvement in myocarditis and has a high sensitivity and specificity (94% and 97%, respectively). Quantitative T2 mapping can also provide diagnostic data in patients who have difficulty with breath holding (eg, patients with neuromuscular disorders), providing better assessment of the extent of involvement compared with wall motion abnormalities (by echocardiography), LGE, and conventional T2-weighted imaging. As the field of CMRI continues to advance, more sophisticated imaging techniques have in addition to quantitative T2 mapping become available, including myocardial T1 mapping and quantification of diffuse interstitial fibrosis.

Management

Treatment of acute myocarditis is controversial and predominantly supportive in the case of a viral cause. Many institutions administer intravenous immunoglobulin, but data regarding the benefit of intravenous immunoglobulin are lacking. Alternatively, corticosteroids are beneficial in some case series and randomized trials, but the fact that many patients recover spontaneously questions whether administering corticosteroids truly improves outcome. In the setting of moderate or severe cardiac dysfunction, inotropic support is warranted. Milrinone is typically used in the acute care setting, and the patient is typically transitioned to an oral regimen that consists of an angiotensin-converting enzyme inhibitor with or without additional heart failure medications (β-blockers or diuretics), depending on the degree of residual ventricular dysfunction. In some cases, mechanical support via extracorporeal membrane oxygenation or left ventricular assist device may be warranted.

Patient Course

Evaluation for a viral cause was unnecessary because the patient's CMRI was diagnostic for acute myocarditis, most likely of viral origin. His troponin I level decreased, and he became asymptomatic during 3 days of hospitalization. At discharge, his troponin I level was 14.5 ng/mL (14.5 mcg/L), and 1 week later, his troponin I level was 0.2 ng/mL (0.2 mcg/L). At that time, his echocardiogram revealed an EF of 57%. Three months after discharge, his EF by CMRI was 55%, and LGE imaging again revealed extensive left ventricular lateral wall epicardial enhancement (see Figure 11.2B). However, his quantitative T2 mapping revealed normalized T2 imaging (53 milliseconds compared to 52 milliseconds in the unaffected interventricular septum), suggesting improvement in the inflammation and injury (see Figure 11.3B). He remained asymptomatic, and no further troponin I levels were measured.

Summary

Our patient's cardiac magnetic resonance imaging (CMRI) findings, in combination with his abnormal electrocardiogram findings and elevated troponin I level, led to the diagnosis of acute myocarditis, and his clinical course was consistent with this diagnosis. This case highlights (1) utility of appropriate screening tests to guide further evaluation, (2) the importance of a high index of suspicion for myocarditis in patients with Duchenne muscular dystrophy with an acute change in symptoms, and (3) the utility of troponin I levels and novel CMRI techniques in establishing the diagnosis. Although dystrophin deficiency may increase the susceptibility to viral myocarditis and myocarditis may hasten the decline in cardiac function, we would caution against the generalization of late-gadolinium enhancement on CMRI as evidence of myocarditis or prognosticating rapid decline in cardiac function in all boys with Duchenne muscular dystrophy. Rather, we believe that it is important to differentiate late-gadolinium enhancement due to fibrosis and late-gadolinium enhancement secondary to active myocarditis.

Philip T. Thrush, MD, Department of Pediatrics, The Ohio State University, Columbus, OH, and The Heart Center, Nationwide Children's Hospital, Columbus, OH

Kevin M. Flanigan, MD, and Jerry R. Mendell, The Center for Gene Therapy, Research Institute, Nationwide Children's Hospital, Columbus, OH; Muscular Dystrophy Cooperative Research Center, Nationwide Children's Hospital, Columbus, OH; and Departments of Pediatrics and Neurology, The Ohio State University, Columbus, OH

Subha V. Raman, MD, Division of Cardiovascular Medicine, The Ohio State University, Columbus, OH

Curt J. Daniels, MD, Department of Pediatrics, The Ohio State University, Columbus, OH; The Heart Center, Nationwide Children's Hospital, Columbus, OH; and Division of Cardiovascular Medicine, The Ohio State University, Columbus, OH

Hugh D. Allen, MD, Associate Editor, Department of Pediatrics, Baylor College of Medicine, Texas Children's Hospital, Houston, TX

CHAPTER 12

Palpitations and Dizziness in an Adolescent Boy

Presentation

A previously healthy 18-year-old boy presents for the evaluation of palpitations and light-headedness, which started after he drove home after finishing his regular work shift. His symptoms were relieved partially by vomiting but then reappeared and worsened progressively, leading to diaphoresis and dizziness, after which he has been brought to an emergency department. There is no history of fever, diarrhea, intake of coffee or caffeinated beverages, or use of illicit drugs.

On arrival, his temperature is 98.6°F (37.0°C); heart rate, 180 beats/min; respiratory rate, 22 breaths/min; blood pressure, 100/50 mm Hg; and oxygen saturation, 99% on room air. His weight is 99 kg (>95th percentile); height, 184 cm (75th–90th percentile), and body mass index, 29.2. He is uncomfortable because of the palpitations, but he is able to follow commands. His cardiac examination reveals tachycardia, regular rhythm, normal S_1 and S_2, no murmurs, and equal peripheral pulses. His breath sounds are clear bilaterally. There are no signs of injury or trauma. Family history is negative for any sudden cardiac deaths, arrhythmias, or structural heart disease.

Laboratory evaluation reveals normal electrolyte levels, thyroid function, urine toxicology, and cardiac enzyme levels. Electrocardiogram (ECG) reveals a left axis deviation (–84°), wide QRS tachycardia at 180 beats/min, and right bundle branch block (Figure 12.1). With amiodarone infusion, he converts to a sinus rhythm. He is admitted to the intensive care unit, a specialist is consulted, and the diagnosis is established.

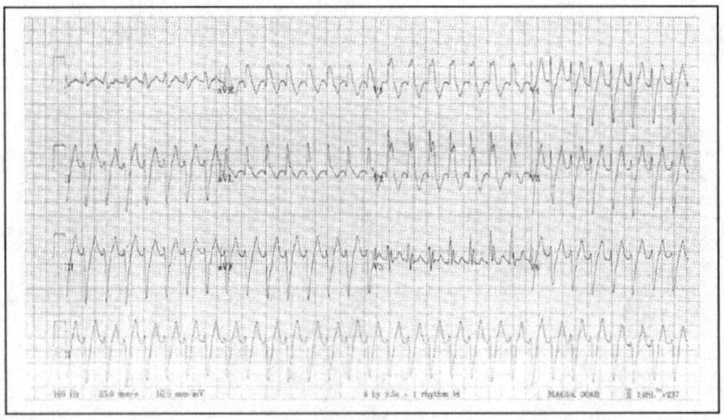

Figure 12.1. Electrocardiogram reveals a left axis deviation (−84°), wide QRS tachycardia at 180 beats/min, and right bundle branch block.

- **What is your differential diagnosis at this point?**
- **Are there any elements of history or physical examination that would help you?**
- **What additional diagnostic studies would you like performed?**

Discussion

Review of the 12-lead ECG at the time of presentation to the emergency department suggested a left ventricular posterior fascicular site of origin of tachycardia, known as Belhassen tachycardia (see Figure 12.1). A 2-D echocardiogram revealed normal structural cardiac anatomy. Because of nonspecific ST segment changes on the ECG, he underwent cardiac catheterization, which revealed normal coronary artery course, caliber, and origins. The patient did well and was discharged home without complications 3 days after admission. He was discharged in stable condition while taking nadolol. At follow-up visits, he denied any similar episodes of perceived tachycardia or palpitations.

Differential Diagnosis

By definition, ventricular tachycardia (VT) is 3 or more premature ventricular contractions at a rate faster than 120 beats/min. In pediatric patients, supraventricular tachycardia is more common than VT, and the two can usually be differentiated by ECG features such as wide QRS complex and atrioventricular dissociation. Depending on the age and mechanism of tachycardia, VT rate can vary and can be as high as 400 beats/min. Ventricular tachycardia can be polymorphic or monomorphic, and if it lasts more than 30 seconds or requires electrical cardioversion, it is labeled sustained VT. Symptoms may range from irritability, feeding problems, and palpitations to syncope and sudden death.

Pediatric patients who have VT may have underlying structural heart disease, such as congenital heart disease, hypertrophic cardiomyopathy, anomalous origin of the left coronary artery, myocarditis, arrhythmogenic right ventricular dysplasia, and coronary heart disease. In the absence of structural heart disease and after excluding electrolyte disturbances or drug ingestion, conditions predisposing to malignant arrhythmias should be considered, such as Wolff-Parkinson-White syndrome, long QT syndrome, Brugada syndrome, Belhassen tachycardia, or catecholamine-induced polymorphic VT.

The Condition

Belhassen, or fascicular, VT is an idiopathic form of VT that occurs in a structurally normal heart. It is a microreentrant tachycardia with its foci in the left posterior fascicle of the left bundle branch. Electrocardiogram characteristically reveals a relatively narrow QRS complex between 100 and 140 milliseconds, a right bundle branch block pattern, and left axis deviation. The first episode of VT usually occurs in healthy young adults. The attack may be precipitated by exercise, excitement, or infection. Patients are typically hemodynamically stable and present with palpitations, dizziness, fatigue, and shortness of breath.

Management

This arrhythmia is generally responsive to calcium channel blockers and thus is known also as verapamil-sensitive tachycardia. Class III antiarrhythmic drugs such as amiodarone can be effective. The arrhythmia does not respond to vagal maneuvers or lidocaine. In some cases, termination with intravenous adenosine has been noted. Postconversion nonspecific ST and T wave changes in inferior and lateral leads may be seen.

Prognosis

Long-term oral calcium channel blockers (such as verapamil) are used to prevent recurrences. In resistant cases, elective catheter ablation can be performed. The success rate for ablation approaches 90%, which is one of the highest for any form of VT encountered in young patients. The long-term prognosis is usually very good.

Lessons for the Physician

- Ventricular tachycardia is an important cause of palpitations and chest discomfort in an apparently healthy young individual with no underlying predisposing condition.
- Belhassen tachycardia is an idiopathic ventricular tachycardia with good prognosis and can be recognized by its typical clinical and electrocardiographic presentation. It responds to calcium channel blockers.

Vaneet Kumar Kalra, MD; Fuad M. Kiblawi, MD; and Dorothy Myridakis, MD, Department of Pediatrics, St. Joseph Children's Hospital, Paterson, NJ

Part 4

Dermatology

CHAPTER 13

Erythematous Papulovesicular Rash in a 3-Month-Old Girl

Presentation

A 3-month-old previously healthy girl presents to the emergency department with a 1-day history of a blistering rash. Her parents noted an erythematous area on her occiput after picking her up from child care yesterday. Overnight, she became fussy, took less orally, and had trouble sleeping. By this morning, the lesions on her occiput had become vesicular, and an erythematous rash had extended down her back. She has had no fever, vomiting, diarrhea, cold symptoms, mucous membrane involvement, decreased urine output, or sick contacts. Her birth history is unremarkable.

Physical examination reveals a nontoxic but fussy infant who is afebrile and whose other vital signs are within normal parameters. Skin examination reveals a 5 × 6–cm, erythematous, boggy area on the occiput (Figure 13.1), with evidence of 3 ruptured vesicles and serosanguineous drainage. A clearly delineated erythematous maculopapular rash is evident on the back of her neck, back, buttocks, and posterior aspects of both the upper and lower extremities (Figure 13.2).

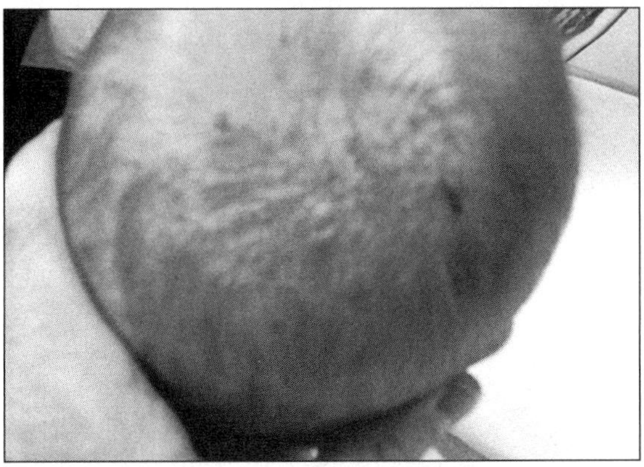

Figure 13.1. Erythematous vesicular lesions with serosanguineous drainage on the infant's scalp.

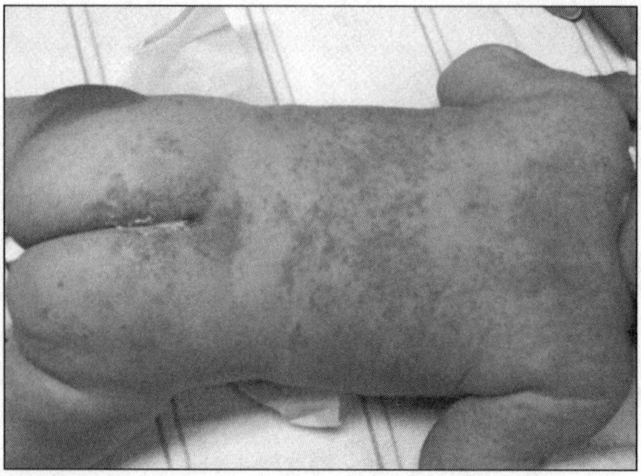

Figure 13.2. Extensive erythematous maculopapular rash on the back.

Laboratory evaluation reveals a white blood cell count of 17.0×10^3/mcL (17.0×10^9/L) with 37% neutrophils, 46% lymphocytes, 11% monocytes, and 6% eosinophils. Serum electrolyte values are normal. Cultures of the blood and lesion are sent. The Gram stain is negative. One day after admission, the 14-month-old sibling of the patient is hospitalized for a similar rash, and 2 days later, 5 of 11 infants and children attending the child care facility present with similar symptoms. The child care facility is closed for inspection by the county health department, which leads to the diagnosis.

- **What is your differential diagnosis at this point?**
- **Are there any elements of history or physical examination that would help you?**
- **What additional diagnostic studies would you like performed?**

Discussion

The investigator from the health department discovered that undiluted bleach (sodium hypochlorite) was being used to clean the diaper changing table without any protective barrier between the children and the table.

Diagnosis

Acute contact dermatitis reactions to strong irritants (eg, acids, alkaline solutions) are equivalent to chemical burns in severe cases and can be graded like thermal burns (ie, first-, second-, or third-degree burns). Contact dermatitis can result from either an allergic reaction or an irritant such as bleach, as in this case. Irritant-induced contact dermatitis accounts for 80% of cases. It often is difficult to distinguish between the 2 entities. Irritant contact dermatitis is due to a physical and chemical change of the epidermis, whereas allergic contact dermatitis is a delayed hypersensitivity reaction. Patients who have preexisting skin conditions (atopic dermatitis, dry skin) and those who have fair skin are more susceptible.

Other possible diagnoses include atopic dermatitis, seborrheic dermatitis, nummular eczema, dyshidrotic eczema, and fungal infections. Violent injury should also be considered in the case of severe dermatitis that has a defined distribution. Patch testing can confirm allergic contact dermatitis if the offending agent is available. Skin biopsy is usually not helpful in these circumstances. Gram stain and culture can identify secondary bacterial infection. Potassium hydroxide examination may be performed to rule out fungal infection, depending on the site and morphology of the lesions.

Clinical manifestations in the acute phase of dermatitis can range from chapped skin, dryness, and fissuring in mild cases to erythema, edema, vesiculation, and serous oozing in more severe cases. Irritant contact dermatitis can cause painful or tender lesions that, unlike allergic contact dermatitis, are usually not pruritic. Chronic exposure can lead to pigmentary changes, lichenification, scaling, and fissuring. The rash is usually well delineated, with sharp demarcations that suggest the application of a toxic substance. Flexural areas are the most susceptible, due to prolonged exposure. Clothing should be examined to ascertain if it has been soaked with the toxic substance.

The Condition

Household bleach contact and ingestion are common causes of childhood poisoning. The most common symptoms are from ingestion and include vomiting, hematemesis, excess salivation, and dysphagia. Systemic effects include hypernatremia and hyperchloremic acidosis. Caustic burns of the facial skin, lips, or oropharyngeal mucosa may appear as white or gray patches with erythematous borders. Irritant contact dermatitis is reported less frequently. The degree of tissue damage caused by a caustic alkali depends on the duration of contact with the tissue and the pH of the product. The mechanism of action is due to the alkalinity of the solution producing edema and saponification and oxidoreduction causing coagulation of cutaneous proteins. Household bleaches contain varying amounts of sodium peroxide, sodium perborate, and sodium hypochlorite. Most contain 3% to 6% sodium hypochlorite. The pH is close to 11, which is less corrosive than other industrial cleaners.

In 2007, the American Association of Poison Control Centers reported that dermal exposures were ranked second behind ingestions in poisoning incidents. Household cleaning substances such as bleach were placed second in terms of substances most frequently involved in pediatric exposures (5 years and younger). During 2007, 14,395 children younger than 6 years were seen for sodium hypochlorite exposure, with 44% requiring treatment in a health care facility.[1]

Treatment and Prognosis

Treatment is primarily supportive and involves dilution of the toxic substance with water to reduce contact time with the skin. Ideally, the substance should be avoided in the future. Healing in irritant contact dermatitis begins immediately after removal of the offending agent, in comparison with allergic contact dermatitis, in which there is a transient increase in the reaction before subsiding.

Topical antibiotics such as silver sulfadiazine, which has activity against *Staphylococcus aureus, Escherichia coli, Klebsiella, Pseudomonas aeruginosa, Proteus,* and *Candida albicans,* can be useful in the prevention of infections. This treatment, however, is contraindicated in preterm infants or infants younger than 2 months because sulfonamides may displace bilirubin from protein-binding sites and cause kernicterus. Leukopenia may occur in 5% to 15% of treated patients, but this occurrence does not increase the risk of infection.

The use of topical corticosteroids and immunomodulators is not proven. Pain control is also necessary. Hospital admission is recommended for severe dermal burns (>10% body surface area), evidence of systemic toxicity, need for pain control, or suspected abuse. Transfer to a regional burn center to optimize care should be considered if the damage is severe. Mild lesions (superficial, <10% body surface area) can be treated in the outpatient setting but must be rechecked frequently. The prognosis is good, with resolution of the rash in the following weeks. No permanent scarring should occur if the dermis is not damaged.

Reference

1. Bronstein AC, Spyker DA, Cantilena JR, et al. 2007 Annual Report of the American Association of Poison Control Centers' National Poison Data System (NPDS): 25th Annual Report. *Clin Toxicol.* 2008;46(10):927–1057

Lessons for the Physician

- The diagnosis of an environmental exposure must be considered a sentinel event, leading to an investigation for other cases and to identify the source of exposure.
- Parents should be asked if they think the illness is related to their home environment, the child care facility, or another location.
- The parents should also be questioned about their work or hobbies, which could lead to exposure.
- It is important to clarify the quantity of the agent; frequency, duration, and intensity of exposure; which parts of the skin surface area are exposed; and if there was occlusive contact with the skin. This important element of the history is key in making the correct diagnosis, starting the appropriate treatment, and preventing additional exposure.

Nadia Bajwa, MD, and Dominique Belli, MD, Hôpital des Enfants, Geneva, Switzerland

CHAPTER 14

Irritability, Vomiting, and a Mildly Reddened Right Eye in a 6-Month-Old Girl

Presentation

A 6-month-old girl presents to the emergency department with irritability, vomiting, and a mildly reddened right eye. The infant was well in the morning, and her parents left her unattended in her playpen. There did not appear to be any hazards in the vicinity of the infant, and the parents had not noticed anything unusual at the time. However, she developed the manifestations several hours after they left her in the playpen.

Physical examination reveals a right eye hyphema completely filling the anterior chamber and an intraocular pressure (IOP) in the high 70s by portable tonometry (normal IOP for most adult patients is <21 and slightly less in pediatric patients). The left eye pressure is normal. External eye examination reveals no evidence of trauma. The right pupil cannot be seen directly; the left pupil shows no relative afferent pupillary defect. Dilated fundus examination is deferred to monitor the patient's pupillary response in the setting of elevated IOP. The patient is admitted for acute management.

- **What is your differential diagnosis at this point?**
- **Are there any elements of history or physical examination that would help you?**
- **What additional diagnostic studies would you like performed?**

Discussion

Hyphema is a common presentation to a children's hospital that has potentially permanent sequelae of blindness or amblyopia. Typically, hyphema is associated with trauma and often includes periocular signs of trauma, such as bruising, skin abrasion, subconjunctival hemorrhage, corneal abrasion, or even an orbital fracture. The hyphema in this case appeared to be spontaneous and without trauma, which suggests a possible underlying condition. Entities that may present as spontaneous hyphema include leukemia, bleeding diathesis, retinoblastoma, and other intraocular tumors or lesions.

Diagnosis

Appropriate evaluation includes a complete blood cell count, ultrasonography of the eye (B-scan), and coagulation studies if a bleeding diathesis is suspected. If there is suspicion of violent trauma, a child abuse team should be notified and the appropriate evaluation, initiated, including a skeletal survey and head computed tomography scan. A dilated fundus examination should be performed by an ophthalmologist and remains an important part of the evaluation for violent trauma. If the patient is African American, a thorough history regarding sickle cell anemia should be obtained, and hemoglobin electrophoresis is recommended if sickle cell disease is considered. Both sickle cell anemia and sickle cell trait can have devastating consequences on an eye with a hyphema. The presence of either condition dramatically changes the treatment plan from noninvasive to surgical on an emergent basis. Patients who have sickle cell anemia have a significantly worse visual prognosis from a hyphema, and the use of acetazolamide is contraindicated.

Treatment and Clinical Course

Acute treatment of hyphema is aimed at lowering the IOP because a high IOP can lead to corneal staining from the iron in hemoglobin, permanent optic nerve damage, and blindness. In this patient, therapy was directed at lowering the IOP with systemic acetazolamide and topical timolol. A β-blocker must be used judiciously in an infant or child who has asthma. Intravenous methylprednisolone was added to control intraocular inflammation (topical prednisolone acetate could also be considered as an anti-inflammatory agent), and atropine eyedrops were instilled to fix and dilate the pupil, theoretically lowering the risk of the iris rebleeding. Prostaglandin analogs and alpha$_2$-adrenergic agonists are not appropriate choices in the pediatric patient but are often used in adults to control IOP. Bed rest is the standard of care for patients who have hyphema, although difficult to enforce in small children. The vomiting reported for the patient may have been related to the elevated eye pressure. Hospitalization with sedation must be considered if the child's activities at home cannot be controlled. The goal is for bed rest to lower the risk of rebleeding and to allow the settling and clearing of the red blood cells from the anterior chamber of the eye.

The next day, this patient's hyphema appeared to have cleared to about 20% to 30% anterior chamber involvement (Figure 14.1), and her IOP improved. Examination of the right eye revealed a small iris lesion partially obscured by the blood in the anterior chamber. Further physical examination revealed two 2.5-mm yellowish pink, smooth papules on the left lateral abdomen and right upper back (Figure 14.2). A dermatologist performed a skin biopsy, and the diagnosis of juvenile xanthogranuloma was established on histopathology.

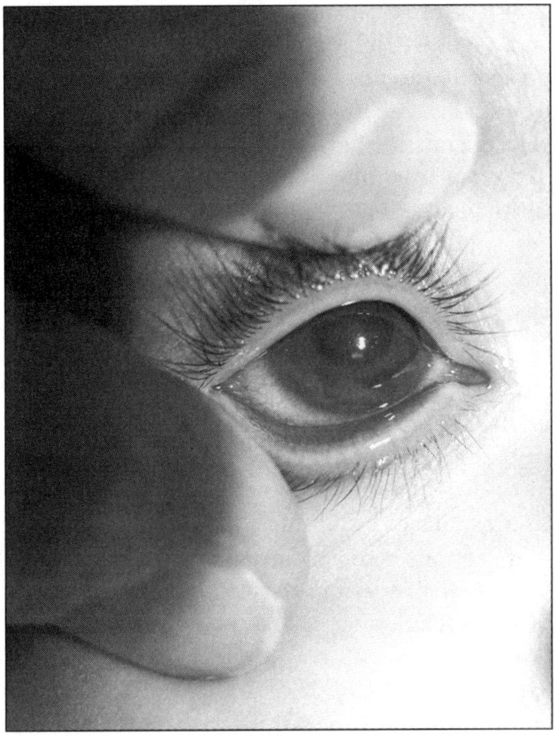

Figure 14.1. Hyphema involving 20% to 30% of the anterior chamber.

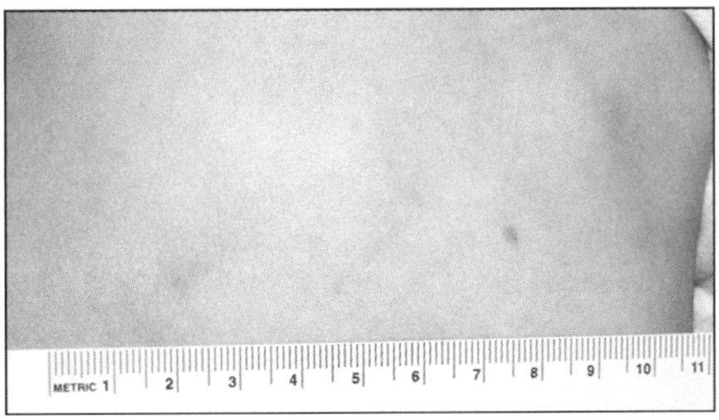

Figure 14.2. A yellowish pink, smooth papule (juvenile xanthogranuloma) on the right upper back.

The Condition

Juvenile xanthogranuloma is a localized, benign, histiocytic infiltrative lesion that appears to affect the pediatric population most commonly. Juvenile xanthogranuloma is primarily a self-limited dermatologic disorder that is associated rarely with systemic manifestations. The nodular lesions are typically cutaneous, arise spontaneously, and typically regress within 2 months. The lesions may also be found in many other locations. Subcutaneous, intramuscular, and visceral lesions may develop and are typically noted incidentally. The eye, particularly the uveal tract (the iris and ciliary body), is the most frequent site of extracutaneous involvement. Approximately 50% of patients who have ocular involvement have skin lesions. Juvenile xanthogranuloma is the most frequent cause of spontaneous hyphema in infants and children and can result in secondary glaucoma and eventual blindness. Ciliary body involvement may also present as a uveitis, with the patient having a painful red eye, photophobia, and tearing.

Prognosis

The prognosis for juvenile xanthogranuloma is excellent. Typically, the lesions resolve with topical steroids but may require systemic or periocular steroids if topical treatment fails. Occasionally, low-dose radiation therapy or surgical excision is recommended for otherwise nonresponsive lesions. Patients should be followed closely and all potential eye complications, managed by an ophthalmologist until the lesions regress. This patient had new skin lesions develop but no further eye involvement, and she continues to do well at home.

Lessons for the Physician

A child who has an ophthalmologic emergency, such as hyphema, can present with the vague complaint of irritability. Although hyphemas are most commonly caused by trauma, uncommon causes may be supported by physical findings. A thorough physical examination is critical when making the diagnosis in a child, especially if violent trauma is part of the differential diagnosis.

Heather Toth, MD; Robert Fish, MD; David Dueker, MD; Raja Sadiq, MD; and Yolanda Wolff, MD, Medical College of Wisconsin, Milwaukee, WI

CHAPTER 15

A 7-Month-Old Who Has a Persistent Rash (Visual Diagnosis)

Presentation

A 7-month-old boy presents to the pediatric infectious diseases clinic with an unusual rash for the past 4 weeks. The rash appeared first on the back of his neck as a reddish brown raised "spot" (Figure 15.1). Over the past month, other reddish brown macules and papules have appeared on his anterior trunk that have later developed a fine scale, followed in some places by erosions and black eschar formation. These lesions were neither vesicular nor pustular in appearance before eroding. The eschars eventually healed, leaving hypopigmented scars.

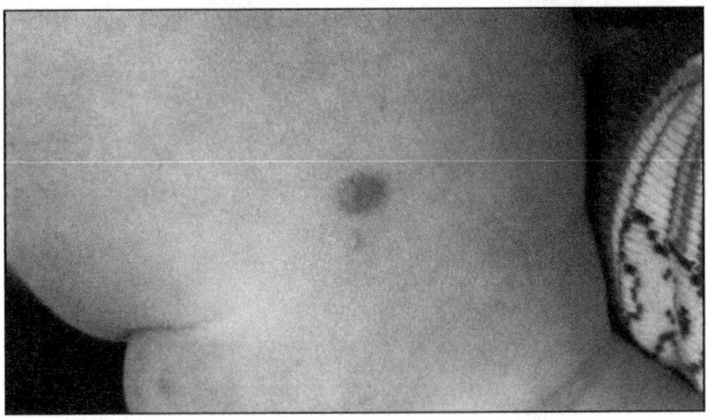

Figure 15.1. Reddish brown raised "spot" on back of thigh similar to the spot that first appeared on the back of infant's neck.

The infant has been asymptomatic otherwise and has gained weight during this time, maintaining his normal appetite and activity. There is no history of fever or discomfort. Initially, a pediatrician thought the infant had scabies and prescribed permethrin cream, but there was no improvement of the infant's condition. The pediatrician then prescribed 2 courses of antibiotics (cephalexin and amoxicillin) for a presumed varicella infection complicated by bacterial superinfection. Again, there was no improvement. Because of the continued appearance of new lesions the infant was referred to a pediatric infectious diseases clinic.

The infant's past medical history is unremarkable. He was delivered vaginally without complications at term and has been healthy otherwise until the rash appeared. There has been no animal exposure or travel. There is no history of a respiratory or gastrointestinal infection or administration of any medications before the onset of the rash. His immunizations are up to date, and he does not have any allergies. The family history is unremarkable.

Physical examination reveals a playful, smiling infant in no distress who has a heart rate of 112 beats/min, respiratory rate of 24 breaths/min, temperature of 97.5°F (36.4°C), and weight of 8.8 kg (75th percentile). Skin examination reveals reddish brown papules and plaques measuring 0.5 to 1.5 cm in diameter (Figure 15.2). The lesions appear to be in different stages of development; some are covered with a fine white scale, while others show erosion and black eschars. There is mild scarring and hypopigmentation where the earliest lesions had appeared. Most of the lesions are localized to the anterior trunk, especially in the periumbilical area and under the right axilla. No involvement of the palms, soles, or mucosal surfaces is appreciated. The posterior torso is spared. The rest of the examination is unremarkable.

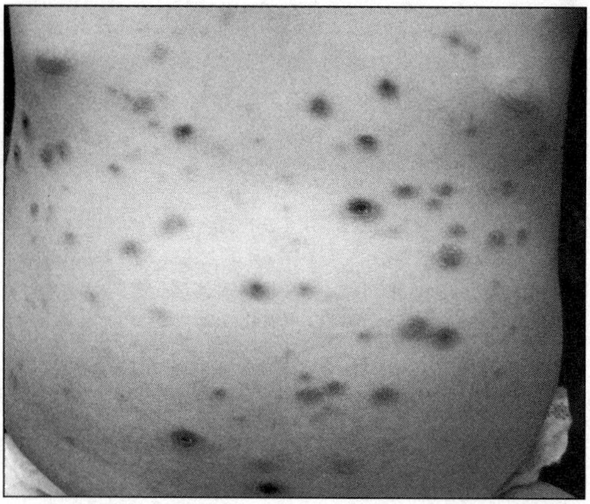

Figure 15.2. Reddish brown papules and plaques with fine scales and eschars on trunk.

A complete blood cell count shows a hemoglobin level of 12.4 g/dL (124 g/L), hematocrit of 35% (0.35), white blood cell count of 6,800/μL (1% bands, 13% neutrophils, 74% lymphocytes, 6% monocytes, 4% eosinophils, and 2% basophils), and platelet count of 434,000/mm^3. C-reactive protein level is less than or equal to 0.5 mg/dL.

Consultation with a pediatric dermatologist and a medical procedure confirm the clinical diagnosis.

- **What is your differential diagnosis at this point?**
- **Are there any elements of history or physical examination that would help you?**
- **What additional diagnostic studies would you like performed?**

Diagnosis

A skin-punch biopsy showed focal parakeratosis overlying a spongiotic epidermis, with occasional dyskeratotic keratinocytes and extravasated red blood cells in the epidermis and papillary dermis (Figures 15.3 and 15.4). The reticular dermis contained a lymphocytic infiltrate that extended to the lower portion of the dermis and surrounding adnexal structures. These findings were compatible with pityriasis lichenoides et varioliformis acuta (PLEVA), an idiopathic-acquired dermatosis characterized by evolving erythematous, scaly papules that develop vesiculation, ulceration, and necrosis.

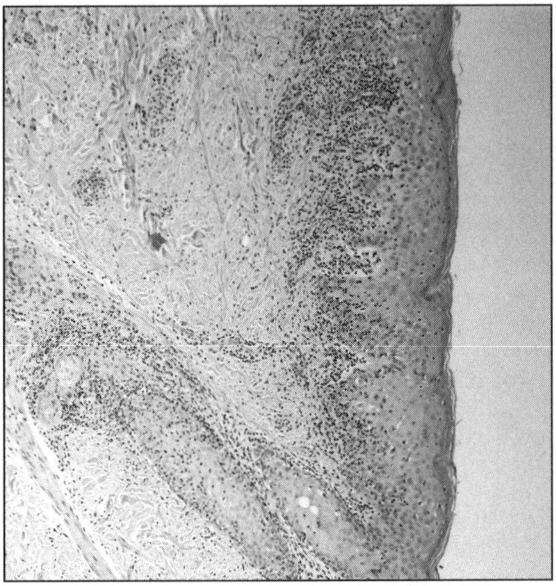

Figure 15.3. Skin-punch biopsy shows lymphocytic infiltration obscuring the dermoepidermal interface. There is extravasation of red blood cells, parakeratosis, dyskeratotic keratinocytes, spongiosis, and basal vacuolar changes.

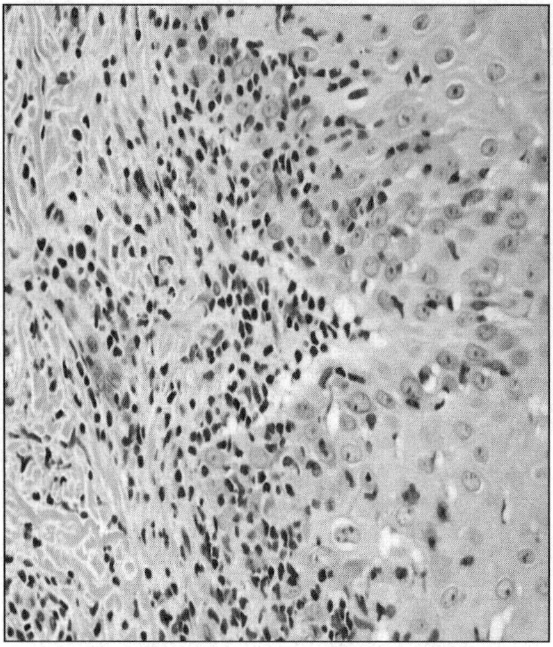

Figure 15.4. High power (40×). Lymphocytic infiltrate at the dermoepidermal interface with rare extravasated red blood cells, dyskeratotic keratinocytes, and basal vacuolar changes.

Discussion

Etiology

Pityriasis lichenoides et varioliformis acuta is commonly preceded by an upper respiratory or gastrointestinal tract infection. Epstein-Barr virus, *Mycoplasma pneumoniae, Streptococcus pyogenes, Toxoplasma gondii,* parvovirus B19, and adenovirus are among the infectious agents associated with the onset of this rash. Other potential triggers include antibiotics, antipyretics, and vaccines. These observations, plus biopsy findings of immune complexes composed of IgM and complement component C3 in the dermoepidermal junction and blood vessels, support the hypothesis that PLEVA represents a hypersensitivity reaction to an infectious or noninfectious antigen. Recently, it has been suggested that in some cases the eruption represents a true cutaneous lymphoproliferative disorder due to the demonstration of monoclonal $CD8^+$ lymphocytes infiltrating the skin.

Epidemiology

Once thought to be uncommon in infants and children, recent reports suggest that the incidence of PLEVA may be underestimated in the pediatric population. The incidence of PLEVA peaks twice during childhood; the first peak occurs at

24 to 36 months of age and the second peak, between 5 and 7 years of age. Pityriasis lichenoides et varioliformis acuta rarely occurs before the second year after birth, although neonatal cases have been described. No ethnic group seems to be affected predominantly over another. Pityriasis lichenoides et varioliformis acuta has a mild male preponderance, with a male to female ratio close to 1.5 to 1. The incidence may be higher during the winter and fall.

Clinical Presentation

Pityriasis lichenoides et varioliformis acuta usually presents acutely with crops of brown or reddish papules about 1 cm in diameter that have surrounding erythema. New lesions appear rapidly, most frequently affecting the trunk, flexor surfaces, and proximal extremities. The soles, palms, and mucosal surfaces are usually spared. Facial and scalp involvement, although rare in adults, occur in 40% of children. Lesions usually change over time, and multiple stages of development coexist at any point. The lesions can acquire white scale; they evolve into vesicles, pustules, and then erosions and ulcers. The ulcer will generally develop a necrotic appearance and finally a black eschar before healing. Healing of the lesion usually results in a scar (varioliform, or resembling smallpox) and hypopigmentation or, less commonly, hyperpigmentation.

The presence of necrosis, vesiculation, and ulceration rather than the duration of symptoms distinguish PLEVA from pityriasis lichenoides chronica (PLC), the chronic form of pityriasis lichenoides. Pityriasis lichenoides chronica is characterized by asymptomatic reddish brown papules with white scale that usually do not erode, ulcerate, or necrose. Histologically, PLC is similar to PLEVA, but the observed changes are milder in PLC. It is common for patients to have lesions of PLEVA and PLC simultaneously. This coincidence suggests that both forms represent different ends of the spectrum of the same disease. Constitutional symptoms accompany PLEVA in two-thirds of cases. Pruritus is the most common symptom, occurring in 50% of cases. Fever, arthralgias, and malaise occur less commonly.

Differential Diagnosis

The differential diagnosis of PLEVA includes scabies, varicella, erythema multiforme, secondary syphilis, Gianotti-Crosti syndrome, tularemia, ecthyma, papular urticaria, and vasculitis. In an immunocompetent host, varicella lesions appear within a 2-week period and usually develop rapidly, evolving from macule to papule to vesicle to crust in 2 to 3 days, whereas PLEVA lesions evolve more slowly. Scabies, secondary syphilis, and Gianotti-Crosti syndrome seldom show necrosis. Lymphomatoid papulosis, a form of cutaneous lymphoma, may be impossible to differentiate from PLEVA on clinical grounds; this distinction is generally made by skin biopsy, which usually shows the presence of $CD30^+$ lymphocytes having the atypical features of lymphomatoid papulosis.

Classification

If PLEVA affects the trunk, head, and inguinal region, it is classified as central; if the eruption affects only the limbs, it is classified as peripheral. Pityriasis lichenoides et varioliformis acuta is classified as diffuse if there is central and peripheral involvement. The diffuse form represents 60% to 74% of PLEVA cases; the central form, 5% to 21%; and the peripheral form, 18% to 20%.

Evaluation

There is often a delay in making the diagnosis of PLEVA because of its polymorphic appearance, indolent course, and broad differential diagnosis. Skin biopsy is the criterion standard for diagnosis and should always be performed when PLEVA is suspected. Inflammatory markers such as C-reactive protein level, erythrocyte sedimentation rate, and white blood cell count can be elevated, as well as liver transaminase levels, but these findings are nonspecific.

Course

Pityriasis lichenoides et varioliformis acuta is considered a self-limited disease. Ersoy-Evans et al[1] reported a median resolution time of 18 months (range, 2–108 months) for PLEVA and 20 months (range, 3–132 months) for PLC. Relapses are common before complete resolution. Although initial reports suggested that the diffuse form had the fastest resolution rate and the peripheral form, the slowest, this distinction has not been corroborated in more recent reports.

Complications

Febrile Ulceronecrotic Variant of Mucha-Habermann Disease

Febrile ulceronecrotic variant of Mucha-Habermann disease is characterized by high fever and progression of the typical PLEVA lesions to larger (5- to 10-cm) and more painful ulcerative lesions with extensive necrosis as well as multiorgan involvement, including liver, central nervous system, and coagulation abnormalities. This condition carries a fatality rate as high as 25%. Sepsis can complicate this presentation because of bacterial superinfection of the lesions. Mucosal involvement is more common in this condition. Skin biopsy is critical for making a timely diagnosis.

Malignancy

Although rare, cutaneous T-cell lymphoma can arise from PLEVA lesions. Some researchers have suggested that PLEVA is a premalignant condition representing the mildest end of a spectrum that includes PLEVA, PLC, lymphomatoid papulosis, and cutaneous T-cell lymphoma.

Associated Conditions

Juvenile idiopathic arthritis, immune thrombocytopenic purpura, nonskin lymphomas, and hemophagocytic syndrome have been associated with PLEVA.

Treatment

Evaluating the efficacy of therapies for PLEVA is difficult because of lack of randomized controlled trials and the relapsing and self-limited nature of the disease. Ultraviolet B phototherapy is the most effective treatment; however, long-term carcinogenic concerns in infants and children preclude this treatment as first-line therapy.

Oral erythromycin at standard doses is the most prescribed medication for PLEVA and has demonstrated a 25% to 87% response rate in children. Tetracyclines have also been used in older children and adults. Clinical response may be obtained within 2 weeks, but it may take up to 2 months. If response is obtained, the antibiotic should be tapered to prevent flares; in most cases, the taper can be completed within 1 to 4 months after clinical response is obtained. There are reports of clinical success with azithromycin in erythromycin-refractory cases. It is unclear why antibiotics are effective in treating PLEVA, but it has been suggested that the immunomodulatory properties of the macrolides may play an important role in the improvement of lesions. Because PLEVA usually follows a benign course, some experts advocate observation without further intervention if antibiotics are unsuccessful.

Therapy with topical tacrolimus, systemic corticosteroids, and methotrexate has been successful in patients.

Symptomatic relief of pruritus with emollients, antihistamines, and topical corticosteroids is an important component of treatment; however, these medications have minimal, if any, effect on the skin lesions' evolution.

In febrile ulceronecrotic variant of Mucha-Habermann disease, methotrexate can be lifesaving. Intravenous immunoglobulin, cyclosporine, and systemic corticosteroids have also been successful.

Patient Course

The patient was started on oral erythromycin 3 times a day and was scheduled for a 1-month follow-up visit with a dermatologist. Unfortunately, the patient did not show up to this appointment. Six months later he was evaluated in the emergency department for a viral gastroenteritis and was found to be free of skin lesions at that time.

Reference

1. Ersoy-Evans S, Greco MF, Mancini AJ, Subasi N, Paller AS. Pityriasis lichenoides in childhood: a retrospective review of 124 patients. *J Am Acad Dermatol.* 2007;56(2):205–210

Summary

- Pityriasis lichenoides et varioliformis acuta should be considered in children who present with coexisting papules, ulcers, and eschars. These skin lesions heal, leaving a hypopigmented scar.
- Most infants and children who have PLEVA are nontoxic in appearance and are healthy otherwise.
- If systemic symptoms are prominent, febrile ulceronecrotic variant of Mucha-Habermann disease should be considered.
- A skin biopsy is mandatory to confirm the diagnosis and exclude more serious conditions, such as malignancy or vasculitis.
- Erythromycin is the medication most commonly used as first-line therapy.
- Most PLEVA cases are self-limited, although some cases can have a relapsing course before resolving.

Angel Alberto Herrera Guerra, MD, Fellow, and Russell J. Osguthorpe, MD, Assistant Professor, Division of Pediatric Infectious Diseases, Department of Pediatrics, University of Utah, Salt Lake City, UT

Angelica Putnam, MD, Department of Pediatric Pathology, University of Utah, Salt Lake City, UT

Sheryll L. Vanderhooft, MD, Professor, Department of Dermatology, University of Utah, Salt Lake City, UT

CHAPTER 16

Perinasal and Perioral Rash in a 2-Year-Old Girl

Presentation

A 2-year-old Caucasian girl presents with a 2-month history of a rash around her mouth and nose. On examination, she has perioral and perinasal pink papules and papulopustules, which coalesce to form thin plaques, as well as occasional periorbital papules and a small area of crusting in the perinasal region (Figure 16.1). The rash is nonpruritic but accompanied by a burning sensation. Notably, the patient's vermilion border is spared.

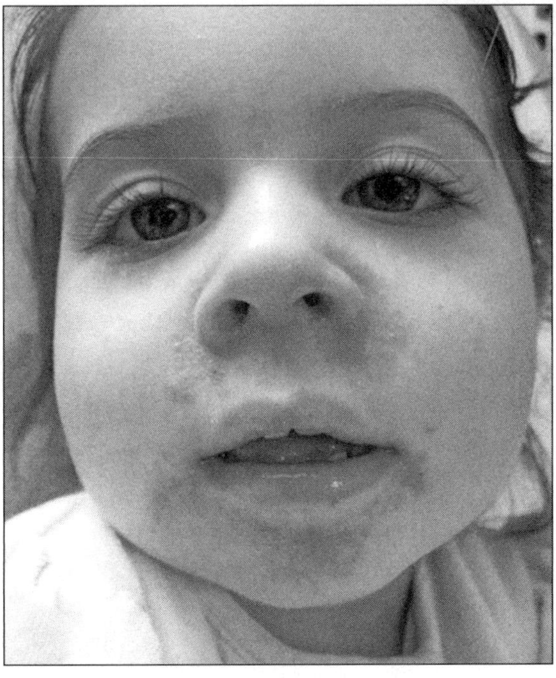

Figure 16.1. Perioral and perinasal pink papules and papulopustules that have coalesced to form thin plaques, occasional periorbital papules, and a small area of crusting in the perinasal region.

Her past medical history is significant for a congenital cystic adenomatoid malformation (surgically resected at 6 weeks of age), atopic dermatitis, seasonal rhinitis, and asthma, requiring fluticasone propionate (44 mcg/puff twice daily) via a metered dose inhaler with spacer and face mask for the past 6 months (Figure 16.2). The dermatitis has been treated with over-the-counter cream and ointment without relief, but no topical products containing hydrocortisone have been used. The patient is seen by a dermatologist for the cause of the persistent facial rash, and her history and findings on physical examination lead to a presumptive diagnosis.

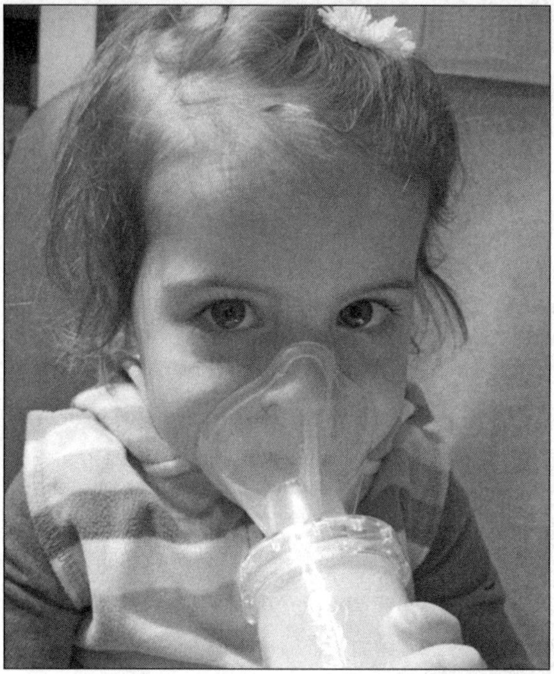

Figure 16.2. Patient using metered dose inhaler with spacer and face mask.

- **What is your differential diagnosis at this point?**
- **Are there any elements of history or physical examination that would help you?**
- **What additional diagnostic studies would you like performed?**

Discussion

The presentation of papulopustular lesions in a periorificial (surrounding an opening) distribution along with a history of routine corticosteroid exposure to the area is characteristic of periorificial (perioral) dermatitis (POD).

The Condition

Perioral dermatitis is a persistent papulopustular eruption that presents as discrete 1- to 2-mm papules irregularly grouped on an erythematous background, primarily around the mouth, with frequent involvement of the perinasal and orbital (especially infraorbital) regions. Sparing of the vermilion border of the lips is characteristic. Histopathologically, the eruption is characterized by subtle eczematous changes in the perifollicular skin.

In adults, POD is most common in females aged 16 to 45, associated with the increased use of cosmetics and other topical facial products in this population. Perioral dermatitis is less well described in the pediatric age group, but recent reviews have revealed a higher incidence of POD in children younger than 6 years as compared with older children. A boy to girl predominance has not been determined in the pediatric population.

The exact cause of POD is unknown; however, an impaired skin barrier has been described as a critical causative factor in its development. Patients who have atopy or other intrinsic causes of skin barrier dysfunction may thus be predisposed to develop POD. Although no large association studies have been performed, a personal or family history of atopy is observed with high frequency in patients who have POD. A variety of extrinsic allergens and irritants, such as cosmetics, moisturizers, sunscreens, and fluoride-containing toothpastes, may trigger the initial epidermal dysfunction.

Perioral dermatitis is typically and markedly aggravated by topical corticosteroids, and exposure to steroids through topical products or inhaled medication, as in this patient, may also precipitate the dermatitis. A common scenario in children is the presence of an initial irritant contact dermatitis, treated with topical corticosteroids by family or physicians, leading to POD as a secondary eruption. Thus, the elimination of irritants and avoidance of all topical skin care products, particularly topical corticosteroids, is essential for healing and prevention of POD.

Differential Diagnosis

The differential diagnosis of POD in the pediatric population includes allergic or irritant contact dermatitis, acne vulgaris, atopic dermatitis, seborrheic dermatitis, and lip licker's dermatitis. Unlike contact dermatitis and lip licker's dermatitis (caused by habitual licking of the lips and surrounding skin), POD rarely involves the vermilion border. An absence of comedones can distinguish POD from acne vulgaris. In atopic dermatitis, pruritus is always present, and the extremities or trunk are usually involved in addition to the face, whereas in POD, pruritus may or may not be present, but a burning sensation or feeling of tightness is reported more commonly.

Seborrheic dermatitis, typically seen in either infants or adolescents, should be considered when the perinasal region is the sole location of involvement; presence of waxy scale near the scalp and eyebrows supports this diagnosis. In cases in which allergic contact dermatitis is suspected, patch testing can help identify causative environmental allergens.

Treatment and Prognosis

To limit skin exposure to the corticosteroid, the patient's parents began washing her face with soap and water after every treatment, and she began the application of topical erythromycin ointment, 2%, twice daily to the affected areas. Although several medications have been used in the treatment of POD, topical metronidazole gel, 0.75%, has been associated with a good clinical outcome in at least one study, although this preparation is not licensed for use in children. These antibiotics are chosen for their anti-inflammatory properties and may prevent secondary infection of the dermatitis; if infection is suspected, appropriate diagnostic procedures should be performed.

Corticosteroids of any potency should be avoided, and patients who have experienced temporary alleviation with steroids should be advised of a rebound flare in erythema, papules, or pustules upon cessation that may continue for days to weeks if not treated otherwise. Families should be aware that the dermatitis commonly takes several weeks to resolve; averages of 7 weeks and 3 to 6 months have been reported. A several week course of topical metronidazole may be used solely or in combination with oral antibiotics (typically erythromycin, or doxycycline and tetracycline in children older than 8 years), particularly in more persistent or severe cases. Perioral dermatitis may recur without obvious cause but improves spontaneously over time.

This patient's lesions began to show improvement within 10 days, and erythromycin was discontinued after 3 weeks. The dermatitis had completely resolved in 1 month. She continued to wash her face after she used the inhaler and has had no recurrence.

Lessons for the Physician

- Perioral dermatitis is a persistent, uncomfortable facial inflammatory condition, caused or exacerbated by glucocorticoids, which can be frustrating for patients and their families because it is misdiagnosed often as a steroid-responsive dermatosis.
- When perioral dermatitis in children is associated with inhaled corticosteroids, the eruption may be prevented simply with thorough cleansing of the facial skin after each exposure to the steroid.

Suzanne J. Tintle, MD, MPH, Columbia University College of Physicians and Surgeons, New York, NY

Richard J. Antaya, MD, Departments of Dermatology and Pediatrics, Yale University School of Medicine, New Haven, CT

Charles L. G. Halasz, MD, Department of Dermatology, College of Physicians and Surgeons, Columbia University Medical Center, New York, NY

CHAPTER 17

5-Year-Old Girl Waking in Morning With Spots of Blood on Her Pillow and Sheets

Presentation

A 5-year-old girl is seen because of a 3-day history of waking every morning with spots of blood on her pillow and sheets. Her mother attributed the blood to epistaxis because of previous epistaxis. Today the child cried, and her mother found blood in her panties. The child says that she "fell on a chair" at school. On physical examination, her labia majora appear irritated, with several areas of purpura and dried blood on the skin.

The child is referred to a specialized clinic for evaluation of suspected sexual abuse. Her mother recalls that a sister, with whom the girl shares a room, said that the girl had been scratching her private parts every night for the past week. The mother also remembers a similar problem of labial irritation and mild scabbing, without excessive bleeding, 6 months ago. The girl denies improper touching of her genital area by others, and her parents deny suspicions of sexual abuse.

Upon examination, there are dark blood blisters along the medial aspects of both labia majora. The medial aspects of both labia majora appear white and thin. She has an annular hymen, which has a continuous inner edge without any transections or hematomas. There is mild friability of the posterior fourchette. The hymen and vestibule appear normal. The history and findings lead to the diagnosis.

- **What is your differential diagnosis at this point?**
- **Are there any elements of history or physical examination that would help you?**
- **What additional diagnostic studies would you like performed?**

Discussion

The pediatrician who assessed the girl initially in her office was concerned about sexual abuse as the cause of the girl's genital bleeding. On further questioning at the children's hospital, the mother's description of a similar episode with genital bleeding and scabbing in the past, as well as the patient's recent history of genital itching, suggested the possibility of a more chronic process. An additional physical finding was the hypopigmented, atrophic skin bilaterally along the medial labia majora, suggestive of the diagnosis of lichen sclerosus et atrophicus. A steroid cream was prescribed, and the appearance of the vulva improved.

The Condition

Lichen sclerosus is a skin condition of the perineum that can cause a variety of lesions in that area. The cause of lichen sclerosus is unknown. In young girls, lichen sclerosus most commonly involves the vulva, perineum, anus, and perianal tissues (Figure 17.1). The hymen and the mucosal surfaces of the vestibule are not involved. The skin becomes white and atrophic in a figure-of-eight pattern around the vulva and anus.

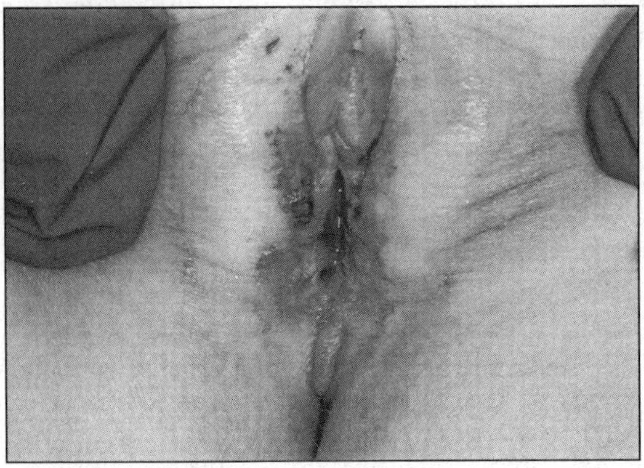

Figure 17.1. Perineum of child who has lichen sclerosus, showing pallor of the labia as well as erythema, hemorrhage, and excoriation.

Pain and itching of the skin lead to excoriation, often causing erythema, bleeding, and secondary infection. The presence of lichen sclerosus increases the susceptibility to vulvar trauma, and minor injuries often cause bleeding and bruising. Subepidermal hemorrhage may occur, leading to the appearance of hemorrhagic blisters or bullae. Problems with defecation, including painful bowel movements, constipation, and anal fissures, may also occur when the anus and perianal tissues are involved.

Lichen sclerosus is diagnosed clinically. A biopsy shows specific and fairly consistent histologic features, including thinning of the epidermis, vacuolar changes at the dermoepidermal border, edema of the papillary dermis, a bandlike lymphocytic infiltrate beneath the edema, and dilated capillaries with hemorrhage. In most cases, however, a biopsy is not necessary, and it is best to avoid the trauma of the procedure, particularly in a young child.

Other Conditions to Consider

The clinical picture of lichen sclerosus can be alarming to parents and physician alike, raising fears and suspicion of possible sexual abuse. Although most sexually abused children have normal physical findings on examination of their genitalia, sexual abuse should be considered in any child who presents with apparent genital trauma. Although she had a history of falling on a chair, the child's findings on examination were not consistent with this mechanism of injury. Trauma to the genitalia from straddle injuries may reveal lacerations and bruising of the anterior aspect of the genitalia between the labia majora and minora and periclitoral area. Injuries from trauma due to sexual abuse are not unique, but they frequently involve the posterior aspect of the genitalia, including penetrating injuries of the hymen and floor of the vestibule.

Complaints of genital bleeding in a young child should always be assessed carefully. This sign is not common in children and deserves careful consideration. If possible, the site of the bleeding should be determined because the blood may arise from the genitalia, urinary system, anus, or gastrointestinal tract. Each site of bleeding suggests its own list of specific causes. Besides lichen sclerosus, unintentional trauma to the genitalia, and injuries due to sexual abuse, other causes of genital bleeding include condyloma acuminata, urethral prolapse, vaginitis due to *Shigella* species or group A streptococci, and vaginal foreign body. Rarer causes include sarcoma botryoides, precocious puberty with menses, hemangioma, and bleeding disorders.

As in all areas of medicine, a careful history is always the best place to start when investigating genital bleeding. There was no history of any behaviors or specific statements to suggest that the child in question had been sexually abused. If the child has other signs of precocious puberty, such as breast tissue or pubic hair, precocious puberty should be considered. A child having no other signs of bleeding, such as epistaxis, petechiae, or purpura, is less likely to have a bleeding disorder. In this case, the girl had a history of genital itching and previous genital irritation, lending support to the diagnosis of lichen sclerosus.

Evaluation

Usually, the physical examination of the young child is performed best with the caregiver present. This support makes the examination less anxiety-provoking for the child and easier for the physician to complete thoroughly. The child should be examined first in the frog leg supine position. If this initial assessment does not yield the diagnosis, as in this case, a prone knee-chest or lateral knee–chest position allows for detailed visualization of the hymen, distal vagina, anus, and adjacent tissues. Any erythema, bruises, lacerations, excoriations, or discharge should be noted in addition to the shape and appearance of the hymen and other tissues. Dried or fresh blood may have to be removed to help identify the source of the bleeding. A thorough examination cannot be emphasized too strongly.

Management

Although there is no definitive cure, topical high-potency corticosteroid cream with careful medical follow-up and appropriate tapering as the condition improves are used to treat lichen sclerosus by ameliorating the symptoms. Recurrences are frequent. Some children experience resolution in puberty. Scarring of the clitoral hood can be a consequence despite treatment.

Lessons for the Physician

- Evaluating a child for possible sexual abuse is one of the most emotionally difficult experiences for a pediatrician. The physician must take a thorough history and perform a complete physical examination. Anogenital examinations in young girls can often be achieved with the least difficulty when a parent or assistant helps distract the child during the examination.
- Lichen sclerosus is a common skin condition that is sometimes mistaken for sexual abuse. Similarly, other conditions, such as urethral prolapse, perineal groove anomaly, or unintentional trauma, can be mistaken as well. Genital bleeding always necessitates a thorough investigation.
- Physicians must realize that lichen sclerosus and sexual abuse are not mutually exclusive diagnoses. A child who has lichen sclerosus can be abused just as any other child, and the finding of lichen sclerosus could simply be incidental during the abuse evaluation.
- This case serves as a reminder to evaluate carefully every suspicious case for sexual abuse, keeping in mind that not all anogenital symptoms and signs are due to sexual abuse.

John C. Browning, MD, and Clifford O. Mishaw, MD, Texas Children's Hospital, Baylor College of Medicine, Houston, TX

COMMENTARY BY DR MIRIAM WEINSTEIN, PEDIATRIC DERMATOLOGIST, SICK CHILDREN'S HOSPITAL, TORONTO, CANADA

Lichen sclerosus remains a rare but important diagnosis to be aware of given the significant morbidity and frequently missed diagnosis. Currently, it is thought to be of autoimmune origin. While seen more frequently in girls, it is important to note it can occur in boys and may involve the glans, foreskin, and urethra, but spare the perianal area. Boys may present with phimosis. While it was often thought that this disorder abated in most girls with the onset of puberty, it is now understood that it may persist as a chronic condition in girls beyond that time. Treatment of lichen sclerosus has typically been with ultra-potent topical steroids. A recent study showed that ultra-potent topical corticosteroids were superior to mild to moderate potency topical steroids with respect to symptom clearance. There is known risk of squamous cell carcinoma developing in adult and postmenopausal lichen sclerosus patients. Childhood lichen sclerosus does not appear to increase this risk, but children who continue to have the condition beyond puberty should be considered at risk for squamous cell carcinoma and monitored appropriately.

CHAPTER 18

Ecchymotic Lesions on the Backs of Asian Boys

Presentation

Two Asian boys, aged 9 and 11 years, who are neighbors, present to the emergency department (ED) 1 day apart complaining of sore throat, fever, headache, and abdominal pain for about 1 week. Both boys are otherwise healthy and have no known chronic illnesses, medication use, or previous hospitalizations.

Physical examination reveals normal vital signs in both boys. However, both boys exhibit an erythematous oropharynx, exudates on tonsils, and bilateral submandibular lymphadenitis. The findings on dermatologic examinations are of concern. The 9-year-old boy has numerous ecchymotic lesions on his back that are approximately 3 × 10 cm (Figure 18.1), and the 11-year-old boy has numerous round areas of ecchymosis approximately 8 cm in diameter across his back (Figure 18.2). All other physical findings are normal.

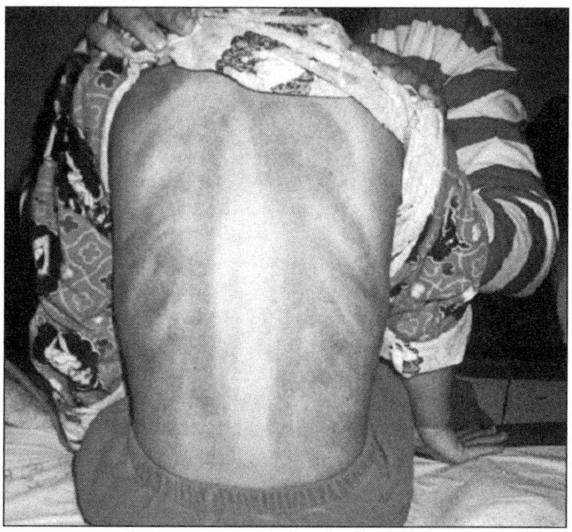

Figure 18.1. Numerous ecchymotic linear lesions on the back.

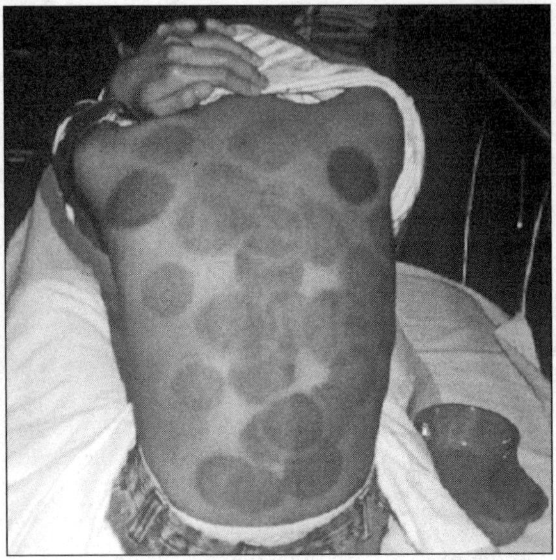

Figure 18.2. Numerous round areas of ecchymosis approximately 8 cm in diameter across the back.

On further questioning, neither boy has a history of epistaxis, bruising, petechiae, hemoptysis, hematochezia, fatigue, or weight loss. When questioned directly about the lesions, neither boy makes eye contact or provides an explanation of how the lesions occurred. Additional history reveals the cause for the findings.

- **What is your differential diagnosis at this point?**
- **Are there any elements of history or physical examination that would help you?**
- **What additional diagnostic studies would you like performed?**

Discussion

Both boys had positive rapid streptococcal latex agglutination tests and were started on penicillin therapy. Because of concern about the ecchymoses, screening coagulation studies were performed, and results were within reference range. Both boys were interviewed without adult supervision and were still not willing to provide an explanation for the bruising on their backs. Child protective services (CPS) was contacted to initiate an evaluation for violent trauma in both cases.

Diagnosis

On further questioning of the parents, it was learned that an Asian folk healer had treated both boys earlier that week. The 9-year-old boy was treated with coining and the 11-year-old boy, with cupping.

The Condition

The practices of cupping and coining are believed to heal individuals affected by respiratory and febrile illnesses. Coining (*cao gao*) is performed by massaging the back or chest with mentholated oil and then aggressively scraping the edge of a coin back and forth linearly until bruising or petechiae develop. Coining is not intended to cause permanent bodily harm and is a widespread practice throughout much of Vietnam and parts of Southeast Asia. Although coining does not typically cause serious harm, there is a reported case of a renal contusion with hematuria following coining.

Cupping is a traditional folk healing practice rooted in Latin American, Asian, and Eastern European beliefs. For cupping, a small amount of alcohol is ignited within a glass cup to heat the air inside the container. The cup is then placed on the bare skin of the affected individual. As the air within the cup cools, a vacuum is created between the cup and the skin, resulting in bruising of the skin.

Several cultural healing methods are mistaken for child abuse, the most common being cupping, coining, moxibustion, and spooning. Moxibustion is a Southeast Asian practice considered to be a variation of acupuncture in which a Chinese herb (*Artemisia vulgaris*) is burned onto the skin using an instrument such as yarn or incense near the affected area to draw out "the evil." Spooning is a practice in China that is similar to coining.

Asian folk healers have been practicing these techniques in major metropolitan cities that have large Asian populations. In both these cases, the ED physicians taking care of these boys were not aware of these healing methods despite practicing medicine in an institution where many of their patients came from ethnic and cultural populations that practice such faith-healing methods. Because the patients had physical findings of bruising in unusual patterns over the back without explanation, the ED physicians suspected violent trauma, thereby warranting reports to CPS, which determined that the bruising was the result of nonharmful attempts to heal the patients.

These procedures had parental consent and therefore did not constitute violent trauma. In both cases, the intent behind the treatment methods was based on culturally accepted traditional beliefs. Thus, it was determined that the injuries were not a result of physical abuse, and CPS released the boys to their parents.

Most bruising in children is due to unintentional trauma, and 93% of unintentional bruises occur over bony prominences. In the ambulatory child, unintentional bruises generally occur on the extensor surfaces of the leg, the anterior thigh, and the forehead. Unintentional bruising on the chest, abdomen, back, buttocks, soft tissue of the face, ears, and "protected areas" such as the neck, genital area, and inner thighs is uncommon in children of all ages. The presence of a bruise in any of these uncommon locations may signal violent injury and possible serious underlying pathology such as intracranial injury, skeletal fracture, or intra-abdominal trauma, particularly in a child younger than 2 years.

Bruises due to violent trauma often assume a pattern that reflects the shape of the impacting object. Common "patterned" violent injuries include pinch marks, human bites, hand slaps, ligature marks around the neck or extremities, and marks from electric cords, belts, brushes, shoes, and kitchen utensils.

In the case of a child younger than 2 years who has suspicious bruises, the physician should consider further evaluation for abuse (such as imaging studies) because 43% of all violent skeletal fractures are unsuspected clinically at the time of the child's evaluation, and approximately 50% of children in whom a violent fracture is diagnosed have more than one fracture at the time of diagnosis. For children older than 2 years, further evaluation for underlying injuries should be initiated if the patient is symptomatic.

The differential diagnosis for bruising includes Mongolian spots, phytophotodermatitis, coagulopathy, Henoch-Schönlein purpura, Ehlers-Danlos syndrome, erythema multiforme, and cultural practices such as coining and cupping. Most of these diagnoses can be distinguished on the basis of the history, physical examination, and laboratory evaluation to rule out bleeding disorders.

Because of the high morbidity and mortality associated with child abuse, physicians need to be sensitive to the possibility of abuse. Although reporting suspected child abuse might cause discomfort for the family, not reporting child abuse may cause significant harm to the child. However, the physician should be aware of cultural practices that may appear to hurt a child but do not.

Lessons for the Physician

- Physicians must consider the possibility of physical abuse when faced with a child who has an unexplained traumatic injury.
- Lack of awareness of the cultural and traditional healing practices used by various communities can lead a physician to suspect potential physical abuse when encountering certain physical findings.
- Although the stigma of suspected child abuse can be painful for families, it is extremely important to investigate fully any suspected violent trauma to prevent further harm to children.

Ryan P. Flanagan, MD, Children's Hospital of Pittsburgh Heart Center, Pittsburgh, PA

Neil Mullen, MD, Department of Pediatrics, Madigan Army Medical Center, Fort Lewis, Tacoma, WA

CHAPTER 19

Petechial Lesions on Toes of an 11-Year-Old Girl

Presentation

An 11-year-old girl presents with a 2-month history of petechial lesions on her toes. The lesions first appeared 2 months ago on the second toe of her left foot, after which the lesions began to spread to her adjacent toes and other foot. The lesions are painful with applied pressure. In the past she was either given a course of antibiotics with no discernable benefit or told that the lesions may have been from a viral illness. She denies any recent cold exposure or trauma to the area, and her only sport participation is in physical education class. Her second left toe has been pale blue and slightly swollen for approximately 1 week, and she started walking on her heels in response to pain. She has no other symptoms. She is allergic to peanuts and has a history of eczema, which was not active or associated with the skin lesions. She is not taking any medicines. There is no family history of bleeding or clotting disorders, thrombosis, recurrent miscarriages, Reynaud disease, or rheumatologic conditions.

Physical examination reveals bilaterally tender tips of toes with scattered purpuric papules, some of which have a 2- to 4-mm erythematous base and a few circular patches of desquamation (Figure 19.1). There are no ulcerations, splinter hemorrhages, masses, or evidence of trauma. Her left second toe is pale, cyanotic in color, and cold to the touch; however, capillary refill is less than 2 seconds. The rest of her physical examination findings are within reference range and unremarkable.

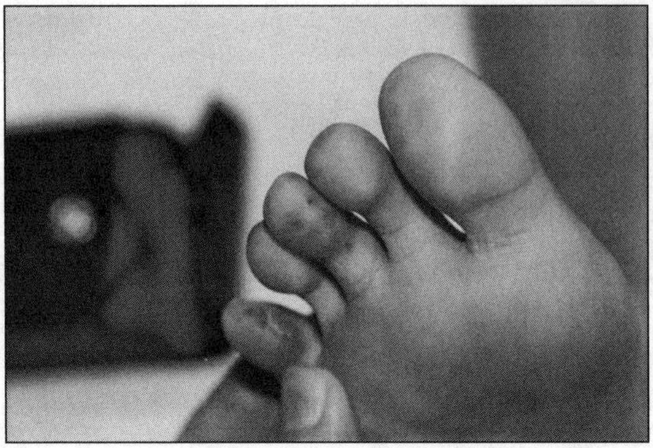

Figures 19.1. Purpuric papules on erythematous bases (A) and a few circular patches of desquamation on the plantar aspect of the toes of both feet (B).

- **What is your differential diagnosis at this point?**
- **Are there any elements of history or physical examination that would help you?**
- **What additional diagnostic studies would you like performed?**

Discussion

The patient was admitted to the hospital, and consultations with the pediatric hematology and dermatology departments were requested. Her complete blood cell count, prothrombin time, partial thromboplastin time, and fibrinogen level were all within reference range. The results of laboratory evaluation of a possible hypercoagulable state, including protein C, antithrombin III, homocysteine, and factor V Leiden, were negative. She had low factor XII (35%; reference range, 50%–150%) and protein S levels (52%; reference range, 60%–140%). Her echocardiogram and computed tomography angiogram results were normal. A consulting dermatologist suggested chilblain on the basis of clinical presentation. On further questioning, she admitted to hiking in the snow the day before onset of lesions. The patient was discharged with close follow-up and instructions to avoid contact sports, keep extremities warm, and limit cold exposure. She was allowed weight bearing as tolerated and treated with acetaminophen as needed for pain. The lesions resolved without intervention before her 2-week follow-up appointment; however, the patient presented a month later with inflammation of her earlobes and cellulitis of her right eyebrow. She was treated with antibiotics, but the lesions were likely recurrent chilblain. The lesions resolved in 7 to 10 days. She denied any cold exposure or trauma. She had a third episode 1 year later with similar lesions on the lateral 2 toes of her left foot after wearing open-toed shoes at an outdoor winter school function. Her lesions resolved after 2 weeks. She was counseled to avoid cold exposure, cigarette smoking, obesity, prolonged sitting, use of estrogens (birth control pills), and other factors that increase the risk for thrombosis.

Differential Diagnosis

The differential diagnoses for purpuric or petechial lesions on bilateral toes are hypercoagulable conditions, thrombotic or embolic process, vasculitis, and chilblain (also known as pernio or perniosis). Perniosis associated with lupus erythematosus is probably the most important condition in the differential diagnosis because the cutaneous lesions are the same, whereas typical chilblain is idiopathic and self-limited. Perniosis associated with lupus erythematosus could be the harbinger of a significant systemic disease. Therefore, it may be beneficial to check an antinuclear antibody titer in patients in whom there is a clinical suspicion or family history of a rheumatologic disorder.

The Condition

Chilblain is itchy and tender red or purple papules that occur in response to prolonged cold exposure. The lesions start as red areas with itching and burning a few hours after cold exposure and typically resolve in 7 to 14 days but may thicken and persist for months. Chilblain is a localized form of vasculitis. Small blood vessels constrict with cold exposure, and blood leaks into the surrounding tissues with rewarming. It is more common in children, women, and elderly people. It is seen almost exclusively in the winter months and in damp or wet, cold conditions. It is associated with positive family history of chilblain, diabetes mellitus, smoking, hyperlipidemia, low body weight, poor nutrition, connective tissue diseases (most commonly lupus), cryoglobulins, and cold agglutinin disease. Lesions most commonly occur on the fingers, toes, nose, and ears.

The patient's low factor XII and protein S levels are not likely to be related to the chilblain. Both of these factors increase the risk for thrombosis, and thrombosis can be seen in patients who present with purpura. There was no proven clinical thrombosis in this patient. Most patients with these hereditary risk factors for thrombophilia do not develop thrombosis, and the condition is asymptomatic. Of patients who present with early thrombosis, there is a high incidence of one or more of the many predisposing laboratory abnormalities.

The origin of chilblain is not primarily related to thrombotic problems. There have not been reports associating the 2 conditions, although chilblain belongs to the vascular acrosyndromes because of its symmetrical lesions and to the dystrophic group because of its organic obstructive and thrombotic microangiopathy, especially of venules. It might be worth probing this association in other patients with chilblain to see whether there might be an as yet unrecognized association.

Diagnosis

Chilblain is usually a clinical diagnosis; however, if necessary, a skin biopsy may be performed. It is also important to rule out associated conditions.

Treatment and Prognosis

Chilblain responds poorly to treatment, but the lesions usually self-resolve in 7 to 14 days. Treatment options include a 2- to 3-day course of topical corticosteroid cream, which may also help with itching and swelling. Topical or oral antibiotics may be used for any secondary infection. For chilblain, prevention is the key, including avoidance of smoking, secondhand smoke exposure, diet aids, or medications that cause blood vessel constriction, such as decongestants. Keeping extremities warm and dry and wearing wool or moisture-resistant socks and mittens may help prevent development of new lesions or exacerbation of existing ones. In extreme cases, nifedipine (vasodilator) may be prophylactically prescribed before the onset of cold weather and taken throughout the winter season. Prognosis is very good in children, most of whom typically enjoy complete recovery, but a small number may still have lifelong cold weather recurrences.

Lessons for the Physician

- Chilblain is typically a benign and self-limiting form of localized vasculitis.
- Chilblain is usually diagnosed clinically, but other causes of vasculitis must be ruled out. Chilblain is more common in those with a positive family history, women, children, and elderly people.
- The mainstay of treatment is prevention, such as limiting cold exposure and any medications or exposures that cause vasoconstriction.
- Most cases of chilblain completely resolve in 1 to 2 weeks; however, a small percentage of patients will continue to have lifelong reoccurrences after cold exposure.

The views expressed in this chapter are those of the authors and do not reflect the official policy or position of the Department of the Navy, the Department of the Army, the Department of Defense, or the US government.

CPT Lera Liv Fina, DO, and CPT Peter Everson, MD, Madigan Army Medical Center, Fort Lewis, WA

CHAPTER 20

13-Year-Old Girl With Pink Papules (Visual Diagnosis)

Presentation

A 13-year-old girl presents to the clinic with pink papules on her abdomen, legs, arms, and the lateral aspects of her cheeks. The lesions have been present for 4 years, always appearing in the same area, with satellite lesions surrounding the primary site. The rash blanches on palpation. The papules are primarily located on her abdomen and become more prominent and pruritic with sun exposure. The rash is most noticeable in the periumbilical region, where the patient's metal pants button comes in contact with her skin. The papules are accompanied by pruritus for which she gets mild relief by taking oral antihistamines and applying topical corticosteroids. However, she has been unable to completely get rid of the rash with this regimen.

The patient has an unremarkable medical history and is developing appropriately. There are no similar skin lesions on any close contacts.

On physical examination, the patient has multiple pink papules on the bilateral aspects of her cheeks, upper arms, elbows, knees, and legs (Figure 20.1). All vital signs are within reference range. There are papules that have coalesced into plaques surrounding her umbilicus (Figure 20.2), with lichenification. There is evidence of excoriation, without any ulcerations or bleeding. The remainder of the physical examination findings are unremarkable.

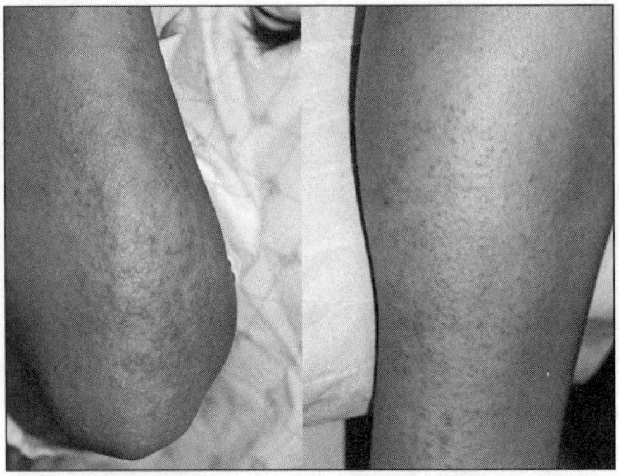

Figure 20.1. Multiple papules were noted on the arms (left) and legs (right) of the patient.

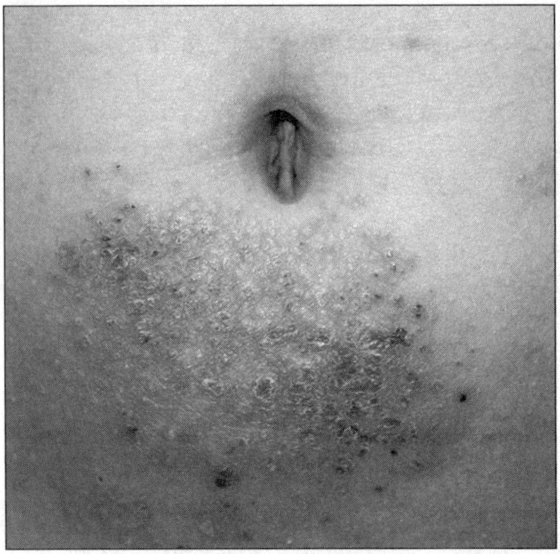

Figure 20.2. The initial location of the rash was on the patient's abdomen. It eventually coalesced into plaques.

The skin biopsy of the rash confirms the suspected diagnosis.

- **What is your differential diagnosis at this point?**
- **Are there any elements of history or physical examination that would help you?**
- **What additional diagnostic studies would you like performed?**

Diagnosis

The biopsy specimen showed perivascular inflammation containing neutrophils and eosinophils. On the basis of these histologic findings and the clinical history and physical examination of the rash, the patient is given a diagnosis of allergic contact dermatitis to nickel with id (autoeczematization) reaction.

Discussion

Nickel exposure is nearly unavoidable in everyday life because it is present in a wide variety of products, such as hairpins, jewelry, coins, spectacle frames, blue jean buttons and zippers, wire clasps, door handles, cosmetics, dental fillings, textiles, foods, and even drinking water. However, for many people this exposure can be problematic. Nickel is one of the most common causes of allergic contact dermatitis worldwide. It is the most frequently detected allergen on patch tests and in 2008 was proclaimed the contact allergen of the year by the American Contact Dermatitis Society.

Nickel allergy is increasing in prevalence among both the general population and children. A total of 26% of all patch tests in the pediatric population have a positive result for nickel sensitivity. This increase may be due to many factors, including changing environmental exposures in childhood, such as the increased incidence of body piercing. Certain cultural practices, such as early ear piercing, may particularly predispose children to nickel allergy. Once acquired, nickel allergy is permanent, and when acquired in childhood or adolescence, it may even affect future career considerations if the hypersensitivity reaction is a severe one.

The clinical presentation of nickel allergy varies widely, depending on both the source of allergen and the severity of the reaction. The typical appearance is that of eczematous, erythematous papules, accompanied by pruritus. Long-term exposure can result in lichenified plaques. Recognizing the clinical patterns of nickel allergy is important in distinguishing it from atopic dermatitis. The history together with the specific anatomic site is particularly important in identifying nickel allergy. The most common presentation is infraumbilical dermatitis, as seen in this case, due to exposure to metal buttons. Other signs include the earlobe sign caused by nickel-containing earrings or earring backs. Bilateral posterior thigh dermatitis is characteristic of school chair dermatitis from chairs with nickel in the hardware fastening the seat to the back. A high index of suspicion is needed; without it, the diagnosis may be delayed by months or even years, resulting in subacute or chronic patterns of dermatitis.

Another important and at times confusing aspect of nickel contact dermatitis is spread of the rash to sites distant from the site of exposure. This finding of an autoeczematous response, also known as an id reaction, is relatively common, estimated to be present in up to 50% of all cases of nickel allergy. It is believed to be due to hematogenous autosensitization by immune cells that are circulating throughout the body. Common sites include the thighs, upper arms, and elbows. Symptoms of the id reaction can be severe and can persist for months even after the allergen has been removed.

The diagnosis of nickel dermatitis can usually be based on the clinical presentation; however, a positive patch test result can be useful. Skin biopsy is not necessarily needed. Even if it is performed, the similarities in the histopathologic features of allergic contact dermatitis with other types of dermatitis may lead to a diagnosis of dermatitis without specifically pointing to nickel as the culprit. Allergic contact dermatitis to nickel is a type 4 delayed hypersensitivity reaction in which small antigens (metal ions) are conjugated with antigen-presenting cells, primarily Langerhans cells, in the epidermis. This complex is presented to T lymphocytes, resulting in downstream increases in inflammatory cytokines that direct the allergic response. The mechanism of sensitization is similar for all types of metals.

Differential Diagnosis

The differential diagnosis of this rash includes atopic dermatitis, cellulitis, herpes zoster, impetigo, and fixed drug eruption.

Management

The mainstay of treatment for any type of allergic contact dermatitis is avoidance of the offending agent. This can be difficult because of the pervasiveness of nickel in everyday life. Patient education should be a central part of treatment and prevention of nickel allergic contact dermatitis. Patients can use over-the-counter dimethylglyoxime kits to test objects for detectable amounts of nickel before purchasing them. Internet searches can point to many sites with information concerning nickel allergy and where dimethylglyoxime kits and low-nickel jewelry and other low-nickel products can be purchased. For symptomatic dermatitis, middle- to high-potency topical steroids or calcineurin inhibitors are useful, and antihistamines can help alleviate pruritus. Rarely, systemic steroids may be needed, especially if widespread autoeczematization is present. In some cases of severe nickel contact dermatitis, symptoms may persist despite nickel avoidance secondary to small amounts of the allergen that occur naturally in foods (eg, chocolate, nuts, seeds, and canned foods). In these cases, dietary nickel avoidance is recommended.

Prognosis

The prognosis for nickel contact dermatitis with id reaction is very good, provided that adequate measures are taken to avoid recurrent nickel exposure. When an id component is present, resolution of the rash can be delayed by many months after the offending agent is removed. However, with strict nickel avoidance and symptomatic treatment of the rash, most patients will have complete symptom resolution.

Patient Course

The patient was counseled extensively on nickel avoidance. She was also encouraged to avoid possible sources of dietary nickel given the severity of her symptoms. In addition, because of the severe id component, the patient was prescribed a 2-week prednisone taper. She was also given topical fluocinonide ointment, 0.05%. The patient's symptoms improved with this multipronged approach.

Summary

Allergic contact dermatitis to nickel is extremely common and is increasing in prevalence. Nickel dermatitis is characterized by an eczematous, pruritic rash at the primary site of contact. In severe cases, direct contact nickel dermatitis is accompanied by cutaneous involvement of other sites not in contact, a development known as an id reaction. Diagnosis is often made on clinical grounds; however, a positive patch test result may be used to confirm diagnosis. The mainstays of treatment are nickel avoidance and topical corticosteroids.

Meghan M. Dickman, MD, and Ilona J. Frieden, MD, University of California, San Francisco, CA

CHAPTER 21

Anterior Chest Pain, Daily Low-grade Fevers, and Worsening Acne in a 14-Year-Old Boy

Presentation

A 14-year-old boy complains of anterior chest pain, daily low-grade fevers, and worsening acne. His dull back pain starts in the left scapular region and migrates to the right anterior chest. His pain is believed to be due to "infected" acne on the chest, and oral cephalexin is administered for 2 weeks. His symptoms worsen despite therapy. He is referred to a dermatologist, who initiates oral isotretinoin therapy at 60 mg/d. The patient declines oral prednisone because he has a history of associated severe mood changes. After 2 days, his pain and acne continue to progress, requiring hospital admission.

Past history is significant for weight loss (4.5 kg in 1 month) and ulcerative colitis (treated with sulfasalazine). He denies trauma, cough, vomiting, shortness of breath, dyspnea on exertion, and palpitations.

Physical examination reveals an afebrile, thin boy who has a blunted affect. Vital signs are normal. He has erythematous papules, pustules, cysts, and scars on his face, chest, and back. His sternum, especially over the manubriosternal, costochondral, and sternochondral joints, is exquisitely tender when palpated. Respiratory, cardiac, and abdominal findings are normal.

He has a normal white blood cell count and differential count, hemoglobin level of 11.3 g/dL (113 g/L) (normocytic), and erythrocyte sedimentation rate of 32 mm/h. Cultures from the skin and blood show no growth. Tests for rheumatoid factor, antinuclear antibody, and human lymphocyte antigen-B27 are negative.

Radiographs of the chest and electrocardiogram yield normal results. Technetium bone scan shows an area of increased uptake in the sternum.

- **What is your differential diagnosis at this point?**
- **Are there any elements of history or physical examination that would help you?**
- **What additional diagnostic studies would you like performed?**

Discussion

Findings on the bone scan suggested a reactive process such as osteomyelitis or acne fulminans. Because no source of infection was found, the combination of joint pain and tenderness plus weight loss in a patient who had acne led to the diagnosis of acne fulminans (Figure 21.1). The boy was treated with open wet dressings and prednisone. The sulfasalazine was continued as maintenance therapy for his ulcerative colitis. After marked improvement over 3 days, he was discharged on oral prednisone (40 mg/d), isotretinoin (60 mg/d), indomethacin, and sulfasalazine. By 2 weeks, his condition had improved significantly. The prednisone was continued for 4 weeks and the isotretinoin for 5 months. He has been doing well without recurrence of his acne fulminans.

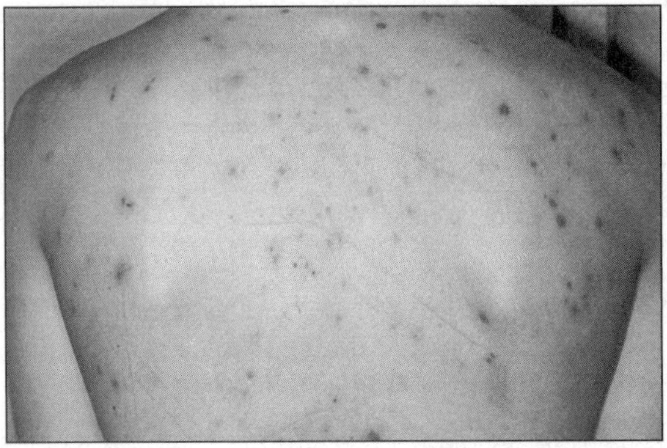

Figure 21.1. Erythematous papules, pustules, cysts, and scars are evident on the patient's back.

The Condition

Acne fulminans is a rare condition characterized by the explosive onset of severe acne. Bright red, weeping cysts coalesce to form ulcerated plaques, especially on the face, chest, and back, and can lead to extensive scarring. Most patients have associated systemic symptoms, including fever, weight loss, arthralgias, and myalgias. Erythema nodosum and hepatosplenomegaly occur in some patients. The large joints tend to be affected primarily, especially the sternum, clavicles, shoulders, and pelvis.

Imaging studies reveal osteolytic lesions with a periosteal reaction, suggesting osteomyelitis. Blood and bone culture results are negative. Laboratory alterations include anemia, hematuria, leukocytosis, hypergammaglobulinemia, and elevations in the erythrocyte sedimentation rate, C-reactive protein level, circulating immune complex titer, and liver enzyme levels. Bone scans often demonstrate increased uptake in affected regions, and radiographs show osteolytic lesions. Adolescent boys seem to be at greatest risk, and many of them are undergoing oral therapy for acne with either an antibiotic or isotretinoin at the onset of the acne fulminans.

Pathogenesis

The pathogenesis of acne fulminans remains obscure but is most likely related to an immune-mediated phenomenon. The rapid response to systemic steroids and the presence of systemic symptoms suggest an immunologic or inflammatory process. Hypotheses include a de novo autoimmune process as well as a reaction caused by an unknown trigger in susceptible individuals. Possible triggers include infection (*Propionibacterium acnes*) and drugs (oral antibiotics and isotretinoin). Antibodies against *P acnes* have been detected in patients who have severe acne and acne fulminans, and *P acnes* has been cultured from bony lesions, supporting the role of this organism as a potential trigger.[1]

Autoimmunity may be a factor because acne fulminans has occurred in patients with inflammatory bowel disease. In these patients, it is unclear if acne fulminans is an extraintestinal feature of inflammatory bowel disease or if they are separate and distinct conditions sharing a common trigger. Because acne fulminans occurs primarily in adolescent boys, androgen excess may be important in the pathogenesis. Certain families appear to have several affected members, although a gene has not been identified. The associated osteolytic lesions have been misdiagnosed as osteomyelitis and osteosarcoma, which can delay prompt diagnosis and treatment.

Therapy

Systemic prednisone is the principal therapy for acne fulminans at doses of 0.5 to 1 mg/kg/d. Skin and systemic symptoms tend to respond readily to prednisone, but treatment should be continued for 2 to 4 months to avoid recurrence. Isotretinoin (1–2 mg/kg/d) can exacerbate acne fulminans, but when used in combination with prednisone, it can control the condition rapidly and prevent recurrence. Following control of the acne fulminans with prednisone, lower doses of isotretinoin (20 mg/d) may be added. Dapsone has also been used as a secondary therapy.

Reference

1. Nault P, Lassonde M, St-Antoine P. Acne fulminans with osteolytic lesions. *Arch Dermatol.* 1985; 121(5):662–664

Lessons for the Physician

Acne fulminans is a rare but important diagnostic consideration in patients who develop flaring of acne in association with fever and muscle and joint aches. Systemic corticosteroids in combination with isotretinoin are the treatment of choice. Patients tend to respond well, although acne fulminans can recur in rare instances.

Myto Duong, MD, and James G. H. Dinoulos, MD, Children's Hospital at Dartmouth, Lebanon, NH

COMMENTARY BY DR JONETTE E. KERI, DERMATOLOGIST, UNIVERSITY OF MIAMI HEALTH SYSTEM

It is postulated that the androgenic or anabolic steroids increase sebum production with a resultant increased population of *Propionibacterium acnes,* which then trigger an immunologic reaction. Support for increased levels of testosterone in the blood causing acne fulminans comes from 2 settings. The use of testosterone for treating certain medical conditions has resulted in acne fulminans. Also, the recent abuse of anabolic steroids to improve strength and body size has been reported to cause acne fulminans.

There has been controversy regarding the overlap between acne fulminans and conditions in which acne and rheumatologic diseases are seen together, such as SAPHO (**s**ynovitis, **a**cne, **p**ustulosis, **h**yperostosis, **o**steitis) syndrome. These conditions may represent part of a disease spectrum.

There is some role for potent topical steroids mixed with 20% to 40% urea in the first 7 to 10 days to help with the explosive crusting. Finally, there are case reports where azathioprine, cyclosporine, and infliximab have been found to be beneficial to patients with acne fulminans.

CHAPTER 22

Rash, Eye Pain, and Lesions in an Adolescent (Visual Diagnosis)

Presentation

A 17-year-old boy presents to his primary care physician with a 3-day history of rash, bilateral eye irritation, and sores in his mouth and on his genitals. He had been seen in the emergency department approximately 1 week ago for fever and a sore throat. A rapid streptococcal antigen test was positive at that time, and he was started on oral azithromycin therapy. Four days later, he developed facial swelling, eye redness, and urticaria, appearing initially on his hands and then spreading to his legs and feet. Although his sore throat resolved, new and different oral lesions appeared, and his lips became chapped and painful, prompting him to go to an urgent care clinic, where his azithromycin therapy was discontinued and he was started on oral prednisone and diphenhydramine. However, his skin lesions and eye pain continued to worsen, and sores appeared on his genitals. When he developed dysuria, he presented to his primary care physician for additional evaluation.

The patient reports a history of allergy to penicillin, manifesting as urticaria in the past. Except for this past week, he takes no medications. There is no family history of skin disease. He is a sophomore in high school and smokes a half pack of cigarettes daily. He acknowledges occasional binge drinking and daily marijuana use but denies the use of other illicit drugs. He has been sexually active since the age of 16 years and has had many female partners, including some intercourse without protection, but denies any history of sexually transmitted infection.

Physical examination reveals an alert, thin, but well-nourished adolescent boy. His temperature is 98.6°F (37.0°C), respiratory rate is 18 breaths/min, oxygen saturation is 100% on room air, heart rate is 65 beats/min, and blood pressure is 134/63 mm Hg. His weight is 58.7 kg (26th percentile for age). Examination of his head, ears, nose, and throat reveals dry, peeling, bleeding lips with erosions (Figure 22.1); erythema of the soft palate with tonsillar erosions and exudates (Figure 22.2); and several palpable 5-mm nontender bilateral submandibular lymph nodes. His conjunctivae are injected. Skin examination shows scattered annular vesicular lesions (5–7 mm in diameter) with surrounding erythema over the palms and dorsal aspects of his hands (Figure 22.3). Similar lesions are present on his forearms and the plantar aspect of his right foot. Examination of his genitourinary system reveals a 2-cm erythematous desquamated area surrounding the urethral meatus (Figure 22.4) and scattered 2- to 3-mm vesicular lesions on his penis and scrotum (Figure 22.5). The remainder of the examination findings are unremarkable.

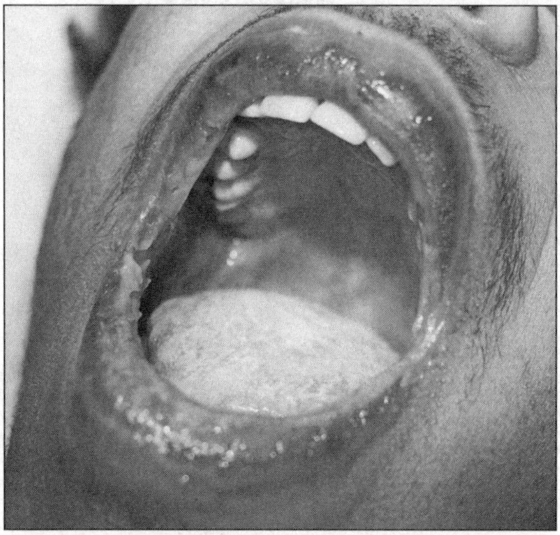

Figure 22.1. Dry, peeling, bleeding lips with erosions.

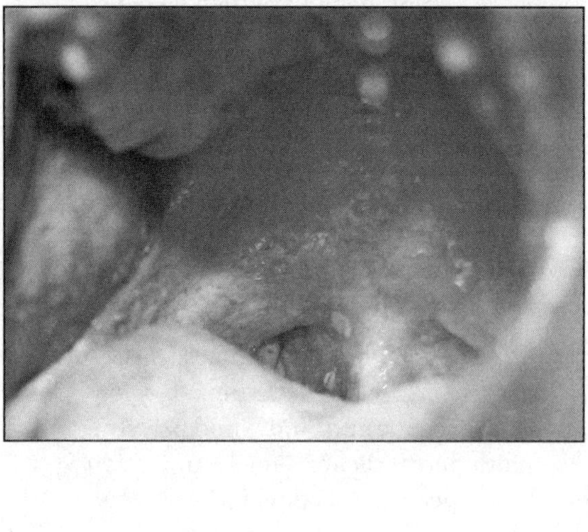

Figure 22.2. Erythema of the soft palate with tonsillar erosions and exudates.

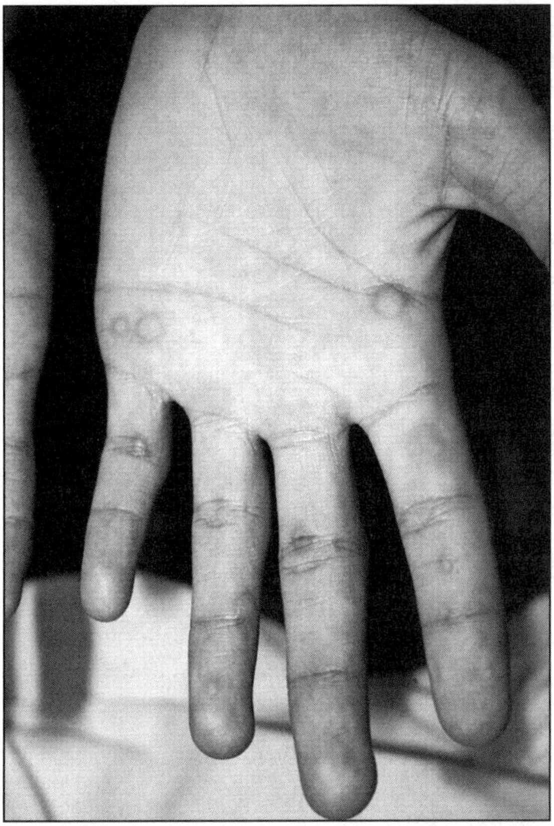

Figure 22.3. Scattered annular vesicular lesions with surrounding erythema over the palms.

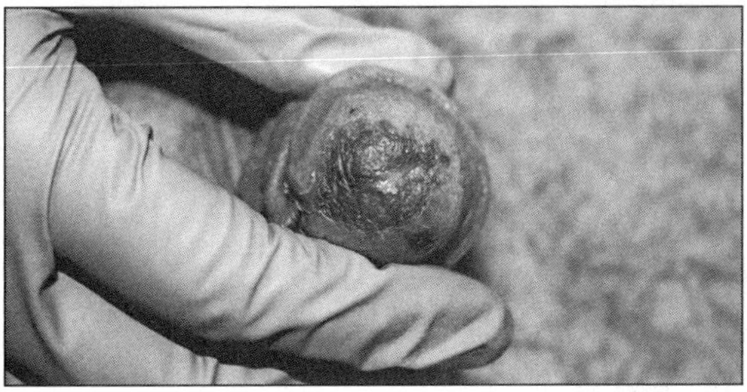

Figure 22.4. Erythematous desquamated area surrounding the urethral meatus.

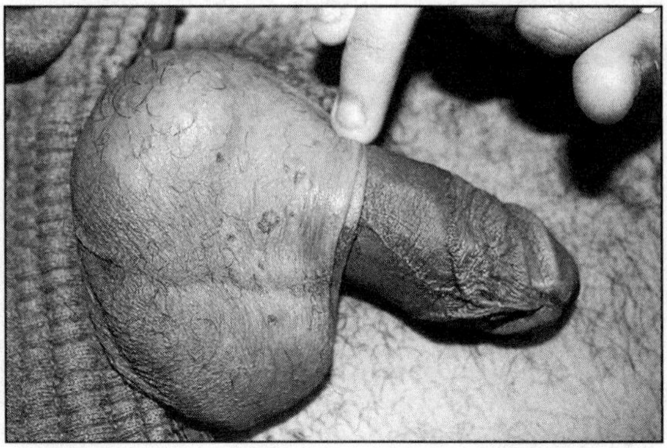

Figure 22.5. Vesicular lesions on scrotum.

A complete blood cell count demonstrates a hemoglobin of 14.3 g/dL (143 g/L); hematocrit of 41% (0.41); and white blood cell count of 13.9 × 10³/mcL (13.9 × 10⁹/L) with 90% neutrophils, 8% lymphocytes, and 2% monocytes. The platelet count is 455 × 10³/mcL (455 × 10⁹/L). Serum electrolyte, blood urea nitrogen, creatinine, alanine aminotransferase, and aspartate aminotransferase values are normal, but the glucose is slightly elevated at 111 mg/dL (6.2 mmol/L). A urine drug screening is positive for cannabinoids but negative for other illicit substances. Laboratory evaluation for sexually transmitted infections, including human immunodeficiency virus, syphilis, hepatitis C, *Chlamydia,* and gonorrhea, is negative.

A punch biopsy of a skin lesion (Figure 22.6) confirms the diagnosis.

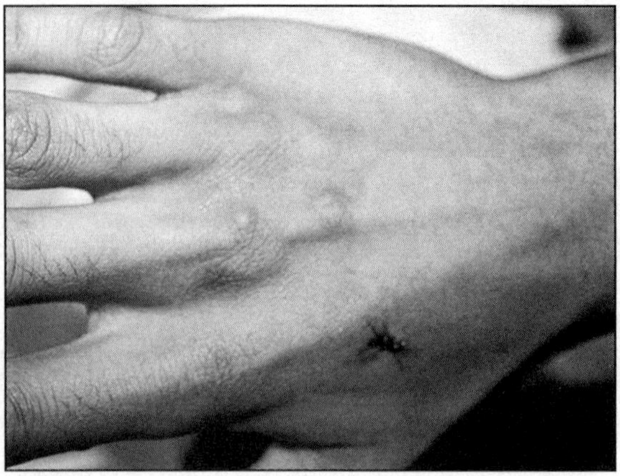

Figure 22.6. Punch biopsy site of skin lesion.

Diagnosis

A clinical diagnosis of Stevens-Johnson syndrome (SJS), based on the targetlike skin lesions and oral mucosal involvement, was confirmed by punch biopsy of one of the hand lesions, which revealed necrosis and vacuolar change along the epidermal basal layer with adjacent subepidermal vesicle and perivascular lymphocytic infiltrate, histologic findings consistent with SJS.

Of note, the history of unprotected sexual activity plus the appearance of palmar and urethral lesions strongly suggested secondary syphilis in the differential diagnosis.

- **What is your differential diagnosis at this point?**
- **Are there any elements of history or physical examination that would help you?**
- **What additional diagnostic studies would you like performed?**

Discussion

Stevens-Johnson syndrome is one part of a spectrum of severe cutaneous reactions characterized by disseminated skin and mucous membrane lesions induced by exposure to drugs or infections. Clinically, this disorder presents as multiple target-shaped erythematous macules, with or without epidermal detachment and necrolysis. Stevens-Johnson syndrome lesions can occur anywhere on the skin, involving up to 10% of the total body surface area. From 92% to 100% of individuals who have SJS experience involvement of the mucous membranes, with 2 or more mucosal surfaces usually affected. Stevens-Johnson syndrome is typically preceded by a prodromal phase consisting of fever, arthralgia, malaise, and myalgia.

Included in this spectrum of severe cutaneous reactions are toxic epidermal necrolysis (TEN) and, in the past, erythema multiforme. However, the World Health Organization has formally distinguished erythema from SJS and TEN, placing it in a separate category defined by its relatively benign nature and lack of mucosal involvement. Toxic epidermal necrolysis is a similar type of eruption that has more extensive skin and mucosal involvement and a more rapidly progressive course that involves exfoliation of the epidermis, producing a positive Nikolsky sign (detachment of epidermis with the application of lateral pressure). The Nikolsky sign may also be seen in SJS to a lesser extent. By definition, SJS must involve less than 10% of the body surface area, TEN must involve more than 30% of the body surface area, and SJS-TEN overlap defines involvement between 10% and 30% of the body surface area (Table 22.1). Toxic epidermal necrolysis has typically more systemic involvement than SJS, and patients may exhibit anemia, lymphopenia, neutropenia, and

Table 22.1. Comparison of Stevens-Johnson Syndrome and Toxic Epidermal Necrolysis

	Histopathology	Lesions	Mucous Membrane Involvement	Frequency	Mortality
Stevens-Johnson syndrome	Perivascular mononuclear infiltrate, eosinophilic infiltrate of dermis	Painful macules with purpuric centers, eventual blister formation with or without progression to epidermal separation (Nikolsky sign), involves <10% body surface area	Mucosal surfaces involved in 92%–100% of cases, typically the conjunctiva, oral, or genital mucosa	1.2–6 cases per million annually	<5%
Toxic epidermal necrolysis	Cleavage in the upper dermis, eosinophilic necrosis of the epidermis	Similar to above with more extensive involvement of epidermal separation, involves >30% body surface area	>2 mucosal sites involved	0.4–1.2 cases per million annually	As high as 44%

Stephanie Todd, MD, Children's National Health System, Washington, DC mildly elevated serum liver enzyme values. Because of the more extensive systemic involvement, TEN has a significantly higher mortality rate than SJS (approximately 40% versus 5%), typically due to sepsis from bacterial entry into exposed dermis.

Stevens-Johnson syndrome occurs more commonly than TEN, with an estimated incidence of 1.2 to 6 cases per million annually. There is an equal girl to boy distribution among children and adolescents, although the syndrome is more common in women among adults. Approximately 15% of cases are caused by infections, most commonly due to *Mycoplasma pneumoniae* and herpes simplex virus types 1 and 2. Another one-third to one-half of cases is attributed to drug exposure, with the most commonly implicated drugs including antibiotics (particularly sulfonamides, cephalosporins, and quinolones); antiepileptic drugs, including carbamazepine, phenobarbital, and phenytoin; and oxicam nonsteroidal anti-inflammatory drugs. Although cases of SJS triggered by azithromycin have been reported in children and adults, azithromycin is a rare cause of this disorder.

The pathophysiology of SJS and TEN is not known definitively, but proposed mechanisms include immunologic reactions, reactive drug metabolites, and interactions between these 2 mechanisms. Features supporting the role of the immune system in these disorders are an immune-mediated keratinocyte apoptosis that precedes the epidermal detachment and an infiltration of the epidermis with activated lymphocytes and macrophages. Some evidence suggests that patients who have SJS and TEN may have an altered ability to metabolize the drugs, leading to increased production of reactive metabolites that cause SJS or TEN. It is likely that interaction between both of these factors may play a role, with epidermal necrosis mediated by an immune reaction to reactive drug metabolites adhering to epidermal cells.

Other disorders to consider in the differential diagnosis include toxic shock syndrome and staphylococcal scalded skin syndrome. Exfoliative erythroderma, paraneoplastic pemphigus, and acute exanthematous pustulosis can also cause mucocutaneous lesions that can be confused with SJS or TEN. Skin biopsy is helpful for definitive diagnosis; full-thickness epidermal necrosis is present in SJS and TEN but not the other disorders.

Management

The standard of care for SJS is supportive therapy, including close monitoring of fluid and electrolyte status, wound care to prevent infection, nutrition support, and pain management. Mucosal involvement can lead to urologic and ophthalmic complications, and appropriate specialists should be consulted if these complications develop. The use of systemic corticosteroids is controversial. Although some have advocated their use early in the course of drug-induced cases, evidence from retrospective studies suggests that corticosteroids may not only fail to improve the prognosis but might increase patient susceptibility to sepsis and gastrointestinal hemorrhage. Off-label use of human intravenous immune globulin (IVIG) has not yet been studied in a well-controlled, prospective, multicenter trial but has been described in a number of case reports. Such therapy appears to result in decreased blister formation and faster recovery with minimal adverse effects. The typical dose of IVIG is 0.5 to 1.0 g/kg administered over 3 days.

Patient Course

The patient was admitted to the hospital and discharged after 24 hours, with instructions to complete the 5-day course of oral prednisone he had started before admission. Because of the association between SJS and infection, titers for *Mycoplasma* and herpes simplex virus types 1 and 2 were drawn, all of which were negative for acute infection. However, his lesions continued to worsen (Figure 22.7), limiting his intake of food and liquids and necessitating readmission 3 days after discharge. At that time, physicians decided to add IVIG at a dose of 1.0 g/kg divided over 3 days to the symptomatic treatment of his pain. Following IVIG administration, he improved significantly and was discharged from the hospital. At follow-up evaluation 1 week later, his lesions had resolved almost completely.

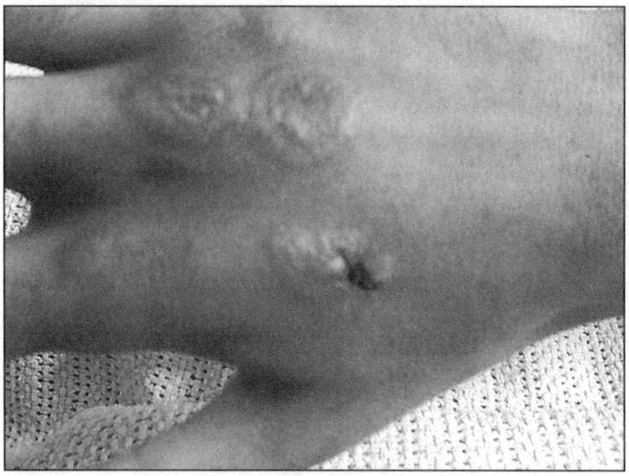

Figure 22.7. Progression of lesions from erythematous vesicles to targetlike plaques on dorsum of hand.

Summary

Stevens-Johnson syndrome (SJS) is part of a spectrum of skin disorders, including toxic epidermal necrolysis, that should be suspected in a child who has fever and mucocutaneous blistering lesions developing soon after recent drug or infectious exposure. Among the common infectious causes for SJS are *Mycoplasma pneumoniae* and herpes simplex virus types 1 or 2. Drugs frequently implicated in the development of SJS include antibiotic and antiepileptic medications and nonsteroidal anti-inflammatory drugs. Treatment of SJS is primarily supportive, including hospitalization and intravenous immune globulin therapy for severe cases.

Sarah Powers, MD, Department of Pediatrics, University of New Mexico School of Medicine, Santa Fe, NM

Gina Carter-Beard, MD, Doernbecher Children's Hospital, Oregon Health & Science University, Portland, OR

Part 5

Emergency Medicine

CHAPTER 23

7-Year-Old Girl Passing Red Urine

Presentation

A previously well 7-year-old girl has been passing red urine. She was born at term, has developed normally, and has experienced no serious illnesses. Over a few days, her parents have noticed yellow discoloration of her conjunctivae and skin. The child reports that she has been passing red urine for a few days without pain, dysuria, or frequency. There was one transient episode of mild dysuria several days before. There is no history of oliguria, fever, or sore throat. The family history is negative for urolithiasis.

On physical examination, the child looks well and is not distressed. Her temperature is 98.1°F (36.7°C), respiratory rate is 25 breaths/min, pulse is 85 beats/min, and blood pressure is 90/60 mm Hg. She appears well perfused, but her skin and sclerae are yellow. Her conjunctivae are not pale, and there is no peripheral edema. Her abdomen is soft, and her liver, spleen, and kidneys are not palpable. The remainder of her examination yields normal findings.

Laboratory findings include hemoglobin, 11 g/dL (6.82 mmol/L); white blood cell count, 8.5 × 10^3/mcL (8.5 × 10^9/L) with 65% neutrophils and 30% lymphocytes; reticulocyte count, 0.5% (0.005); platelet count, 200,000/mcL (200 × 10^9/L); and normal red blood cell morphology, with no schizocytes, target cells, or Heinz bodies. The direct Coombs and sickling tests are negative. Her level of glucose-6-phosphate dehydrogenase is normal, as are findings on hemoglobin electrophoresis. Serum bilirubin level is 1 mg/dL (17 mcmol/L), plasma glucose concentration is 90 mg/dL (5.0 mmol/L), and serum urea nitrogen, creatinine, electrolyte, and liver enzyme levels all are normal.

The urine is red, but it tests negative for blood, urobilinogen, and protein. There are no casts, but there is mild glycosuria. Urine culture shows no growth. The child is observed for 24 hours, she remains well, and her blood and urine test results remained unchanged except that her glycosuria disappears. After the diagnosis is made, she is discharged, having clear urine and normal color in her skin and sclerae. She remains well.

- **What is your differential diagnosis at this point?**
- **Are there any elements of history or physical examination that would help you?**
- **What additional diagnostic studies would you like performed?**

Discussion

Diagnosis

A detailed history was taken again from her parents. The mother stated that she herself had been treated for urinary tract infection a few days before, and when her daughter complained of dysuria, she medicated her with the same drug at half dosage. She was requested to bring in this medication, which consisted of 100 mg phenazopyridine hydrochloride tablets. It was calculated that the child had received the equivalent of 100-mg 3 times daily for 4 days. Methemoglobin levels were monitored along with the other tests mentioned earlier, and all results remained normal prior to discharge.

Differential Diagnosis

The changes in the color of the child's skin and conjunctivae led her physicians initially to suspect anemia or hyperbilirubinemia. The red color of the urine made hemolysis or hepatitis possible diagnoses; hemolytic uremic syndrome and acute glomerulonephritis were other possibilities. The normal hemoglobin and bilirubin levels ruled out anemia and hyperbilirubinemia as well as a hemolytic process, especially in the absence of reticulocytosis, abnormal red blood cell morphology, or Heinz bodies and in the presence of a negative Coombs test and a normal glucose-6-phosphate dehydrogenase level and hemoglobin electrophoresis pattern. The absence of pharyngitis, oliguria, edema, and hypertension made glomerulonephritis very unlikely, especially in the absence of hematuria, proteinuria, and abnormal renal function. The absence of oliguria, hypertension, hematuria, proteinuria, thrombocytopenia, and microangiopathic red blood cell changes and the presence of normal renal function also ruled out hemolytic uremic syndrome.

Pathogenesis

Phenazopyridine hydrochloride is an azo dye and urinary tract analgesic. It exerts a topical analgesic effect on the urinary tract mucosa and relieves the pain, discomfort, and dysuria associated with urinary tract infections. The exact mechanism of action is unknown. It is excreted rapidly by the kidneys (within 20 minutes), and 65% is excreted unchanged. The drug is used in adults to treat dysuria at the same time that antibacterial agents are used to control the urinary tract infection.

Treatment should be limited to the duration of symptoms (approximately 2 days); there is no reason to continue for the duration of antibiotic therapy. The adult dose is 200 mg 3 times daily.

Although adverse effects are more common in patients who have impaired renal function or in situations of overdosage, such effects may occur in patients taking normal doses and include lemon-yellow discoloration of skin and sclerae and orange-red discoloration of urine due to pigment deposition and excretion. Staining of underwear and contact lenses is possible. Hemolytic anemia, with the presence of Heinz bodies and bite cells indicative of oxidative hemolysis, has also been described but was absent in this patient.

Methemoglobinemia may also occur, usually in patients who have taken an overdose or in individuals with renal failure. Methemoglobinemia appears to result from metabolic overload of the normal reductase pathways in the red blood cells by phenazopyridine, which is an oxidant. Nephrotoxicity has also been reported, presenting as acute renal failure. Urinary phenazopyridine stones may also occur. Hepatotoxicity, with hyperbilirubinemia and hepatomegaly, has been reported and is probably due to a hypersensitivity reaction. Other adverse effects include headaches and aseptic meningitis. This medication has been found to give false-positive urine glucose measurements, as in this patient, and false-negative white blood cell esterase dipstick test results.

There is no known toxic range for the drug or known serum level that correlates with toxicity. Although hemolytic anemia may occur in cases of overdosage, it may occur even when the patient is given therapeutic doses and in individuals who have normal renal function. Liver toxicity and other adverse effects seem to be idiosyncratic, unrelated to dosage, and most likely due to hypersensitivity reactions. Close monitoring for renal, hepatic, and hematologic complications, including methemoglobinemia, is essential.

Therapy

Treatment of phenazopyridine toxicity is primarily supportive. There is no specific antidote or specific elimination enhancement mechanism, such as dialysis or hemoperfusion, that is known to be effective. There are no data to support lavage or the administration of charcoal, probably because of the very rapid absorption and speed with which renal elimination begins. Management includes the obvious expedient of stopping the offending drug, blood transfusion for severe anemia, and conventional therapy for renal failure and its complications, including dialysis when needed. Treatment of methemoglobinemia includes the administration of oxygen and methylene blue or ascorbic acid.

Lessons for the Physician

- Lemon-yellow skin, scleral discoloration, and orange-red urine in the absence of anemia or hyperbilirubinemia should lead physicians to consider the possibility of phenazopyridine hydrochloride toxicity. Suspicion is necessary, and the importance of taking a detailed history cannot be overemphasized.
- This medication is not approved for pediatric use by the US Food and Drug Administration. As a general principle, parents must be taught not to medicate their children with any agents unless advised by a physician to do so. Physicians treating adults with this medication should prescribe only enough tablets for a 2-day treatment to avoid the risk of having remaining tablets in the household. As with all medications, patients for whom phenazopyridine is prescribed should be informed about its adverse effects.

Hassib Narchi, MD, Saudi Aramco Al-Hasa Health Center, Mubarraz, Saudi Arabia

Part 6

Endocrinology

CHAPTER 24

Seizure in an 8-Month-Old Boy

Presentation

An 8-month-old boy presents to the emergency department after having a seizure. His mother found him in his crib with both arms and legs shaking symmetrically. He appeared pale and had a glazed look on his face. The episode lasted 10 minutes. En route to the hospital, his blood glucose concentration measured 39 mg/dL (2.2 mmol/L), and he was given intravenous dextrose solution.

According to his mother, he had a similar episode 1 month earlier when his blood glucose concentration was found to be 40 mg/dL (2.2 mmol/L). Laboratory evaluation, including complete blood cell count and basic metabolic panel, at that time yielded otherwise normal results, and he was discharged with no clear explanation of his condition. His mother reports that he has had seizurelike episodes with increasing frequency over the past month.

The infant was born vaginally at term, and his birth was complicated by abruption during delivery that resulted in perinatal asphyxia and hypoxic-ischemic encephalopathy. He has been taking oxcarbazepine for petit mal epilepsy and has had no breakthrough seizures until 1 month ago. He has also taken growth hormone (GH) since 3 months of age, when his GH deficiency was diagnosed. He has global developmental delay.

Physical examination reveals a postictal boy in no apparent distress. His vital signs are stable. Except for the decreased muscle tone, his physical findings are normal.

An additional element of the history leads to discovery of the cause of his hypoglycemic seizures.

- **What is your differential diagnosis at this point?**
- **Are there any elements of history or physical examination that would help you?**
- **What additional diagnostic studies would you like performed?**

Discussion

The infant was admitted to the pediatric critical care unit for closer monitoring. He underwent an extensive laboratory evaluation that included complete blood cell count; complete metabolic panel (basic metabolic panel plus liver function tests); urinalysis; urine organic acids; serum amino acids; thyroid function tests; and serum concentrations of insulin, lactate, pyruvate, cortisol, insulinlike growth factor-1, insulinlike growth factor–binding protein, ammonia, and oxcarbazepine. All results were essentially within reference range.

Interventions such as changing the frequency of his nighttime gastrostomy tube feedings to every 2 hours and administering hydrocortisone despite normal cortisol values were undertaken to maintain his blood glucose concentrations. In spite of these therapies, his blood glucose values continued to remain low. He was referred for a GH challenge in which his blood glucose would be monitored for 24 to 26 hours after discontinuing his GH. The test was interrupted at 12 hours because his blood glucose value decreased to 18 mg/dL (1.0 mmol/L). At this time, multiple laboratory tests were performed, yielding the following results: GH value was low at 5 ng/mL (5 mcg/L) (reference range, >10 ng/mL [10 mcg/L]), cortisol concentration was high-normal at 20 mcg/dL (552 nmol/L) (reference range, 7–22 mcg/dL [193–607 nmol/L]), β-hydroxybutyrate value was appropriately elevated at 4.3 mmol/L (reference range, 0–0.3 mmol/L), free fatty acids were appropriately elevated at 1,505 mcEq (reference range, <730 mcEq), the insulin value was low at less than 2 U/mL (reference range, 1–21 U/mL), urine ketones were positive, C-peptide was less than 0.5 ng/mL (0.17 nmol/L) (reference range, 1.0–5.2 ng/mL [0.33—1.72 nmol/L]), and plasma carnitine and ammonia values were normal.

Thus, the only abnormal laboratory value was a low GH value, despite the patient being on an optimal dose of GH.

What Went Wrong?

An explanation for the problem was found after approximately 4 to 5 months of continuous efforts to elucidate the cause of the boy's hypoglycemia. A review of his records documented that just before he started having seizures, his GH administration was switched from disposable syringes to cartridge-filled pens. His daily dose of GH was supposed to be 0.3 mg administered subcutaneously each day. However, with the new prescription employing cartridge-filled pens, he was receiving only 0.1 mg of GH. Instead of the 5-mg cartridge being used with its appropriate color-coded pen, a 5-mg cartridge was being placed into a pen designed for 15-mg cartridges, contrary to the manufacturer's directions. Because the mother was using the wrong pen, she was actually injecting only 0.1 mg of GH, which explains the partial GH deficiency.

The Condition

Hypoglycemia is defined as a blood glucose concentration of less than 50 mg/dL (2.8 mmol/L). Three mechanisms can cause hypoglycemia: defective glucose production, increased glucose utilization, or any combination of the 2. Examples of defective glucose production are defects in carbohydrate metabolism, as seen in disorders of glycogenolysis, gluconeogenesis, amino acid metabolism, and fatty acid metabolism. Hypoglycemia in these disorders usually occurs after a period of fasting or exercise.

Increased utilization of glucose is caused by hyperinsulinism of various causes, including exogenous administration of insulin or hypoglycemic agents and conditions associated with increased metabolic rates (sepsis, burns, hyperthyroidism). Ketotic hypoglycemia, which is believed to be caused by the suppression of glucose utilization by ketone bodies and a limited rate of hepatic glucose production, is an example of hypoglycemia resulting from the combination of the 2 mechanisms. Ingestions of ethanol, salicylates, β-blockers, and pentamidine and deficiencies of GH or cortisol may also cause hypoglycemia.

The Underlying Problem

The underlying problem in this case was a medical error, which resulted in harm to the patient and added stress to the family. Examples such as this, unfortunately, are common. Studies by Folli and colleagues[1] demonstrated that no physician, from intern to attending physician, is immune to medical error. Ordering, dispensing, administering, and monitoring medications for infants and children can be challenging because all of these tasks require more calculations. In addition, pharmacists often prepare the correct doses by diluting stock solutions, which could result in errors in dispensing drugs. Finally, children taking the medications are not in a position to check the accuracy of the prescription.

Medical errors can be divided into 3 groups. The first category is skill-based error, which results from automatic behaviors without a conscious level of control. Examples include putting milk in the cupboard and sugar in the refrigerator or taking a medication without confirming that it is the correct one. The second type is rule-based error, which results when someone fails to apply a rule in a specific setting or applies a rule suitable for a different circumstance. Examples include failure to check if an endotracheal tube is positioned correctly or failure to make sure that the intravenous line is in the vein before injecting medication. The third category is cognitive-based error, which results from a lack of knowledge, overwhelming input, or inadequate problem-solving ability. Examples of this type of error include prescribing the wrong medication, incorrect dosing, or having inadequate knowledge of potential drug interactions or adverse effects of a medication. Among the common examples of these medication errors are prescribing medication in volumes without stating the concentration of the drug, misunderstanding instructions, or using abbreviations for medications. Such errors can result in dispensing and administering a potentially lethal drug, such as using morphine sulfate when magnesium sulfate was to be used.

Medical errors are inevitable in the medical world, but many systems are in place and are being improved continually to identify and prevent such errors.

Reference

1. Folli HL, Poole RL, Benitz WE, Russo JC. Medication error prevention by clinical pharmacists in two children's hospitals. *Pediatrics.* 1987;79(5):718–722

Lessons for the Physician

Hypoglycemia has many causes. Therefore, a systematic approach is required to identify the mechanism in a specific case. Perhaps the biggest challenge in dealing with patients who have significant past medical histories, as in this case, is to avoid becoming distracted by the complexity of the patient. Rather, physicians must learn to take each problem and break it down into its simplest form. Medical errors do occur in health care; they should be recognized and efforts, continued to minimize such errors.

Sara Moussa, MD, Oakwood Healthcare System, Dearborn, MI

Cheryl Huffman, MD, Caughman Health Center, Findley, OH

CHAPTER 25

12.7-kg Weight Gain in 7 Months and Recurrent Fevers

Presentation

A boy aged 5 years and 7 months presents for a second opinion because of a 12.7-kg weight gain in 7 months and recurrent fevers. Other than the new onset of a voracious appetite, the boy has been asymptomatic and has no findings of note on his past medical history. He has had normal development, including verbal and motor skills. The family history includes thyroid disease, celiac disease, and obesity.

On physical examination, the boy looks well, with a weight of 32.2 kg (>95th percentile), height of 116.8 cm (75th–90th percentile), and body mass index of 23.6 (>95th percentile). All findings are normal except for obesity.

Laboratory results include thyroid-stimulating hormone of 1.72 IU/mL (reference range, 0.35–5.50 mIU/mL), free thyroxine of 0.87 ng/dL (11.2 nmol/L) (reference range, 0.90–1.40 ng/dL [11.6–18.0 nmol/L]), serum prolactin of 91.5 ng/dL (reference range, 2.0–20.0 ng/dL), serum morning cortisol of 9.6 mcg/dL (264.8 nmol/L) (reference range, 4.3–22.4 mcg/dL [118.6–618.0 nmol/L]), fasting serum glucose of 85 mg/dL (4.7 mmol/L), sodium of 150 mEq/L (150 mmol/L), potassium of 3.3 mEq/L (3.3 mmol/L), chloride of 114 mEq/L (114 mmol/L), and carbon dioxide of 27 mEq/L (27 mmol/L). A complete blood cell count reveals normal results.

Suspicion of a central nervous system (CNS) tumor such as a craniopharyngioma leads to obtaining magnetic resonance imaging (MRI) of the head, but no tumor is found. During the MRI, the sedated boy experiences hypoxic episodes, and a subsequent sleep study reveals sleep apnea. Expert consultation determines the boy's diagnosis.

- **What is your differential diagnosis at this point?**
- **Are there any elements of history or physical examination that would help you?**
- **What additional diagnostic studies would you like performed?**

Discussion

The 2 most likely diagnoses in a child who exhibits the rapid onset of obesity and hypothalamic dysfunction are CNS tumor and Prader-Willi syndrome (PWS). No tumor was found on MRI, and several features of PWS were absent. An example of genetic imprinting, PWS is a disorder resulting from a deletion of a paternally derived allele within chromosome 15q11–13. Prader-Willi syndrome is associated with hyperphagia, obesity, and sleep disorders, as were present in this patient. However, other features of PWS, such as short stature, hypotonia, mild intellectual disability, and hypogonadism, were not present.

The Condition

This patient exhibited rapid-onset obesity, fevers, hyperprolactinemia, hypernatremia, and a borderline low thyroxine concentration. The expert consultant, a pediatric endocrinologist, diagnosed rapid-onset obesity with hypothalamic dysfunction, hypoventilation, and autonomic dysregulation (ROHHAD).[1] This recently described disorder of unknown cause presents in the first decade of life with rapid weight gain as the initial feature. Hypothalamic dysfunction follows but can occur simultaneously and may manifest as hypernatremia, growth hormone deficiency, hyperprolactinemia, hypothyroidism, adrenal insufficiency, or pubertal irregularity.

Other features of autonomic dysregulation that may manifest are ophthalmologic dysfunction, gastrointestinal dysmotility, thermal dysregulation, and neural crest tumor formation. Hypoventilation is the last feature of the disorder to appear and may lead to death.

The underlying pathophysiology involved in ROHHAD is unclear. The wide spectrum of involved organ systems suggests a genetic defect in the development of the autonomic nervous system. However, a specific mutation has yet to be identified, and imaging studies have been unsuccessful in detecting a structural abnormality.

Differential Diagnosis

Although the endocrinologist determined the presence of this relatively newly described disorder for this child, each of his features generates a long list of potential diagnoses. Obesity is most likely due to nonorganic causes, such as overeating and decreased energy expenditure, and often accompanied by a sedentary lifestyle, increased television or video game viewing, and unhealthy eating habits. Children who have exogenous obesity also typically have linear growth acceleration.

Obesity in a short child raises suspicion of an endocrine disorder such as thyroid disease, growth hormone deficiency, or cortisol excess. The short child who has delayed bone age and rapid weight gain should undergo evaluation of thyroid function. An excess of exogenous or endogenous corticosteroids (Cushing syndrome) should be suspected when moon facies, striae, hypertension, glucose intolerance, muscle weakness, and fatigue are associated with the weight gain. A dexamethasone suppression test and growth hormone stimulation tests can help to rule out Cushing syndrome and growth hormone deficiency, respectively.

Along with PWS, other genetic syndromes such as Lawrence-Moon-Bardet-Biedl and Beckwith-Wiedemann syndrome are also associated with childhood obesity. Other features of the autosomal recessive disorder Lawrence-Moon-Bardet-Biedl include retinal degeneration, supernumerary digits, and intellectual impairment. Beckwith-Wiedemann syndrome is associated with both prenatal and postnatal overgrowth, large tongue, abdominal wall defects, and an increased risk of developing hypoglycemia, hemihypertrophy, and Wilms tumor. When genetic causes of obesity are suspected, genetic consultation is prudent to determine the appropriate testing.

The finding of a high prolactin value must be interpreted carefully because release of prolactin is pulsatile, and elevations can occur with sleep and stress. Hyperprolactinemia can be caused by a prolactin-secreting adenoma, hypothyroidism, pregnancy, chest wall trauma, and exposure to various medications. Hyperprolactinemia in conjunction with visual field defects raises high suspicion for a pituitary adenoma. Acute elevations of prolactin may also occur in the first 20 minutes following a seizure. Brain imaging, thyroid function testing, and urine pregnancy testing are reasonable.

Hypernatremia is defined as a sodium concentration higher than 145 mEq/L (145 mmol/L) and may be caused by too little water, too much salt, or a combination of the two. Determination of the underlying cause is aided by obtaining the following results: urine specific gravity and urine osmolality, the fractional excretion of sodium, and serum osmolality and glucose concentration. Volume contraction results in a fractional excretion of sodium of less than 1%.

Loss of water can occur with diarrhea, vomiting, insensible water loss, or diuretics, leading to a high urine osmolality. A high serum glucose concentration due to diabetes mellitus leads to an osmotic diuresis and hypernatremia. Water intake may be inadequate if a patient's thirst drive is impaired or inhibited. Excess sodium can be ingested through improperly prepared formula or by iatrogenic administration of hypertonic saline or sodium bicarbonate. Elevated sodium concentrations from an increased mineralocorticoid effect can occur in Cushing syndrome.

Another cause of hypernatremia is central or nephrogenic diabetes insipidus (DI). Without antidiuretic hormone, polyuria develops, leading to dehydration and hypernatremia. Urine specific gravity and osmolality are low, while serum osmolality is high. Possible causes of central DI include trauma, tumor, drugs, infections, vascular anomalies, and granulomatous diseases. Magnetic resonance imaging of the brain can determine if central DI is caused by a CNS tumor. Consultation with an endocrinologist and a carefully monitored water deprivation study should also be part of the evaluation for DI.

Sleep apnea beyond the neonatal period is most often due to airway obstruction during sleep. Tonsillar and adenoidal hypertrophy leading to apnea can cause snoring and daytime sleepiness or irritability. Obesity, anatomically narrow airways, enlarged tongue, and craniofacial abnormalities can also cause airway obstruction. Patients who have neuromuscular diseases (spinal muscle atrophy, muscular dystrophy, cerebral palsy, and various causes of brainstem dysfunction) can experience sleep apnea due to their inability to maintain a patent airway while asleep. Polysomnography is the key to evaluation of sleep apnea.

Recurrent fevers should prompt initial evaluation for infection. Recurrent viral infections are the most likely cause of recurrent childhood fever. Noninfectious causes, including malignancy, rheumatologic disease, inflammatory bowel diseases, medications, and other autoimmune diseases, are pursued on a case-by-case basis. Central nervous system tumors can also affect the thermoregulatory center and cause temperature instability.

Management

Multidisciplinary care is critical in the treatment of ROHHAD because of the many abnormalities associated with the condition. The hypoventilation requires immediate evaluation, and referral to a respiratory physiology laboratory for studies performed during wakefulness and sleep should be arranged. The patient may require early ventilatory support and close monitoring with pulse oximetry and measurement of end-tidal carbon dioxide concentrations. If treated inadequately, the alveolar hypoventilation can lead to cardiorespiratory arrest. Tonsillectomy may be required for obstructive sleep apnea.

The endocrinologist helps establish a treatment plan for the underlying hypothalamic-pituitary axis and water balance abnormalities. Psychiatric and psychological interventions and support are needed for both patient and family. Chest and abdominal imaging with computed tomography or MRI should be performed every 12 to 18 months as surveillance for neural crest tumors.

Over the past 6 months, this boy has been treated for DI with oral desmopressin, and his serum sodium values have remained in the range of 140 to 144 mEq/L (140–144 mmol/L). The sleep apnea improved following tonsillectomy. The development and worsening of behavioral abnormalities have posed the biggest challenge. Because of severe temper tantrums and violent outbursts, the boy has required treatment with haloperidol and trazodone. He has been thoroughly reevaluated at another academic medical center by a multidisciplinary team, and no underlying cause of his syndrome has been discovered.

Reference

1. Ize-Ludlow D, Gray JA, Sperling MA, et al. Rapid-onset obesity with hypothalamic dysfunction, hypoventilation, and autonomic dysregulation presenting in childhood. *Pediatrics.* 2007;120(1):e179–e188

Lessons for the Physician

A syndrome must be considered when a patient presents with multiple abnormalities involving different systems. Finding links among the multiple features can be difficult. Expert consultation is necessary when a patient experiences an unusual constellation of signs and symptoms, as occurs in the uncommon disorder rapid-onset obesity with hypothalamic dysfunction, hypoventilation, and autonomic dysregulation.

Brian A. Ely, MD, and Linda S. Nield, MD, West Virginia University School of Medicine, Morgantown, WV

CHAPTER 26

6-Year-Old Boy With Delayed Walking and Partial Primary Dentition

Presentation

A 6-year-old boy comes for an initial health supervision visit after the family relocated from Maine. He has received timely medical care and all immunizations. All developmental milestones were reached on schedule except for the ability to walk, which was delayed to 18 months of age. The boy uses an albuterol inhaler for mild, intermittent asthma. Recurrent acute otitis media since 7 months of age has necessitated bilateral myringotomy and pressure-equalization tube placement. Recently, a tonsillectomy was performed because numerous episodes of bacterial tonsillopharyngitis had occurred in the preceding year. Since surgery, the child has felt fine.

Physical examination reveals a well-nourished, short boy (2nd percentile). He has brachycephaly and symmetric facial features. Pressure-equalization tubes are present bilaterally, and no effusion is noted. His oropharynx is clear. Cervical lymphadenopathy is not present. No oral soft-tissue lesions are noted. A partial primary dentition is visible, with 3 mandibular and 2 maxillary incisors missing. He has no dental caries, and satisfactory oral hygiene is evident. His mother states that all primary teeth once were present, but tooth loosening began at age 3 years. All teeth exfoliated with fully formed roots. Dental trauma is denied. Additional physical examination findings include bowed legs and complaints of joint and muscle pain, and there is a history of limited exercise tolerance. As the boy leaves the office, he exhibits a waddling gait.

- **What is your differential diagnosis at this point?**
- **Are there any elements of history or physical examination that would help you?**
- **What additional diagnostic studies would you like performed?**

Discussion

The pediatrician took 3 courses of action before discharging the boy from his office. He ordered laboratory tests to measure serum alkaline phosphatase (ALP) and plasma pyridoxal 5′-phosphate as well as 24-hour urinary phosphoethanolaminuria excretion. He referred the boy to a community pediatric dentist for oral assessment, extraction of a highly mobile mandibular incisor, and histopathologic study of the tooth and its periodontal ligament. He planned a genetics consultation with pedigree analysis and gene testing pending the results of these preliminary measures.

The Signs

Exfoliation of primary (deciduous or "baby") teeth with fully formed roots constitutes a pathologic finding because the roots are normally resorbed by odontoclasts during the shedding process. This finding, coupled with delays in the ability to walk, presence of a waddling gait, short stature, joint and muscle pain, and limited exercise tolerance, suggests a generalized disorder of bone metabolism. Laboratory test results for the boy were abnormal when calibrated appropriately for age and sex. The serum ALP value was markedly subnormal. Urinary phosphoethanolaminuria excretion was elevated after 24-hour assay with creatinine normalization. Plasma pyridoxal 5′-phosphate was present in excess.

The pediatric dentist found no evidence of other causes of tooth loss, including aggressive periodontitis. A mobile primary incisor was extracted, and the external surface of the root was noted to be free of connective tissue. The tooth specimen was sent for histopathology. A root free of acellular cementum (the surface of the root in contact with the periodontal ligament that usually contains cementocytes) and Sharpey fibers (collagen fibers connecting tooth to bone) was seen by using microscopy. The triad of musculoskeletal findings, classic laboratory values, and notable histopathologic results confirmed the diagnosis of hypophosphatasia.

The Condition

Hypophosphatasia is a rare metabolic disease that occurs in 1 in 100,000 individuals. The disease, transmitted through autosomal dominant or recessive inheritance patterns, is defined by mutation of the liver/bone/kidney type ALP (*ALPL*, Online Mendelian Inheritance in Man 171760) gene. Although *ALPL* encodes for tissue nonspecific ALP in the liver, kidney, and adrenal tissues, its primary deleterious effects occur in bone and the dentition. Genetic testing for tissue nonspecific ALP mutation on chromosome 1p36.1 is available commercially and can be performed as early as the prenatal period to detect infantile forms of the disease.

This discussion focuses on the childhood form of hypophosphatasia, characterized by premature primary tooth loss; rachitic "tongues" of radiolucency within the costochondral junctions of long bones; flared metaphyses in the wrists, knees, and ankles; and the presence of calvarial deformities displaying a "copper beaten" skull appearance. Such bony changes are diagnosed readily through skeletal survey.

Differential Diagnosis

Childhood hypophosphatasia must be differentiated from other local and systemic disorders responsible for premature tooth exfoliation with fully formed roots. If teeth are not extracted because of dental caries or subjected to profound dental trauma, local sources of aggressive periodontitis must be excluded. Gingival crevicular fluid (inflammatory exudate located in the pocket around the tooth) can be acquired in the dental office for identification of known periodontal pathogens, including *Porphyromonas gingivalis* and *Actinobacillus actinomycetemcomitans* by polymerase chain reaction–based methods. When identified, these organisms are usually treated through nonsurgical scaling and root planning (mechanical debridement of plaque and calculus) of the affected periodontal sites, along with adjunctive antibiotic.

Periodontal disease in children tends to be acute and aggressive. Disorders that affect the ability of the body to fight infection can encourage periodontitis and lead to exfoliation of primary teeth that have fully formed roots. Disorders in neutrophil numbers, chemotaxis, and phagocytosis, including Chediak-Higashi syndrome, severe congenital neutropenia, cyclic neutropenia, and Papillon-Lefèvre syndrome, must also be considered. In this case, the boy had a significant history of bacterial infections. However, he had no opportunistic infections that would have raised greater suspicion for neutrophil abnormalities. These conditions can be excluded formally through a complete blood cell count with differential and, if needed, neutrophil function studies.

White blood cell adhesion deficiency, a very rare primary immunodeficiency, also promotes rapid destruction of the periodontal tissues and premature tooth loss. White blood cell adhesion deficiency should be explored when more likely causes are not found. Of note, white blood cell adhesion deficiency has been implicated in cases of odontohypophosphatasia, a condition in which dental manifestations are present without any rachitic changes in the skeleton.

In addition to periodontitis, collagen defects seen in diseases such as Ehlers-Danlos syndrome type VIII, vitamin D–resistant hypophosphatemic rickets, scurvy, and osteogenesis imperfecta can cause similar tooth loss and should be considered when musculoskeletal findings and dental anomalies are diagnosed. Of note, premature tooth loss is not a typical finding in patients who have osteogenesis imperfecta.

Poorly controlled diabetes mellitus and Langerhans cell histiocytosis can also induce rapid periodontal bone loss and premature tooth exfoliation. These conditions can be excluded by using various laboratory tests and gingival biopsy in the case of Langerhans cell histiocytosis. Enzyme deficiencies such as acatalasia are also possibilities when oral gangrene is present.

Therapy and Prognosis

Childhood hypophosphatasia remains untreatable. Nonsteroidal anti-inflammatory drugs can palliate pain from metabolic inflammation. The prognosis for a normal life span remains promising. Remission of the bone disease often occurs in adolescence, only to regress in middle to late adulthood. Tooth loss occurs more frequently in the primary dentition than in the permanent dentition, despite similar histologic findings. Primary incisors are often exfoliated, while primary molars are spared. However, widespread exfoliation of all primary teeth has been reported.

Lessons for the Physician

All children who have a full complement of developing permanent teeth undergo exfoliation of the primary dentition following parameters of their dental developmental age. Normally, the roots of primary teeth resorb slowly over time as the permanent tooth emerges through the alveolar bone and overlying gingival tissue. Premature exfoliation of teeth that still have substantial root structure constitutes a pathologic finding requiring clinical investigation. Exfoliated teeth of children suspected of having hypophosphatasia can undergo histopathologic examination after prolonged dry storage and desiccation when 10% formalin is not readily available. Multidisciplinary case management by pediatricians and pediatric dentists is necessary to permit diagnosis and treatment of the underlying systemic disease and to foster optimal outcomes for the remaining dentition. Pediatricians should suspect hypophosphatasia in healthy nonsyndromic children who have very early tooth loss (a primary incisor with intact root) in the absence of any trauma to the dentition.

Jeffrey M. Karp, DMD, MS, University of Rochester School of Medicine and Dentistry, Rochester, NY

CHAPTER 27

15-Year-Old Girl With No Menstrual Periods for 7 Months

Presentation

A 15-year-old girl who experienced menarche at age 13 years has had no menstrual periods for 7 months. Her only symptom is an occasional headache occurring at the end of the day. She denies sexual activity, medication use, and substance abuse and has had no recent weight change, heat or cold intolerance, skin or hair problems, difficulties with vision, or fainting. The patient's family history includes a granduncle who has acromegaly.

On physical examination, she looks well. Her height is in the 50th percentile, weight is in the 75th percentile, blood pressure is 113/62 mm Hg, and pulse is 90 beats/min. Her skin is not flushed or dry, and she has no rashes or abnormalities of hair pattern or hirsutism. Extraocular movements, visual fields by confrontation, and pupils all are normal. Heart, lung, abdominal, and neurologic examinations yield normal findings. Breasts and external genitalia are at Sexual Maturity Rating 4 and normal, with a patent vagina and palpable uterus.

Normal laboratory findings include follicle-stimulating hormone, 4.5 mIU/mL (4.5 IU/L); luteinizing hormone, 6.6 mIU/mL (6.6 IU/L); testosterone, 46 ng/dL (1.6 nmol/L); dehydroepiandrosterone sulfate, 122 mcg/dL (3.3 mcmol/L); thyroid-stimulating hormone, 1.28 mcIU/mL; thyroxine, 8.9 mcg/dL (114.5 nmol/L); and total cholesterol, 186 mg/dL (4.8 mmol/L). A pregnancy test is negative. Pelvic ultrasonography reveals a normal uterus and no free fluid. Two final studies reveal the origin of the patient's amenorrhea.

- **What is your differential diagnosis at this point?**
- **Are there any elements of history or physical examination that would help you?**
- **What additional diagnostic studies would you like performed?**

Discussion

The patient's prolactin level was 120 mcg/L (120 ng/mL) (reference range, 1–20 mcg/L [1–20 ng/mL]). Magnetic resonance imaging of her head revealed a 1-cm low-signal area in the midline extending eccentrically to the left, consistent with an adenoma within the pituitary fossa. Cabergoline was administered to treat the presumed prolactinoma. The prolactin level normalized, and menses resumed after initiation of therapy.

The Hormone

Prolactin is a hormone that is produced and stored by the anterior pituitary gland. It stimulates human milk production after childbirth and the production of progesterone by the corpus luteum. Prolactin is produced intermittently, with peak production occurring during sleep. Secretion is inhibited by dopamine concentrations. As the dopamine concentration rises, the prolactin level falls. Excessive prolactin secretion may cause galactorrhea.

Hyperprolactinemia occurs in normal states, including during pregnancy and the initial postpartum period, when there is stress, with breast stimulation, after eating, and with exercise. It is seen with the use of drugs such as risperidone, phenothiazines, amitriptyline, cimetidine, and haloperidol. Hypothyroidism, polycystic ovary syndrome, pituitary tumor, hyperplasia of lactotropes, and hypothalamic disease are among the endocrinologic causes of hyperprolactinemia. Chronic renal disease, renal and bronchogenic carcinomas, herpes zoster, atopic dermatitis of the chest, and chest wall trauma are other causes. In some patients, hyperprolactinemia is idiopathic.

The Underlying Cause

Prolactinomas are pituitary tumors that produce prolactin. They are the most common type of pituitary tumor in adolescents but occur infrequently in children and are more common in girls than boys. Boys more often have a macroadenoma at presentation. Prolactinomas in girls of reproductive age may become symptomatic earlier because of the disruption of normal menses and presentation with amenorrhea.

Clinical Presentation

The functional effects of a prolactinoma result from increased serum levels of prolactin and from the mass effect of the tumor on nearby structures and pituitary function. The mass effect of the tumor can suppress gonadotropin secretion as well as locally compress or destroy pituitary tissue. This destruction may create other hormonal effects, including growth changes and delayed or arrested puberty.

Prolactinomas are rare in prepubertal children and may present with headache, visual problems, and growth failure. Pubertal girls display amenorrhea, galactorrhea, headache, halted pubertal development, and, rarely, visual problems. Pubertal boys who have prolactinomas may present with headaches, visual disturbances, gynecomastia, and hypogonadism.

Diagnosis

Clinical evaluation of a patient who has secondary amenorrhea should include discussion of menstrual history, pregnancies, drug use, acne, hirsutism, symptoms of thyroid disease, headaches, and vision difficulties. The physical examination should focus on signs of thyroid disease, hirsutism, visual field defects, breast discharge, funduscopic findings, neurologic signs, evidence of androgen excess, and vaginal estrogenization.

Hyperprolactinemia may indicate a range of problems, including pituitary hyperplasia, tumors, and cysts. A pituitary tumor is suggested by blood prolactin levels greater than 100 mcg/L (100 ng/mL). The level of serum prolactin often corresponds to the size of the prolactinoma. A large tumor associated with minimal elevation of prolactin is consistent with a nonprolactin-secreting tumor causing pituitary stalk compression. Insulinlike growth factor-1 concentrations should be measured if acromegaly is present. Other neuroendocrine testing is indicated for macroprolactinomas and preoperatively. Estrogen status should be evaluated because of the risk of low bone density in patients who have hyperprolactinemia and low serum estradiol levels.

Pituitary lesions are visualized best by using magnetic resonance imaging, which allows clear views of the pituitary region and depicts anatomy of the region in 3 dimensions. Prolactinomas are classified based on diameter as either microadenomas (<1.0 cm) or macroadenomas (>1.0 cm).

Management

Several different strategies are employed to control growth of prolactinomas, to reverse or halt deleterious hormonal effects and to restore vision and menses. The modality used is based on the clinical presentation. Important considerations include tumor size, estrogen status, presence or absence of galactorrhea, contraception use, and desire for fertility.

Medical management employing dopamine agonists is the treatment offered most commonly for macroadenomas. A lack of treatment risks an increase in the size of the tumor, pituitary dysfunction, and visual problems. Common dopamine agonists include bromocriptine and cabergoline. These medications decrease tumor volume and prolactin levels. They are also effective in treating estrogen deficiency, promoting fertility, and stopping galactorrhea. Although tumor size is generally reduced with these medications, dopamine agonists must be used continuously. The primary disadvantages of bromocriptine are nausea, vomiting, headache, fatigue, and postural hypotension. Cabergoline requires administration only once or twice per week and has fewer adverse effects than bromocriptine.

Adolescents who have microadenomas may be estrogen deficient, which creates a high risk for bone loss. These patients are usually treated with dopamine agonists to restore normal menses. Some patients can discontinue dopamine agonists after 2 to 4 years of therapy. Treatment with cyclic conjugated estrogens and medroxyprogesterone or low-dose oral contraceptives may be an alternative, but close follow-up is required. Patients desiring pregnancy are treated with bromocriptine or cabergoline. Dopamine agonists should be stopped once the patient becomes pregnant. Patients having microadenomas are unlikely to experience adverse effects, but those having macroadenomas may have a more complicated pregnancy course. After delivery, prolactin levels decline and breastfeeding may occur; patients may need to resume dopamine agonist medications.

If a patient cannot tolerate the adverse effects of dopamine agonist medication, if the tumor grows or fails to shrink after a medication trial, if the patient has visual loss and chiasmal compression, or if sudden pituitary failure occurs, physicians may consider surgery. Transsphenoidal surgery is the favored surgical strategy for prolactinomas. Radiotherapy is used infrequently to treat prolactinomas. When used, it is reserved for large prolactinomas that have failed to respond to medical and surgical therapy.

Lessons for the Physician

When evaluating a patient who has secondary amenorrhea, it is important to look for hyperprolactinemia. Prolactinomas are diagnosed by serum prolactin testing and radiologic studies and are usually treated with dopamine agonist medication. Long-term follow-up includes monitoring prolactin levels as well as performing serial examinations and magnetic resonance imaging. Treatment may need to be lifelong, but it can afford patients more comfortable lives.

Stacey Maslow, MD, Southboro Medical Group, Framingham, MA

CHAPTER 28

16-Year-Old Girl Who Has Not Achieved Menarche

Presentation

A 16-year-old Caucasian girl comes in for a health supervision visit. She has been in good health, although she is concerned that she has not achieved menarche. Both her mother and sister attained menarche at age 13 years. She denies any unusual dieting patterns and has not been sexually active.

On physical examination, she is a pleasant girl whose height is far above the 97th percentile, weight is at the 10th percentile, and body mass index is 14.8. Her thyroid gland is not palpable. Her breasts are at Sexual Maturity Rating 3. She has normal abdominal findings when examined supine, but when standing and coughing, a 3.5-cm mass is palpable in her left inguinal canal. Her external genitalia have a normal female appearance, without clitoromegaly. She has minimal coarse pubic hair and no facial or axillary hair. The remainder of her physical findings are normal. Further testing reveals the reason for her delayed menarche.

- **What is your differential diagnosis at this point?**
- **Are there any elements of history or physical examination that would help you?**
- **What additional diagnostic studies would you like performed?**

Discussion

In this patient, the main concern was primary amenorrhea. A pelvic examination revealed absence of a uterus. Chromosomal analysis revealed a 46,XY karyotype. Androgen insensitivity was suspected, and hormone testing was performed. The girl's follicle-stimulating hormone level was 1.4 mIU/mL (1.4 IU/L) (male reference range, 1.4–18.1 mIU/mL [1.4—18.1 IU/L]). Her luteinizing hormone level was 35 mIU/mL (35 IU/L) (male reference range, 1.5—9.3 mIU/mL), and her testosterone level was 1,088 ng/dL (37.8 nmol/L) (reference range, 241–827 ng/dL

[8.4–28.7 nmol/L]). A low follicle-stimulating hormone level and high levels of luteinizing hormone and testosterone are consistent with androgen insensitivity. Complete androgen insensitivity syndrome (CAIS) was diagnosed. Pelvic ultrasonography was performed to locate the testes.

The Condition

In 1950, Wilkins described a 30-year-old patient who was phenotypically female but lacked pubic and axillary hair.[1] She was interested in growing body hair, but despite the local application of testosterone, there was neither growth of sexual hair nor any other androgenic effects. Wilkins concluded that her syndrome was related to an "insensitivity of end organs to androgen." Since that time, androgen insensitivity syndromes have become recognized as clinical entities, with the incidence of CAIS estimated to be as high as 1 in 20,000.

Pathogenesis

Testosterone is the primary androgen synthesized and secreted by the testes. Tissue-specific expression of the enzyme 5α-reductase converts testosterone to its active metabolite, dihydrotestosterone. Within target cells, dihydrotestosterone and, to a lesser extent, testosterone bind to androgen receptors. In CAIS, there is a resistance to androgens due to defects in the androgen receptor. Some patients have no detectable androgen receptors, while others have a near-normal number of androgen receptors but abnormal androgen-receptor binding. Less commonly, both the number and the function of the androgen receptor are diminished.

The chromosomal basis of androgen insensitivity is a loss-of-function mutation in the *AR* gene that has been localized to Xq and affects all receptors. Although numerous deletions have been described, including complete and partial gene deletions, more than 80% of patients have a single amino acid substitution.

Clinical Features

In patients who have CAIS, although the labia majora and minora sometimes may appear slightly underdeveloped, the general appearance of the external genitalia is unquestionably female. A clitoris is present always, but never enlarged. Both the urethral and vaginal openings are always in the normal position. Although the length of the vagina may be normal, often it is short. The vagina ends blindly, and neither a cervix nor a uterus can be palpated during a bimanual examination.

Because of the generally normal secretion of müllerian-inhibiting factor by Sertoli cells of the testes, development of the müllerian ducts is usually suppressed. Patients who have CAIS never menstruate because they do not possess a uterus nor can they become pregnant. Because of the absence of scrotal development, the testes are located in the abdomen or at various levels in the inguinal canal, attempting to descend into the labial folds. Complete androgen insensitivity syndrome should be suspected in phenotypically normal girls who have inguinal hernias or labial masses. As many as 1% to 2% of girls who develop inguinal hernias have this disorder.

Despite normal androgen synthesis, typical androgen effects, such as acne and voice changes, are blunted because of androgen resistance. Patients who have CAIS are usually taller than unaffected girls, suggesting that the Y chromosome may have effects not mediated by androgens.

Adolescents with CAIS have a normal female body habitus, often with well-developed breasts. Testosterone is converted to estradiol-17β by aromatase in the adrenal gland, testes, and adipose tissue, providing a source of estrogen that can bind to estrogenic receptors and promote breast and bone development.

Partial androgen insensitivity syndrome can also occur in individuals who have a 46,XY genotype. Affected patients are born with ambiguous external genitalia due to their partial ability to respond to androgens. The genital tubercle is larger than a clitoris but smaller than a penis. Often, partially fused labia or a scrotum are present. The testes may be undescended, and hypospadias is often present. Wolffian duct development is either minimal or nonexistent, and the müllerian duct system does not develop.

A Similar Condition

Gonadal dysgenesis is another disorder resulting in a female phenotype despite a male genotype. Unlike androgen insensitivity, in which functional testes can produce testosterone, patients born with gonadal dysgenesis have abnormal testes that are incapable of producing androgens. Complete gonadal dysgenesis affects 46,XY individuals and is characterized by abnormally formed gonads that originally were on the path to testis differentiation. External genitalia are female, and there is müllerian duct development and wolffian duct regression. Female external genitalia develop because of the failure of the gonadal streaks to produce androgens to masculinize the genital tubercle and genital swellings.

Therapy

All patients who have androgen insensitivity syndromes should undergo gonadectomy, the timing of which is controversial. Postpubertal gonadectomy enhances bone maturation as well as body development, but delaying the removal increases the risk of testicular malignancy. After the testes are removed, hormone therapy begins with estrogen replacement. Because of the short length of the vagina, some patients require vaginal lengthening. Most patients report satisfactory outcomes after vaginoplasty.

Psychological support is probably the most important aspect of care for affected patients. Psychosexual development in patients who have CAIS is female. Patients having this condition view themselves as being entirely female, as do other people. The overwhelming number of patients report being attracted to males. The resistance to testosterone does not appear to affect sexual drive adversely. Long-term psychological care should be provided to patients who have androgen insensitivity syndromes and their families by those trained in the fields of intersexuality and psychosexual development.

Reference

1. Wilkins L. *The Diagnosis and Treatment of Endocrine Disorders in Childhood and Adolescence.* Springfield, IL: Charles C. Thomas; 1950

Lessons for the Physician

Androgen insensitivity must be considered in the evaluation of girls who have primary amenorrhea or labial or inguinal masses and in patients who have ambiguous genitalia. This condition should also be suspected in infants who have inguinal or labial masses. A combination of karyotyping, hormone studies, and imaging allows definitive diagnosis. Treatment consists of removal of the testes and hormone replacement therapy in addition to the critical element of psychological support and counseling for patient and family.

Pranita Tamma, MD, and Claude Migeon, MD, Johns Hopkins School of Medicine, Baltimore, MD

COMMENTARY BY DR JENNIFER MILLER, PEDIATRIC ENDOCRINOLOGIST, UNIVERSITY OF FLORIDA

A multidisciplinary approach is recommended for the management of complete androgen sensitivity syndrome (CAIS). The issues are wide ranging and include providing information about the condition in an appropriate manner, monitoring puberty, consideration about the need and timing for gonadectomy, and aiming to support the affected adult to achieve adequate sexual function and optimal quality of life. Psychological support is essential from the time of diagnosis and throughout critical periods in decision making. Key members of the multidisciplinary team include an endocrinologist, urologist, gynecologist and clinical psychologist.

Review of the existing literature revealed a low rate of malignant tumors in women with CAIS, most often in the form a seminoma and usually after adolescence. As hormone replacement therapy is needed following gonadectomy, current recommendations are that if gonadectomy is desired, this should be delayed until after puberty. The optimal doses of hormone replacement therapy for women with CAIS are unknown.

Many clinicians are using testosterone supplementation in complete androgen insensitivity syndrome because it seems to give the individuals an improved sense of well-being. The mechanisms for this is not understood at this time. The thought is that the exogenous testosterone must be aromatized to estrogen and that, plus the supplementary estrogen they are on, must be working to make them feel better.

Part 7

Gastrointestinal

CHAPTER 29

Hematochezia in a Neonate

Presentation

A 25-day-old girl presents with 3 days of dark black stools. The mother mentions that that the girl has been looking pale since yesterday. She has a history of gastroesophageal reflux and suspected allergic proctitis with hemoccult-positive stools. Upper gastrointestinal series was performed, and the results were found to be normal. She is currently taking lansoprazole and an amino acid–based formula. She was born term by spontaneous vaginal delivery and was an appropriate weight for her gestational age. She has had progressive failure to thrive, and weight percentile has decreased from the 50th percentile to the 5th. Her family history is significant for celiac disease.

On physical examination her weight for length is less than the 5th percentile. Vital signs reveal the following values: temperature, 98.8°F (37.1°C); pulse, 111 beats/min; respirations, 21 breaths/min; blood pressure, 100/72 mm Hg (patient crying); and capillary refill, 2 to 3 seconds. She appears very pale, is alert, and has a 2/6 systolic murmur. There is no abnormality noted on rectal examination, and the abdomen is soft with appropriate bowel sounds. There is a small, pink, unraised discoloration of her skin above her upper lip.

Initial laboratory examination reveals a hemoglobin level of 3.8 g/dL (38 g/L) with normochromic and normocytic indices and a red blood cell count of 0.84×10^6/mcL (0.84×10^{12}/L), a platelet count of 401×10^3/mcL (401×10^9/L), a white blood cell count of 30×10^3/mcL (30×10^9/L) with normal differential, a reticulocyte count of 6.24% (0.062), a negative direct Coombs test result, normal lactase dehydrogenase level, and normal liver panel and coagulation study results. The results of abdominal radiography are also normal. The patient requires 2 packed red blood cell transfusions for anemia. The gastrointestinal and surgery services are consulted, and further studies reveal the diagnosis.

- **What is your differential diagnosis at this point?**
- **Are there any elements of history or physical examination that would help you?**
- **What additional diagnostic studies would you like performed?**

Discussion

The differential diagnosis of hematochezia and melena should include intestinal ischemia secondary to intussusception, midgut volvulus, incarcerated hernia, mesenteric thrombosis, Meckel diverticulum, swallowed blood, vasculitis, polyps, peptic ulcer disease, inflammatory bowel disease, vascular anomaly, varices, allergic colitis, coagulopathies, hemophilia, vitamin K deficiency, liver disease, or infectious colitis.

Diagnosis

The first consideration must be the severity of bleeding. The progressive increase in melena with severe anemia is a sign of significant gastrointestinal bleeding that necessitates a brisk and thorough evaluation. The next consideration should be the location of bleeding. A Meckel scan was performed and showed no evidence of a Meckel diverticulum. Esophagogastroduodenoscopy and colonoscopy were performed next, which revealed black, tarry stool in the colon but no specific site of bleeding. Biopsy specimens of the rectum showed eosinophilic infiltrate, diagnosing allergic proctitis, but because of her severe anemia further evaluation was continued. Abdominal ultrasonography was performed to look for a duplication cyst, and the result was normal. Abdominal magnetic resonance imaging results were also normal. This case was now, by definition, considered obscure gastrointestinal bleeding, which is apparent bleeding not identified by esophagogastroduodenoscopy or colonoscopy. The focus of the investigation shifted to the small intestine, which is harder to evaluate. Choices include small bowel follow-through, computed tomography (which may show mucosal irritation but not vascular anomalies), computed tomography enterography or magnetic resonance enterography, push enteroscopy, double-balloon enteroscopy, capsule endoscopy, and surgical exploration. She again had increased fussiness; she passed a large, bright red stool; and her hemoglobin level decreased to 4.7 g/dL (47 g/L), requiring transfusion. Chest and neck magnetic resonance imaging was performed to evaluate the vascular stain above her lip, which showed a small hemangioma in her chest. Because of the severity of her symptoms, an exploratory laparoscopy was performed to evaluate the small intestine, which showed abnormal ileal serosal vasculature but no site of bleeding. Further exploration by small bowel endoscopy during laparotomy showed purple discoloration of mucosa in the midileum, edema, and inflammation. Biopsy specimens taken from this region showed a capillary hemangioma, which stained positive for glucose transporter 1 (GLUT-1). Her hemoglobin level again decreased to 7.4 g/dL (74 g/L) after a large, red stool. She was given prednisone to treat her hemangioma and has had no further bleeding.

The Condition

Vascular anomalies are divided into vascular tumors and vascular malformations. Vascular tumors include hemangiomas and are benign endothelial tumors that grow rapidly. Vascular malformations include port wine stains, are present at birth, and grow proportionally to the neonate's growth. Vascular malformations are defined by abnormal blood vessel development as opposed to vascular tumors, which consist of rapid proliferation of endothelial cells.

Cutaneous infantile hemangiomas commonly affect 1% to 2.6% of neonates and infants, with girls being more frequently affected than boys. They are usually present on skin and soft tissue with uncommon visceral and rare gastrointestinal involvement. Hemangiomas generally follow a 3-stage pattern of growth. The first stage is proliferation, which starts after birth and continues for 6 to 10 months. The second stage is the stationary stage, during which the hemangioma stops growing. The third stage is involution, during which the size of the hemangioma decreases. At 5 years of age and at 9 years of age 50% and 90% of hemangiomas, respectively, have reached the involuted phase and are no longer visible.

Specific pathologic features of hemangiomas include multilaminated basement membranes and GLUT-1 positivity. There are 2 other categories of hemangiomas, including noninvoluting congenital hemangiomas and rapidly involuting congenital hemangiomas. These are both present at birth, do not proliferate, and do not express GLUT-1.

Hemangiomas of the gastrointestinal tract are rare and account for only 0.05% of all gastrointestinal tumors, but when present more than 80% are symptomatic. Hemangiomas are prone to bleeding only in the proliferating phase, making bleeding rare after 1 year of age. Symptoms include bleeding, which manifests depending on the site of the hemangioma, abdominal pain, anemia, obstruction, or intussusception. The presence of multiple hemangiomas or ones in unusual locations, such as the small intestine, should raise the possibility of a syndrome. Syndromes include blue rubber bleb nevus syndrome, Klippel-Trenaunay syndrome, and PHACES (**p**osterior fossa malformations, **h**emangiomas, **a**rterial anomalies, **c**ardiac defects, **e**ye abnormalities, **s**ternal cleft and supraumbilical raphe) syndrome. In blue rubber bleb nevus syndrome, patients have numerous intestinal and cutaneous hemangiomas. In Klippel-Trenaunay syndrome, patients have port wine stains, varicose veins, and bony or soft-tissue hypertrophy. In PHACES syndrome, patients have hemangiomas associated with posterior fossa brain abnormalities and cardiac and eye abnormalities. This patient did not fit any syndrome.

Management

Most infantile hemangiomas are treated with observation and resolve spontaneously. Some require intralesional or systemic corticosteroids. For resistant hemangiomas, vincristine and interferon-α can be used. Propranolol has also shown promise. Surgical removal is rarely indicated.

Lessons for the Physician

- Small intestine hemangiomas are rare but can cause significant bleeding.
- Small intestinal hemangiomas are difficult to diagnose.
- Small intestinal hemangiomas must be kept in the differential of gastrointestinal bleeding.

Marisa M. Fisher, MD, and Pablo Palomo, MD, University of Nebraska Medical Center, Omaha, NE
Fernando Zapata, MD, Children's Hospital and Medical Center, Omaha, NE

CHAPTER 30

2-Month-Old Boy With 6-Day History of Increasing Irritability, High-pitched Cry, and Nonbloody, Nonbilious Vomiting

Presentation

You are evaluating a 2-month-old boy who has a 6-day history of increasing irritability, high-pitched cry, and nonbloody, nonbilious vomiting. He is a term infant, and his mother noted that he was fussier and spit up more than her other 3 children, despite the use of milk-based, soy-based, and elemental formulas. Three weeks ago, they changed to whole cow's milk, alternating daily with 2% cow's milk. Over the past week, the infant has become increasingly irritable and has been vomiting all feedings for 2 days. He has lost 0.5 kg since birth. He is having regular bowel movements, with no blood in his stool. There has been no fever or contacts with sick people.

On physical examination, the infant is alert, responsive, and in no acute distress. His vital signs are within reference range for age. His abdomen is not tender but is distended. No organomegaly is noted, but a large mass is palpated in the midepigastric region.

The results of multiple investigations, including measurement of serum electrolytes and calcium, complete blood cell count, and urine toxicology screening for opiates, barbiturates, cocaine, and amphetamines, are normal. Blood and cerebrospinal fluid cultures are negative for bacteria.

An abdominal radiograph shows a 5-cm mass in his stomach. A barium-enhanced upper gastrointestinal series reveals a 5-cm filling defect in his stomach, which leads to the diagnosis.

- **What is your differential diagnosis at this point?**
- **Are there any elements of history or physical examination that would help you?**
- **What additional diagnostic studies would you like performed?**

Discussion

This infant had a lactobezoar, which is a concretion of undigested milk curds that can cause mechanical obstruction of the gastrointestinal tract. A bezoar is a concretion of foreign materials found anywhere in the gastrointestinal tract, most commonly within the stomach. Bezoars can consist of plant material (phytobezoar), ingested hair (trichobezoar), persimmon fibers (diospyrobezoar), milk products (lactobezoar), or medications, such as aspirin. Bezoars are found commonly in children and adults who have neuropsychiatric disorders, pica, or mental retardation. Patients who have delayed gastric emptying are also at risk for developing bezoars. In adults, bezoars may develop after gastric operations.

The word *bezoar* is derived from a Persian word for "counterpoison" because animal bezoars were believed to be antidotes for poisonous substances.

Although lactobezoars were initially believed to occur in only preterm neonates, a current review of the literature has shown them to occur in children up to 3 years of age. Individual case reports have also demonstrated that lactobezoars may form with any type of neonatal or infantile alimentation, including human milk, traditional formulas, soy-based formulas, lactose-free formulas, and cow's milk. Formula gastric bezoars are rare these days because of the method by which modern formulas are blended. Risk factors, such as milk protein intolerance, low birthweight, and a diet of overconcentrated milk formula, have been associated with specific cases. Foregut anomalies, such as duodenal stenosis and duodenal webs, can result in gastric bezoars. Most cases, however, are presumably due to mixed causes affecting gastric secretion, motility, and emptying.

Clinical Features

A neonate or infant who has a lactobezoar can present with a variety of nonspecific findings that can make prompt diagnosis difficult. The most frequent presenting signs include abdominal distention, vomiting, and diarrhea. In one review, 46% of patients had abdominal distention, 34% had nonbilious vomiting, and 26% had diarrhea. Other common presenting symptoms were gastric residuals in 18%, palpable mass in 13%, and dehydration in 6%.

These infants often become intolerant of their feedings and may develop anorexia, which can cause significant weight loss. It is also important to recognize that signs may be intermittent due to a mobile lactobezoar that causes transient gastric outlet obstruction. Of note, 6% of cases are identified by routine chest radiography in the absence of gastrointestinal symptoms.

Differential Diagnosis

The differential diagnosis of a neonate or infant presenting with abdominal distention, vomiting, or diarrhea is extensive.

Disorders to consider in an infant who has vomiting are gastroesophageal reflux, intoxication, inborn errors of metabolism, urinary tract infection, meningitis or encephalitis, and anatomic obstruction. For an infant having diarrhea, antibiotic-associated diarrhea, postinfectious lactase deficiency, celiac disease, and cystic fibrosis should be considered. The differential diagnosis for gastric obstruction alone includes antral webs, pyloric stenosis, pyloric stricture, and foreign body.

The most common conditions associated with all 3 of these signs are gastroenteritis, systemic infection, overfeeding, and milk protein intolerance. Although lactobezoar is not a common cause of gastrointestinal signs in infants, it must be considered in cases eluding diagnosis.

Diagnosis

Lactobezoar has been diagnosed most commonly by barium-enhanced upper gastrointestinal series. With this study, the bezoar appears as a filling defect or a radiolucent cast within the gastric bubble. An upper gastrointestinal series can also detect any associated congenital foregut anomalies or conditions. On radiographs without contrast, visualizing a bezoar depends on an adequate amount of air being present in the stomach. For either type of imaging, a lateral decubitus film helps confirm the intraluminal location and mobility of the mass.

Some institutions employ ultrasonography to confirm the presence of a lactobezoar to avoid exposing neonates and infants to radiation. A clear-water feeding is given before ultrasonography to delineate the borders of the mass. The mass itself is hyperechoic, with a heterogeneous echo texture. Regardless of the method of imaging used, follow-up imaging is advised to verify dissolution of the lactobezoar.

Treatment and Prognosis

No randomized controlled trials have compared treatments for lactobezoar. Currently, a common treatment regimen combines bowel rest with parenteral fluids for several days. In some cases, gastric lavage with saline via nasogastric tube has been used to help break up the bezoar.

For this patient, enteral feedings were not discontinued; rather, they were switched to a water-based solution containing sugar and electrolytes, given on demand. This regimen avoided the need for intravenous fluids. Further, a nasogastric tube was placed, through which hourly gastric lavage was performed. Over the next few days, he began passing small, white pieces of the lactobezoar in his stool, at which point he was given predigested elemental formula. One case review of lactobezoar purported that a formula change may not be necessary because there are no cases of lactobezoar recurring in neonates and infants.

If a lactobezoar is not diagnosed and treated promptly, the infant is at risk for metabolic and hemodynamic derangements due to vomiting, diarrhea, or anorexia. Gastric perforation is a less common but potentially dangerous consequence of untreated lactobezoar. Both perforation and acute obstruction are complications of a lactobezoar that require immediate surgical intervention.

Lessons for the Physician

By including lactobezoar in the differential diagnosis of gastrointestinal disturbances with feeding intolerance, physicians can identify cases without an extensive evaluation and can prevent complications by initiating early conservative treatment.

Sonja Colianni, MD; Jennifer Ping, MD; Philip R. Fischer, MD; and Deborah Freese, MD, Mayo Clinic College of Medicine, Rochester, MN

CHAPTER 31

3-Month-Old Boy Admitted for Poor Feeding and a Distended Abdomen

Presentation

A 3-month-old African American boy is admitted for poor feeding and a distended abdomen. During pregnancy, polyhydramnios was detected; ultrasonography suggested intestinal obstruction. At birth, the infant's abdomen was distended, with visible and palpable loops of bowel. Barium enema showed normal findings, and a barium study demonstrated gastroesophageal reflux.

The infant breastfed 6 to 8 times a day but for only 5 minutes per side. When offered pumped milk, he took only 30 to 60 mL per feeding. He passed 4 yellow, seedy stools and had 6 wet diapers per day. On oral feedings with human milk and predigested formula, the infant maintained a weight gain of 0.02 to 0.03 kg/d until 7 weeks of age, but by 3 months, he had gained only an additional 0.28 kg.

On physical examination, he is irritable and has a high-pitched cry and a protuberant abdomen with a small umbilical hernia. He weighs 4.06 kg (<5th percentile). His birthweight had been at the 5th percentile.

The infant's serum sodium concentration is 122 mEq/L (122 mmol/L), potassium is 2.8 mEq/L (2.8 mmol/L), chloride is 61 mEq/L (61 mmol/L), bicarbonate is 40 mEq/L (40 mmol/L), urea nitrogen is 9 mg/dL (3.2 mmol/L), and creatinine is 0.3 mg/dL (26.5 mcmol/L). Serum osmolality is 244 mOsm/kg (244 mmol/kg), and urine osmolality is 122 mOsm/kg (244 mmol/kg). Urinalysis shows specific gravity of 1.010, pH 7, and 3 to 5 red blood cells and 0 to 2 white blood cells per high-power field. The urine is negative for ketones, bilirubin, nitrite, protein, glucose, white blood cell esterase, and urobilinogen.

After serum electrolyte concentrations are corrected with intravenous fluids, urinary electrolyte concentrations are sodium, less than 10 mEq/L (10 mmol/L); potassium, 20 mEq/L (20 mmol/L); and chloride, less than 15 mEq/L (15 mmol/L). Serum aldosterone is 64 ng/dL (1.8 nmol/L) (reference range, 3–33 ng/dL

[0.08–0.91 nmol/L]). Serum renin is 149 ng/mL (114.7 nmol × L^{-1}). A sweat chloride level is 17 mEq/L (17 mmol/L). Stool electrolyte concentrations are chloride, 105 mEq/L (105 mmol/L); sodium, 28 mEq/L (28 mmol/L); and potassium, 78 mEq/L (78 mmol/L). Hyponatremia and alkalosis recur when the infant is fed predigested formula in the hospital. The suspected diagnosis is confirmed by a special test.

- **What is your differential diagnosis at this point?**
- **Are there any elements of history or physical examination that would help you?**
- **What additional diagnostic studies would you like performed?**

Discussion

This 3-month-old boy presented with hyponatremia, hypochloremia, hypokalemia, alkalosis, growth failure, and abdominal distention. Loss of chloride and potassium in the stool was excessive. Polyhydramnios had been present during pregnancy. Bowel obstruction had been suspected previously but ruled out by contrast radiography. There was no history of persistent vomiting, formula dilution, or diarrhea.

Stools were loose, seedy, and yellow to green. Because the mother was breastfeeding, most observers believed that the stools did not represent a true diarrhea.

Differential Diagnosis

The differential diagnosis of infants and children presenting with hyponatremia, hypochloremia, and growth failure includes renal and adrenal disease, inadequate sodium and calorie intake, Bartter syndrome, and congenital malabsorptive disorders of the gut, such as cystic fibrosis and chloridorrhea. The low urinary sodium concentration, lack of protein or glucose in the urine, and normal renal function test results ruled out renal causes. A low serum potassium concentration made an adrenal disorder unlikely. The alkalosis without vomiting made inadequate sodium and calorie intake improbable.

Bartter syndrome is a rare condition characterized by muscle weakness, growth retardation, polyuria, polydipsia, constipation, and normal blood pressure. A hypokalemic, hypochloremic alkalosis with hyperkaluria, hyperchloruria, isosthenuria, hyperactivity of the renin-angiotensin-aldosterone system, and increased excretion of prostaglandin E_2 is present in the condition. The low urine potassium and chloride concentrations reported for the infant in this case, after serum electrolyte concentrations were corrected, excluded Bartter syndrome. Suspicion of Bartter syndrome prompted the measurement of an aldosterone level, which was elevated.

This infant had secondary hyperaldosteronism. Hypertension, hypokalemia, kaliuresis, and suppressed plasma renin activity are usually present with primary aldosteronism. This infant was normotensive, had no kaliuresis, and had an elevated plasma renin concentration.

Intrinsic abnormality of human milk electrolytes, which is uncommon, was ruled out when the hyponatremia persisted while the infant was fed prepared predigested formula.

Sodium and chloride loss through the gastrointestinal tract was an alternate possibility. Tufting enteropathy, microvillus inclusion disease, pseudo-obstruction syndrome, and cystic fibrosis are known to cause chloride loss. In 15% to 20% of infants who have cystic fibrosis, the ileum is obstructed completely at birth. Soon after birth, infants who have cystic fibrosis and severe transmembrane conductance regulator mutations may develop dehydration with hyponatremia, hypochloremia, and alkalosis. A normal sweat chloride and negative DNA mutation analysis for cystic fibrosis genes made cystic fibrosis unlikely.

The elevated chloride and potassium loss in this infant's stool suggested chloridorrhea, or congenital chloride diarrhea (CCD). Congenital chloride diarrhea is a rare autosomal recessive disorder caused by a selective dysfunction of a chloride-bicarbonate exchange mechanism located in the brush border of the ileum and possibly in the colon. A resultant marked loss of chloride in the stool occurs, and metabolic alkalosis ensues because of failure to excrete bicarbonate into the bowel lumen. The decrease in stool bicarbonate concentration acidifies the bowel contents, which subsequently limits the absorption of sodium further through decreased sodium-hydrogen exchange.

Genetics

A locus for the affected gene in CCD has been mapped by Kere and associates in proximity to, yet distinct from, the locus for the cystic fibrosis transmembrane regulator gene on chromosome 7.[1] This gene encodes a transmembrane protein belonging to 1 of 3 known members of the sulfate transporter family. More than 20 mutations in the gene deemed responsible for CCD, also known as *SLC26A3* (formerly *CLD* or *DRA* [downregulated in adenoma]), have been identified. Results of nucleotide sequencing confirmed the diagnosis of CCD in this infant.

Clinical Features

Polyhydramnios often heralds the birth of an infant who has CCD, suggesting that the diarrhea begins in utero. Intestinal dilation has also been noted on prenatal ultrasonography of fetuses affected with CCD. Surgeons are often asked to evaluate these infants for possible bowel obstruction, an aganglionic segment of colon, or a vesicorectal fistula.

Neonates who have CCD usually experience diarrhea in the first few postnatal days and occasionally, delayed passage of meconium. In addition to abdominal distension, there are evolving electrolyte abnormalities, including a hyponatremic, hypochloremic metabolic alkalosis. Hyperbilirubinemia is a common finding, hypothesized to be due to poor hydration.

The diagnosis can be delayed, and some infants have been diagnosed as late as 6 months of age following marked retardation in growth, development, and activity. There is a report of a 31-year-old man who presented with recurrent diarrhea exacerbated by viral illnesses and was found to have CCD. The diagnosis can be elusive, especially if the infant presents with a complication of the disease, such as volvulus. This complication is believed to occur because of the constant voluminous filling of intestinal loops. Other mechanical disorders of the gastrointestinal tract are very infrequent.

Growth retardation and motor delay are common observations and were the primary stimuli for further evaluation in this case. Diarrhea was not reported, which made diagnosis more difficult. Stools observed on repeated follow-up visits were documented as yellow and seedy. In a Finnish series, only two-thirds of affected patients had diarrhea documented in the first few postnatal weeks.[2] In some neonates, the stools are so watery in the neonatal period that they are mistaken for urine.

Another observed association is enamel hypoplasia of the teeth.

Diagnosis

Congenital chloride diarrhea is diagnosed by measuring the stool chloride concentration; a chloride concentration of more than 95 to 100 mEq/L (95–100 mmol/L) is definitive. Nucleotide sequencing performed in research laboratories can prove mutations in the *SLC26A3* gene on chromosome 7. High renin and aldosterone levels are common and probably due to a relative hypovolemia coupled with poor sodium absorption and high water losses in the intestine. Hypertension is not a feature of CCD.

Treatment

Treatment is simpler than arriving at the diagnosis. Oral supplements of sodium chloride or potassium chloride are administered to maintain normal serum concentrations. Replacement therapy should be initiated as soon as possible. The diarrhea is lifelong because the intestinal transport defect cannot be corrected. Some increase in the volume of stool has been shown to occur with respiratory tract infections.

Most of the patients in the Finnish study were shown to have an initial growth retardation that corrected over time with adequate electrolyte replacement. This patient's growth improved remarkably after electrolyte supplementation. He has achieved normal growth milestones. Mental retardation has been associated with CCD. Adequate treatment from birth may improve intellectual and psychomotor development.

References

1. Kere J, Lohi H, Höglund P. Genetic disorders of membrane transport. III. Congenital chloride diarrhea. *Am J Physiol.* 1999;276(1 Pt 1):G7–G13
2. Holmberg C, Purheentupa J, Launiala K, Hallman N. Congenital chloride diarrhea. *Arch Dis Child.* 1977;52(4):255–267

Lessons for the Physician

When a neonate or young infant has poor weight gain, abdominal distension, and a history of polyhydramnios, the first step in evaluation should be to obtain basic laboratory studies, such as measurement of serum electrolyte concentrations. Contrast radiography should be performed next to search for an anatomic lesion of the gut. If the diagnosis continues to be unclear, congenital malabsorptive disorders should be considered. If a patient has persistent or recurring hyponatremia, hypokalemia, and hypochloremia while provided with normal feedings, measurement of both urinary and stool electrolyte concentrations may be necessary.

Sujaja Sadiq, MD; Mitch Harris, MD; and John Gaebler, MD, Riley Hospital, Indianapolis, IN

COMMENTARY BY NEAL S. LELEIKO MD, PHD, DIRECTOR, DIVISION OF PEDIATRIC GASTROENTEROLOGY, NUTRITION AND LIVER DISEASES, DEPARTMENT OF PEDIATRICS HASBRO CHILDREN'S HOSPITAL, PROFESSOR OF PEDIATRICS, THE WARREN ALPERT SCHOOL OF MEDICINE AT BROWN UNIVERSITY

Congenital chloride diarrhea (CLD) is a rare disease with approximately 250 reported cases world-wide. It is an autosomal recessive disorder caused by mutations in the gene designated as SLC26A3 (solute carrier family 26 member 3 gene). At least 55 different mutations have been identified. They result in the disruption of the transport of Cl'/HCO3 in the intestinal epithelium. In addition to the genetic mutations, there are several pathogens associated with alterations in the function of this gene. Additionally, there is evidence that there is an interaction with the CFTR in patients affected with CLD. There is no evident association between any of the known mutations and the clinical presentation of patients.

While CLD is classically described as presenting in the neonatal period with polyhydramnios and profuse watery diarrhea, there is clearly a wide variety of presentations, including one adult with chronic watery diarrhea. Many of the reported cases have been diagnosed only after months of investigation. Patients can be successfully treated with oral electrolyte supplements, but will continue to have chronic diarrhea for their entire lives.

The critical finding in CLD is the presence of a high fecal Cl^- (>90 mmol/l). As a practical matter, it is often a challenge to get a hospital lab to assess fecal liquid for Cl^- and the diagnosis is generally first considered when a very abnormally low serum Cl^- is discovered on routine serum electrolyte testing. When this finding is accompanied by metabolic alkalosis, documenting stool Cl^- becomes very relevant. Many of the diseases considered to be part of the differential diagnosis can be excluded on the basis of metabolic acidosis, i.e defects in carbohydrate absorption, lysinuric protein intolerance, microvillus inclusion disease, and acrodermatitis enteropathica. In general, these are diarrheas of malabsorption rather than of secretion. Unusual and unexplained presentations of infantile diarrhea should prompt questioning about non-traditional treatments. For example, hypochloremic, metabolic alkalosis (with hypernatremia) has been noted in a baby with magnesium oxide ingestion (given as a folk remedy for diarrhea).

Genetic testing has, until recently, only been available in the research laboratory, it is now commercially available. Genetic confirmation should be obtained, not only to document CLD, but to exclude other causes of diarrhea. To date, all parental samples have been found to have heterozygote changes. It seems likely that as more and more studies are done, more mutations will be discovered and a much broader spectrum of disease will be recognized.

CHAPTER 32

2-Year-Old Boy With "Yellow Eyes" and Dark-Colored Urine

Presentation

A 2-year-old boy is admitted to the hospital because of "yellow eyes" and dark-colored urine for 7 days. There has been no change in stool color, rash, abdominal pain, diarrhea, lethargy, mental status change, or medication use. There is no history of hemolytic blood disorder, liver disease, or other serious illness. Family history is negative for liver disease.

The child is afebrile and looks well. Findings on physical examination, including the evaluation of the abdomen, are normal except for scleral icterus.

Findings on complete blood cell count are normal, as are levels of serum alkaline phosphatase, amylase, and lipase, as well as a coagulation profile. The child's serum total bilirubin level is 5.0 mg/dL (85.5 mcmol/L), direct bilirubin is 4.0 mg/dL (68.4 mcmol/L), alanine aminotransferase is 300 U/dL, and aspartate aminotransferase is 248 U/dL. Additional results include negative serum viral titers for hepatitis and Epstein-Barr viruses and normal levels of serum ceruloplasmin and alpha$_1$-antitrypsin. Additional radiologic findings and additional history lead to the diagnosis.

- **What is your differential diagnosis at this point?**
- **Are there any elements of history or physical examination that would help you?**
- **What additional diagnostic studies would you like performed?**

Discussion

The initial focus of the evaluation was to consider the various causes of conjugated hyperbilirubinemia. Findings on ultrasonography and computed tomography established the diagnosis, revealing a liver laceration to be the cause of this child's hyperbilirubinemia. Further questioning disclosed that the child had been spanked by his mother prior to the onset of the hyperbilirubinemia. The patient was taken into protective custody and had an uncomplicated recovery.

Pathogenesis and Clinical Picture

Blunt abdominal trauma can cause injury to many organs in the abdomen, including liver, spleen, pancreas, and intestines, without causing any external evidence of trauma. These injuries can result from motor vehicle crashes, falls, bicycle injuries, and physical abuse. Blunt hepatic injury (BHI) occurs as a spectrum ranging from a minimal parenchymal hematoma to massive disruption of the organ. After the injury, the liver heals through stages of coalescence, resorption, and remodeling prior to final healing.

Isolated BHI can present a clinical spectrum extending from an absence of symptoms to mild abdominal discomfort to catastrophic bleeding and shock. Additional injuries inside as well as outside of the abdomen also influence the clinical course and outcome.

Diagnosis

The diagnosis of BHI should be suspected in the presence of conjugated hyperbilirubinemia and elevated levels of liver enzymes in association with a history of trauma or in the absence of other causes. Computed tomography or radionuclide scintigraphy are the appropriate tools for identifying hepatic trauma at initial presentation. Ultrasonography, although not as accurate in making the diagnosis, can be very useful in documenting subsequent progress and eventual healing of the lesions. There is no correlation between the levels of transaminases or bilirubin and the type of hepatic injury, the degree of severity, or the clinical course. Levels of transaminases and bilirubin gradually decrease over 4 to 6 weeks.

The Organ Injury Scaling Committee of the American Association for the Surgery of Trauma has proposed a scaling method for hepatic trauma employing computed tomography that ranges from grade 1 to grade 4, the most severe category. Grade 1 is assigned to subcapsular hematoma, grade 2 refers to a 1- to 3-cm simple laceration or contusion, a laceration greater than 3 cm constitutes a grade 3 lesion, and grade 4 applies to an extensive laceration or transection. The primary determinant of the prognosis in patients who sustain hepatic trauma is hemorrhage due to vessel injuries.

Management

The hemodynamic stability of the patient is the critical factor in determining the success of nonoperative management of hepatic injuries. As well as being physically different from adults, children are injured differently, which supports the appropriateness of a high rate of nonoperative management. As in blunt splenic and renal injuries in children, most hepatic injuries are minor and can be managed nonoperatively. Intensive monitoring for at least 48 hours, with bed rest, repeated clinical assessments, serial laboratory studies, and blood replacement, is the major component of nonoperative treatment of splenic and hepatic injuries in stable patients, which is standard practice in children's trauma centers and has a success rate of 90%. Complete bed rest is prescribed for at least 10 days, depending on the type of injury, with restricted activities up to 3 months postinjury.

Major hepatic injuries can be life threatening and may require immediate operation. The principal indicator for immediate surgery is hemodynamic instability. These patients may demonstrate the following characteristics: a significantly lower Pediatric Trauma Score (the lower the score, the worse the injury) due to multisystem injury; the need for transfusion within 2 hours of admission; and a major retrohepatic vena caval injury on initial computed tomography. A transfusion requirement in excess of 40 mL/kg within the first 6 hours of admission is highly predictive of the need for operative intervention.

Prognosis

Mortality and morbidity rates in pediatric patients who have hepatic injuries of grades 1 to 4 are correlated with the associated injuries rather than the degree of hepatic damage. Low-grade and isolated high-grade hepatic injuries seldom require transfusion. Patients who were abused tend to have high-grade hepatic injuries and significant laboratory and clinical findings. Patients with hepatic trauma due to abuse are younger and have an increased incidence of high-grade hepatic injuries as well as significantly increased transaminase levels compared with other patients. Diagnosis in these patients tends to be delayed.

The mortality associated with serious hepatic injuries in children is about 10%, usually from associated injuries, but it exceeds 50% if major lacerations or juxtahepatic venous injuries are present. In children, most deaths from blunt trauma to the liver are caused by large stellate fractures of the posterolateral aspect of the right lobe of the liver, with extension into the hepatic veins. Late complications include hemobilia, bile peritonitis, abscesses, and bleeding. These complications may occur in patients who do not undergo surgery but are more likely to affect those who have had operations. Late hemorrhage—heralded by persistent right abdominal and shoulder pain—may occur in children who have severe hepatic trauma and high injury severity scores. Ultrasonography or computed tomography is recommended 3 to 6 months after BHI for patients who have grade 3 and 4 injuries. If no cholelithiasis or alteration of the biliary tract is present, no other follow-up is necessary.

Lessons for the Physician

This case illustrates the importance of considering blunt hepatic injury, including injury from abuse, in any child presenting with conjugated hyperbilirubinemia and elevated levels of liver enzymes, even if there is no history or physical evidence of trauma.

Parthak Prodhan, MD, and Anjubal Riar, MD, Cook County Hospital, Chicago, IL

Priya Mendiratta, MD, Beth Israel Deaconess Medical Center, Boston, MA

CHAPTER 33

Intermittent Epigastric Pain, Nausea, and Vomiting With Progressive Abdominal Distension in a 4-Year-Old Boy

Presentation

A 4-year-old boy has experienced intermittent epigastric pain, nausea, and vomiting with progressive abdominal distension over the past week. The vomiting is nonbilious and nonbloody, consisting of food and mucus. Stools are brown, softer than usual, but not watery, and they contain no mucus or blood. He has not consumed large amounts of cow's milk, and urine color and output have not changed. His eyes have looked puffy. He has been taking amoxicillin for 1 week for otitis media.

The physical examination reveals a well-developed child in no apparent distress. His temperature is 99.4°F (37.4°C), pulse is 101 beats/min, blood pressure is 99/70 mm Hg, and respiratory rate is 24 breaths/min. He has moderate periorbital edema and mild dependent edema of the lower extremities. His breath sounds are slightly decreased at the bases. A grade 2/6 ejection murmur, heard previously, is audible at the left sternal border. His abdomen is full, soft, and free of organomegaly but diffusely tender without guarding or rebound. Shifting dullness and a fluid wave are elicited by percussion.

He has a white blood cell count of 9.3×10^3/mcL (9.3×10^9/L) with 13% neutrophils, 3% bands, 36% lymphocytes, 36% atypical lymphocytes, 7% mononuclear cells, and 4% eosinophils. Hemoglobin level is 14.0 g/dL (140 g/L), and mean corpuscular volume is 70.9 mcm^3 (70.9 fL). His calcium level is 6.8 mg/dL (1.7 mmol/L). Total protein and albumin levels are markedly decreased at 3.3 g/dL (33 g/L) and 1.3 g/dL (13 g/L), respectively. Liver enzymes, bilirubin levels, prothrombin time, and partial thromboplastin time all are normal, as are findings on urinalysis. The stool is free of occult blood and white blood cells but has an $alpha_1$-antitrypsin level that is more than twice the upper range of reference. A chest radiograph reveals small bilateral pleural effusions with a normal cardiac silhouette. Computed tomography of his abdomen reveals massive ascites with normal-appearing viscera except for thickened folds in the stomach. An additional test reveals the diagnosis.

- **What is your differential diagnosis at this point?**
- **Are there any elements of history or physical examination that would help you?**
- **What additional diagnostic studies would you like performed?**

Discussion

This previously well child experienced the acute onset of severe hypoproteinemia that resulted in generalized edema (anasarca). The most common causes of this presentation in children are hepatic (cirrhosis, cystic fibrosis), renal (nephrotic syndrome), and gastrointestinal (protein-losing enteropathy [PLE], allergic gastrointestinal reactions, gastroenteropathy). Congestive heart failure can cause significant edema but not through the mechanism of hypoproteinemia. Another common cause of severe edema and hypoproteinemia with associated profound anemia is excessive cow's milk intake. It is believed that excessive amounts of milk in the diet damage the gut, with resulting blood loss. Treatment is reduction of milk intake.

In the absence of hepatosplenomegaly, proteinuria, hematuria, and laboratory evidence of renal failure, coagulopathy, or hyperbilirubinemia, loss of protein from the gastrointestinal tract becomes the most likely source of this patient's hypoproteinemia and edema. An upper gastrointestinal series revealed enlarged rugae in the fundus and body of the stomach. Esophagogastroduodenoscopy showed hypertrophic gastric folds, with a biopsy specimen revealing foveolar hyperplasia of the gastric antrum and body and dilated glands filled with mucus and inspissated secretions. There were areas of focal acute inflammation, with evidence of gland destruction and several cells that had an appearance suggestive of possible viral inclusions, although viral culture and immunostaining for cytomegalovirus (CMV) of gastric tissue were negative. Mild eosinophilia of the gastric body and duodenum was also present. The esophagus appeared normal. These findings, along with the patient's symptoms, are classic features of benign hypertrophic gastropathy of childhood.

The Condition

Hypertrophic gastropathy of childhood is an uncommon, self-limited form of an adult disorder known as Ménétrier disease, which was described first in 1888. This transient, benign entity in pediatric patients consists of significant hypertrophy of the mucus-secreting cells of the stomach, with resultant gastrointestinal protein loss and hypoalbuminemia. The average age of presentation in childhood is approximately 6 years, with relative sparing of adolescents. Adult cases outnumber childhood cases nearly 6 to 1, with more than 300 adult and only 50 childhood cases reported. There is a male predominance in both populations.

The classic presenting signs and symptoms in order of frequency are nausea, vomiting, peripheral edema, abdominal pain, anorexia, ascites, and occasionally hematemesis. In contrast with adults, children often present with complications of the protein-losing gastropathy, such as ascites, pleural effusions, and periorbital or peripheral edema in addition to nonspecific gastrointestinal complaints. Children also tend to have a more favorable clinical course than adults, with complete, spontaneous resolution of disease in several weeks to 6 months. Adults who have Ménétrier disease typically have a more chronic and difficult course that may require partial gastric resection to minimize persistent protein loss or gastric hemorrhage. There is a 10% risk of carcinoma in adults, a complication not often seen in the pediatric population.

Pathogenesis

Although no definitive cause has been discovered for Ménétrier disease, allergy or infection seem to be the most likely possibilities in the pathogenesis of childhood disease. At least one-third of all pediatric cases have been linked to acute CMV infection diagnosed by serology (elevated concentration of CMV IgM), gastric biopsy studies (positive CMV culture, cytomegalic intranuclear inclusion bodies), or urine CMV culture. Of note, results of all 3 of these tests were negative in this patient's case. The frequent association with peripheral eosinophilia and mucosal infiltration with eosinophils may favor an allergic component. Other proposed potential causes include autoimmune disorders, toxins, and dietary factors.

Recent studies using transgenic mice revealed a possible role for transforming growth factor-α in the pathogenesis of Ménétrier disease. Transforming growth factor-α is a polypeptide growth factor that stimulates cell proliferation, inhibits acid secretion, and enhances mucus secretion. Its expression in the transgenic mice was highest in the glandular cells of the stomach at the base of the crypts and in surface mucus cells. The transient disease seen in children who have hypertrophic gastropathy may represent a transient increase in transforming growth factor-α levels due to activation of the *ras* oncogene by a viral infection (such as CMV). Adults, on the other hand, may have a mutation in the *ras* oncogene that would explain their more chronic disease course. Others have proposed that primary CMV infection of the gastric mucosa may induce local production of tumor necrosis factor-α, which subsequently induces mucosal hyperplasia.

Diagnosis

In the presence of edema or ascites and hypoalbuminemia, hepatic and renal disorders must be considered in addition to gastrointestinal disease.

The diagnosis of pediatric hypertrophic gastropathy depends ultimately on visualization and biopsy of the stomach. The characteristic histologic findings include foveolar hyperplasia with hypertrophy of the gastric mucosa. Additional histologic findings may include hypertrophied gastric glands; interstitial inflammatory reaction of eosinophils, lymphocytes, and plasma cells; glandular atrophy; and cysts lined by mucous cells. These findings are generally more pronounced in the body and fundus of the stomach, with relative sparing of the antrum. There also may be focal areas of gastritis, and in some cases, CMV inclusions may be seen.

In addition to the profound hypoalbuminemia (usually <2.0 g/dL [20 g/L]) present in almost all cases of hypertrophic gastropathy of childhood, other laboratory abnormalities may include mild normochromic, normocytic anemia in one-third of cases (due to gastric blood loss) and peripheral eosinophilia.

Additional gastrointestinal causes of hypoproteinemia include inflammatory bowel disease, gluten-sensitive enteropathy, cystic fibrosis, Shwachman syndrome, and trypsinogen or enterokinase deficiency.

Measurement of stool alpha$_1$-antitrypsin levels can be used to screen for protein-losing enteropathy. This test is a sensitive, naturally occurring marker for the presence of PLE, whatever the cause. The test's only limitation is a possible falsely normal result in cases of PLE due to hypertrophic gastropathy and inactivation of the alpha$_1$-antitrypsin itself.

The finding of hypertrophy of the rugal folds on computed tomography and upper gastrointestinal series is suggestive, although not diagnostic, of hypertrophic gastropathy. The differential diagnosis of enlarged rugal folds includes lymphoma, eosinophilic gastroenteritis, gastric varices, Zollinger-Ellison syndrome, lymphangiectasia, and polyps. Among the infectious processes that have been associated with the pathogenesis of hypertrophic gastric rugae are tuberculosis, syphilis, and histoplasmosis.

Endoscopic appearance, histologic findings, laboratory studies, and clinical follow-up are essential to differentiating among these potential causes. Biopsies of the stomach and duodenum are necessary to distinguish hypertrophic gastropathy from lymphoma, lymphangiectasia, and eosinophilic gastroenteritis; all can present similarly to PLE and can mimic hypertrophic gastropathy radiographically. Radiologic and endoscopic appearance rules out the thick folds associated with peptic ulcer disease, Zollinger-Ellison syndrome, hamartomas of Peutz-Jeghers syndrome, or gastric varices.

Management

Because pediatric hypertrophic gastropathy is generally a benign, self-limited illness, supportive treatment is often all that is required. Patients are started on a high-protein, low-fat diet as soon as they are able to tolerate oral intake. Some patients may require albumin transfusion initially if they are severely hypoalbuminemic and symptomatic. Medications to decrease acid secretion and promote healing of stomach ulcerations can also be helpful in managing gastrointestinal complaints. Iron supplementation may be required for those who are anemic because of blood loss. Most patients recover spontaneously within weeks to months, making a minimalist approach with subsequent follow-up appropriate in most cases.

Lessons for the Physician

When evaluating a patient who has edema or ascites, measurement of serum albumin should be an initial step, followed by measurement of stool alpha$_1$-antitrypsin as a screening test in cases of unexplained hypoproteinemia or suspected protein-losing enteropathy. Additional testing will determine if the hypoalbuminemia is due to renal, hepatic, or gastrointestinal causes. Hypertrophic gastropathy of childhood is a benign, self-limited cause of hypoalbuminemia that is diagnosed by findings on endoscopy and biopsy.

Betty LoBlais, MD, and Jay Hescock, MD, Louisiana State University School of Medicine, New Orleans, LA

CHAPTER 34

14-Year-Old Girl Experiencing Vomiting, Abdominal Pain, and Weight Loss Over the Past 11 Months

Presentation

A 14-year-old girl has experienced vomiting, abdominal pain, and weight loss over the past 11 months. The symptoms were initially associated with consumption of dairy products, and a switch to soy-based products led to temporary improvement. However, she continues to have nonbloody, nonbilious vomiting. She has restricted her intake for fear of vomiting. Four months earlier, an evaluation that included abdominal and pelvic ultrasonography and head computed tomography scan was performed by a gastroenterologist and yielded normal results. Trials of prochlorperazine, metoclopramide, and proton pump inhibitor were unsuccessful. She denies diarrhea, headache, fevers, chills, dysuria, dysmenorrhea, binging, purging, and dieting, as well as the use of laxatives, diuretics, tobacco, alcohol, or drugs. She reports regular menstrual periods monthly. Past medical history is significant for 2 episodes of urinary tract infections. Family history is noncontributory. She lives with her parents and siblings. She is in the ninth grade, has a grade point average of 4.0, and remains active in dance. She denies body dissatisfaction or pressure to lose weight.

On physical examination, the girl's body mass index is 17.3 kg/m^2 (10th–25th percentile for age), temperature is 96.1°F (35.6°C), and heart rate is 44 beats/min. She looks tired but is not in acute distress. Cardiovascular examination reveals bradycardia. Abdominal examination findings are unremarkable. She is admitted to the hospital for bradycardia and malnutrition. Results of complete blood cell count, serum electrolyte panel, and liver and thyroid function tests are normal. An additional study reveals the cause of her vomiting.

- **What is your differential diagnosis at this point?**
- **Are there any elements of history or physical examination that would help you?**
- **What additional diagnostic studies would you like performed?**

Discussion

Upper gastrointestinal (GI) series with small bowel follow-through showed a decrease of peristalsis in the stomach, and 2 hours after the initial ingestion of contrast, the second portion of the duodenum was found to be dilated with to-and-fro passage of contrast without significant antegrade passage into the third and fourth portions of the duodenum (Figure 34.1). This picture was consistent with superior mesenteric artery syndrome (SMAS). The girl was placed on a 1,400-kcal meal plan, which was titrated slowly up to 2,800 kcal, while being monitored for refeeding syndrome. She was also started on metoclopramide. After 8 days in the hospital, she had gained weight and was eating well, with only mild nausea. At 1-year follow-up, she had gained weight without recurrence of her symptoms.

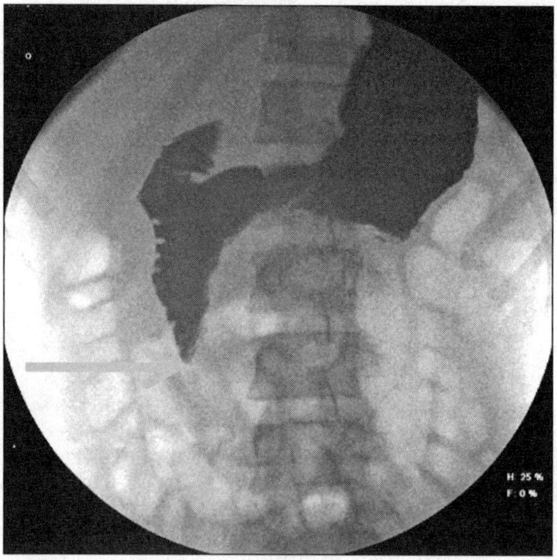

Figure 34.1. Upper gastrointestinal series with arrow showing abrupt cutoff of flow of contrast at third portion of the duodenum.

The Condition

Superior mesenteric artery syndrome is caused by compression of the third portion of the duodenum between the superior mesenteric artery (SMA) and the aorta. It is seen most frequently in individuals who have experienced rapid weight loss. It is also referred to as Wilkie disease, arteriomesenteric duodenal compression, chronic duodenal ileus, or cast syndrome. The disorder was described initially in the 1800s by von Rokitansky and later by Willet, who associated the disorder with prolonged fasting. Superior mesenteric artery syndrome is a rare but clearly defined cause of abdominal symptoms, including pain, and is frequently difficult to diagnose, often being a diagnosis of exclusion. Superior mesenteric artery syndrome is typically seen in older children and adolescents and is more common in girls. Symptoms may be chronic, acute, or intermittent.

Clinical Presentation

The most common symptoms of SMAS are epigastric pain, postprandial vomiting, and distension. Other symptoms include nausea, bloating, early satiety, and vomiting, which may be bilious. Pain is often worse in the supine position and is relieved by assuming the lateral decubitus or knee-chest position. If not diagnosed, SMAS can lead to malnutrition, dehydration, electrolyte disturbances, and death.

Pathophysiology

Superior mesenteric artery syndrome is caused by mechanical compression of the duodenum between the SMA and aorta due to a decrease in the angle of the artery, which should normally be approximately 45 degrees. This outcome can occur when there is loss of retroperitoneal fat, a short ligament of Treitz, or a low origin of the SMA. The decrease in angle between the aorta and SMA can result in chronic, intermittent, or acute duodenal obstruction, leading to the symptoms.

Well-described precipitating factors include thin build, increased lumbar lordosis, abdominal wall laxity, decrease of mesenteric fat, prolonged bed rest, eating disorders, rapid linear growth, spinal deformity, confinement in a body cast, and anatomic abnormalities of the SMA. Rapid weight loss is the most common cause and may occur in the setting of burns, neoplasia, malabsorptive disorders, or eating disorders such as anorexia nervosa and bulimia. Predisposing conditions include cerebral palsy, brain injury, and spinal fusion. Low body mass index and weight loss are not essential for the diagnosis.

Differential Diagnosis

The differential diagnosis for vomiting, abdominal pain, and weight loss in this patient included anorexia nervosa, bulimia, other eating disorders, gastric ulcers, inflammatory bowel disease, pancreatitis, biliary disease, hepatitis, gastrointestinal tract infections, diabetes mellitus, and collagen vascular disease. An extensive evaluation earlier had ruled out these conditions.

Imaging

Diagnosis requires confirmation by imaging studies such as upper GI series, hypotonic duodenography, or computed tomography. The most useful study in diagnosing SMAS is a upper GI series, which can show dilatation of the first and second part of the duodenum with an abrupt vertical or linear cutoff at the third part. Fluoroscopy shows peristalsis of the barium in the dilated portions.

Treatment

The goal of treatment is to address the precipitating factor. Conservative medical management is usually successful. Enteral feedings and metoclopramide are often helpful, and nasojejunal feeding may be necessary to bypass the obstruction. Surgical intervention may also be necessary in cases of failed conservative management, chronic disease states, and complicated peptic ulcer disease.

Lessons for the Physician

- Superior mesenteric artery syndrome should be considered in the differential diagnosis of abdominal symptoms in an adolescent who has lost significant weight.
- High clinical suspicion is needed for the diagnosis of superior mesenteric artery syndrome.
- Once suspected, confirmation can be obtained with a upper gastrointestinal series, computed tomography scan, or endoscopy to rule out other mechanical causes of obstruction and provide direct evidence.
- Superior mesenteric artery syndrome has a good outcome with proper management.

Sara Buckelew, MD, MPH, UCSF, Division of Adolescent Medicine, San Francisco, CA

Melissa Slivka, MD, Kaiser Permanente, Vallejo, CA

CHAPTER 35

Ecchymoses on Legs and Refusal to Walk in a 16-Year-Old Boy With Autism

Presentation

A 16-year-old boy is admitted to the inpatient ward with a 5-day history of worsening lower-extremity ecchymoses and refusal to walk. No trauma, recent illnesses, or fever are reported. Medical history is only significant for nonverbal autism and aggression treated with risperidone.

On examination, his weight is 84.2 kg (90th–95th percentile), height is 178 cm (50th–75th percentile), and body mass index is 26.6 (90th–95th percentile). He displays shortness of breath and tachycardia only with exertion, but vital signs are otherwise normal. In addition to the lower-extremity ecchymoses, extensive purpura are noted from the right posterior thigh to the right posterior calf, with sparing of the popliteal region. Petechiae are present on both lower extremities and the back. No oral lesions are appreciated, and the remainder of the physical examination findings are normal.

A complete blood cell count reveals the following values: hemoglobin, 8.9 g/dL (89 g/L); hematocrit, 30% (0.30); platelet count, 252×10^3/mcL (252×10^9/L); white blood cell count, 9,900/mcL (9.9×10^9/L) with normal differential; mean corpuscular volume, 84.9 mcm^3 (84.9 fL); red blood cell distribution width, 13.2%; and reticulocytes, 3.05% (0.03). Coagulation study results are within reference range. Radiograms of his lower extremities reveal no fractures, and the result of Doppler ultrasonography is negative for deep venous thromboses. Computed tomography of the lower extremities reveals evidence of diffuse hemorrhage in the superficial soft tissues and deep investing layers.

An extensive rheumatologic evaluation was unremarkable. Similarly, evaluation for hematologic and bone malignancies, including whole body positron emission tomography, does not reveal pertinent findings. The diagnosis is eventually made on the basis of observation of his daily habits in the hospital.

- **What is your differential diagnosis at this point?**
- **Are there any elements of history or physical examination that would help you?**
- **What additional diagnostic studies would you like performed?**

Discussion

New ecchymoses appeared on the right thigh and foot, and his hematocrit decreased to 18% (0.18) in 4 days. The hematocrit increased with packed red blood cell transfusions but then decreased again in the following days. During his hospital stay, the patient refused to eat the foods that were provided. A subsequent interview with his mother revealed that his diet at home consisted exclusively of frozen cheese pizza and water due to an extreme aversion to all other foods and beverages. This history raised concern for severe nutritional deficits, and laboratory testing revealed a serum vitamin C level of less than 0.12 mg/dL (7 mcmol/L). After initiating treatment with ascorbic acid (1 g/d orally), his hematocrit stabilized, his musculoskeletal symptoms improved markedly in 2 days, and his ability to ambulate returned to normal. The profoundly low serum vitamin C level, pattern of clinical manifestations, and resolution of these manifestations with vitamin C supplementation led to a diagnosis of scurvy. He was discharged with a prescription for high-dose vitamin C supplementation for an additional week and then prescribed a maintenance dose of 200 mg/d in conjunction with a multivitamin. His hematocrit remained stable after the last transfusion, and his vitamin C level has been normal since discharge.

Differential Diagnosis

This boy's inability to communicate verbally made it difficult to obtain a comprehensive review of systems. However, physical examination and laboratory results suggested that his refusal to walk was due to leg pain around the hemorrhage sites and the dyspnea and tachycardia with exertion were due to anemia.

Disorders in the differential diagnosis for unexplained ecchymoses with anemia include autoimmune diseases (eg, Henoch-Schönlein purpura, systemic lupus erythematosus, and Sjögren syndrome), trauma (including abuse), clotting factor deficiencies, disseminated intravascular coagulation, hematologic malignancies, hypersensitivity vasculitides, platelet dysfunction (eg, immune thrombocytopenic purpura), medication adverse effects, and nutritional deficiencies. Because of the rarity of scurvy in developed nations and clinical overlap between scurvy and other more common diseases, a broad differential should be maintained until successful treatment has occurred.

The Condition

Scurvy (also called scorbutus) is the clinical presentation of severe vitamin C deficiency. It is an ancient illness that has historically been associated with sea voyagers and other populations with restricted diets. Sir James Land, a ship's surgeon for the British Navy, discovered in 1753 that citrus fruits could prevent and treat the illness. It was not until 1931 that Albert Szent-Gyorgyi identified the "antiscorbutic factor" now called vitamin C.

Scurvy occurs when the total body pool of vitamin C decreases below 25% of normal and is usually fatal if untreated because of hemorrhage into vital organs or congestive heart failure. Vitamin C is a cofactor for multiple enzymes, but severe deficiency manifests as scurvy because of its role as a cofactor in collagen synthesis. As a result, collagen-containing tissues, such as skin, cartilage, dentine, osteoid, and capillary blood vessels, are most severely affected. The associated normochromatic-normocytic anemia occurs secondary to hemorrhage and altered iron absorption (because of vitamin C's role in enhancing absorption of iron in the small intestine). Bone radiography may reveal metaphyseal and epiphyseal abnormalities and scorbutic rosary (similar to rachitic rosary), but these findings are mostly seen in young children. Clinical symptoms include weakness, edema, spongy gums with ulceration and loosening of the teeth, mucocutaneous hemorrhages, and induration of the muscles of the legs. Spontaneous hemorrhage into crucial or fragile organs, such as the brain or eyes, can also occur. Although common, the classic oral findings are not universally present in patients with severe vitamin C deficiency.

Infantile scurvy can occur in infants between the ages of 6 and 12 months who are fed a diet deficient in vitamin C or in infants younger than 6 months fed condensed milk formulas. These infants are irritable and adopt a mostly stationary frog leg position due to pain. Radiographs can be diagnostic and may reveal subperiosteal elevation consistent with hemorrhages, alveolar bone reabsorption, or ground-glass–appearing cortex, indicating osteopenia.

Diagnosis

A serum vitamin C level less than 0.11 mg/dL (6 mcmol/L) suggests a diagnosis of scurvy. However, a serum level tends to reflect recent intake rather than total body levels. White blood cell vitamin C levels are more accurate in representing tissue stores, but this test is not readily available. An ascorbic acid tolerance test can be performed in which a loading dose is given and urinary excretion is measured. However, a dietary history consistent with vitamin C deficiency combined with resolution of symptoms after correction of the deficit is sufficient for the diagnosis of scurvy.

Treatment

Scurvy is effectively treated by oral vitamin C replacement. Recommendations in the literature vary regarding dosages and regimens. However, high-dose initial therapy typically results in quicker resolution of symptoms and is recommended when severe symptoms are present. With high-dose therapy, spontaneous hemorrhage usually stops within 1 day, other symptoms resolve in 3 to 5 days, and resolution of physical findings occurs in 1 to 2 weeks. The patient should then meet recommended daily intake according to sex and age. For adolescent boys between ages 14 and 18 years, the recommendation is 75 mg/d.

Lessons for the Physician

- Scurvy still occurs sporadically in developed nations, primarily in patients with restricted diets. Physicians should be aware of the risk of nutritional deficiencies in children and adolescents with unusual diets (such as autism-associated food aversion) and the potentially devastating consequences of vitamin C deficiency.
- Scurvy should be included in the differential diagnosis when unexplained ecchymoses or mucosal bleeding occur in nutritionally at-risk patients.
- Oral vitamin C supplementation leads to rapid improvement in the clinical symptoms of scurvy.

The views expressed in this chapter are those of the authors and do not reflect the official policy or position of the Department of the Navy, the Department of the Army, the Department of Defense, or the US government.

Marilisa Elrod, MD, PhD, Department of Pediatrics, Madigan Army Medical Center, Tacoma, WA

Christina Olson, MD, Department of Pediatrics, Naval Medical Center, San Diego, CA

CHAPTER 36

Lactic Acidosis and Cardiovascular Collapse in an Adolescent With Ulcerative Colitis

Presentation

A 16-year-old boy with ulcerative colitis undergoes total colectomy with ileostomy at an outside facility. Postoperatively, he continues to receive total parenteral nutrition (TPN) for persistent ileus. On hospital day 32, he develops ataxia, tremor, and hallucinations. Two days later, he becomes hemodynamically unstable and acutely decompensates. Vasoactive drips are initiated, and he is intubated for impending respiratory failure. He then transfers to our pediatric intensive care unit for escalation of care.

On physical examination, he is afebrile, his extremities are cool but well perfused, his abdomen is soft, the ostomy site is pink with serosanguinous output, and he is actively bleeding from his oral mucosa.

Laboratory evaluation reveals pH 6.8, anion gap of 33 mEq/L (33 mmol/L), lactate level greater than 270.3 mg/dL (30 mmol/L), mixed venous oxygen saturation of 99%, and bicarbonate level of 4 mEq/L (4 mmol/L), despite multiple doses of sodium bicarbonate. The international normalized ratio is 1.9 (reference range, 0.8–1.2), white blood cell count is 9,300/mcL (9.3×10^9/L) with a normal differential, hemoglobin level is 8.5 g/dL (85 g/L), platelet count is 79.0×10^3/mcL (79.0×10^9/L), C-reactive protein level is 2.0 mg/L (19.0 nmol/L), and creatinine level is 2.6 mg/dL (230 mcmol/L). Broad-spectrum antibiotics, packed red blood cells, fresh frozen plasma, and cryoprecipitate are given. There is concern for necrotic bowel, but emergency exploratory laparoscopy reveals no evidence of ischemia.

He returns to the pediatric intensive care unit with a presumptive diagnosis of septic shock from a central venous catheter–associated infection. He continues to take sodium bicarbonate, dopamine, norepinephrine, vancomycin, piperacillin-tazobactam, and metronidazole. Continuous venovenous hemodialysis is initiated for refractory acidosis. His condition continues to deteriorate despite aggressive resuscitative measures, and alternative causes of lactic acidosis are sought. The diagnosis is made on further discussion with the transferring hospital.

- **What is your differential diagnosis at this point?**
- **Are there any elements of history or physical examination that would help you?**
- **What additional diagnostic studies would you like performed?**

Discussion

The most likely cause of lactic acidosis in a patient with an indwelling central venous catheter is septic shock. However, several aspects of this case were not consistent with sepsis. First, the patient was never febrile, and his examination findings were notable for cool extremities. Septic shock is associated with systemic inflammatory response syndrome and dilatation of peripheral vasculature, known as warm shock. Note that cold shock may occur in younger children with sepsis, due to decreased cardiac output and increased systemic vascular resistance, but older children and adults are much more likely to present with warm shock. Second, laboratory study results were inconsistent with an infectious cause, including normal white blood cell count and normal C-reactive protein level, although C-reactive protein may be a poor biomarker for serious bacterial infection in certain pediatric populations. Third, the neurologic changes before decompensation were not fully explained by sepsis. Last, the extent of lactic acidosis was out of proportion to the patient's clinical status. As a result, we continued to look for an alternative explanation for the patient's condition.

We contacted the transferring hospital and discovered that the patient had been receiving TPN without multivitamins for the past month because of a national shortage of intravenous (IV) adult multivitamins. The patient's lactic acidosis and cardiovascular collapse were caused by thiamine (vitamin B_1) deficiency. His initial neurologic changes were consistent with Wernicke encephalopathy, another manifestation of thiamine deficiency. The patient was given 2 doses of 400 mg of IV thiamine 2 hours apart, followed by dosing every 4 hours. Within 6 hours, vasoactive drips were discontinued, serum pH and bicarbonate level normalized, and the coagulopathy resolved. He was extubated the following day and appeared neurologically intact.

The Condition

Thiamine is an essential vitamin involved in aerobic cellular metabolism. It functions as a coenzyme for pyruvate dehydrogenase, which converts pyruvate to acetyl coenzyme A before entering the Krebs cycle. Without thiamine, cellular metabolism becomes anaerobic, and lactic acid is produced. The half-life of thiamine is approximately 10 to 20 days. Without regular intake of thiamine, which is present in legumes, rice, pork, and enriched cereals, the body will use up its stores in a matter of weeks, which was the case for our patient.

Thiamine deficiency is classically associated with malnourished alcoholic patients, patients with gastrointestinal or oncologic conditions, and patients with Wernicke encephalopathy—a triad of encephalopathy, oculomotor dysfunction, and gait ataxia. Brain lesions in Wernicke encephalopathy primarily occur in the mammillary bodies, dorsomedial thalamus, and oculomotor nuclei, among other regions. In addition to neurologic changes, thiamine deficiency can cause heart failure (wet beriberi), fluid refractory shock, and profound lactic acidosis.

Thiamine deficiency is exceedingly rare in pediatric populations. However, during a previous national multivitamin shortage in the 1990s, there were multiple case reports of acute thiamine deficiency characterized by shock and lactic acidosis. There was also a recent outbreak of thiamine deficiency in Israel among infants who were fed soy-based formula deficient in thiamine.

Diagnosis of thiamine deficiency is generally clinical because serum laboratory evaluation is often unavailable, slow, or unreliable. Clinical improvement after thiamine administration is highly suggestive of thiamine deficiency, which was the case for our patient. Radiologic workup of Wernicke encephalopathy is also useful, primarily to rule out other causes of encephalopathy.

Differential Diagnosis

The differential diagnosis of anion gap metabolic acidosis includes renal failure, diabetic ketoacidosis, lactic acidosis, and ingestions. Many physicians use the mnemonic MUDPILES (**m**ethanol, **u**remia, **d**iabetic ketoacidosis, **p**ropylene glycol, **i**soniazid, **l**actic acidosis, **e**thylene glycol, and **s**alicylates). Thiamine deficiency is notably absent from this mnemonic, although it belongs in a subset of causes of lactic acidosis.

Lactic acidosis is most commonly caused by cardiogenic shock, distributive shock, hypovolemia, or ingestion (eg, metformin). However, knowledge of the biochemical pathway that surrounds lactic acidosis reveals a much broader differential diagnosis, including mitochondrial disorders, cyanide poisoning (blocks electron transport chain), or any other process that interferes with aerobic metabolism, including thiamine deficiency. Given the current national shortage of IV multivitamins, thiamine deficiency should remain on the differential diagnosis for patients receiving long-term TPN.

Treatment

Thiamine deficiency should be treated with IV thiamine, which is generally safe and well tolerated. We gave our patient 400 mg of IV thiamine every 4 hours for several days, on the basis of data that parenteral doses less than 200 mg may be ineffective in adults. We recommend consultation with a pediatric gastroenterologist and a pediatric pharmacist at your institution before dosing IV thiamine.

Lessons for the Physician

- Signs and symptoms of thiamine deficiency may include encephalopathy, lactic acidosis, and cardiovascular collapse.
- Thiamine deficiency diagnosis should be based on the differential diagnosis for unexplained anion gap metabolic acidosis.
- It is important to recognize thiamine deficiency in patients receiving long-term total parenteral nutrition, particularly in the setting of a national multivitamin shortage.
- Early diagnosis of thiamine deficiency is essential for prevention of irreversible damage.

Matthew B. Wallenstein, MD; Elizabeth B. Burgener, MD; Jenna Klotz, MD; and John A. Kerner, MD, Department of Pediatrics, Stanford University School of Medicine, Palo Alto, CA

Part 8

Genetics

CHAPTER 37

A Male Neonate Who Has a White Hair Tuft and Hypopigmented Macules (Visual Diagnosis)

Presentation

A male neonate is born at 39 weeks' gestation to a 25-year-old *ADAR* (formerly *G1P1*) African American woman. The pregnancy was uncomplicated and the mother received appropriate prenatal care. Results for maternal group B *Streptococcus* colonization and standard viral serologic testing were negative. Delivery is via cesarean delivery because of breech presentation at onset of labor. At delivery, initial examination reveals a prominent tuft of white hair at the forehead hairline (Figure 37.1) as well as large hypopigmented macules with well-defined borders covering significant areas on the torso and the middle upper and lower extremities (Figure 37.2). The remainder of the physical examination findings is normal. Apgar scores are 9 and 9 at 1 and 5 minutes, respectively, and vital signs are normal for age. Weight, length, and head circumference are between the 25th and 50th percentiles. On the second day of life, the neonate fails his click auditory brainstem response hearing screening in the left ear, suggesting a preliminary diagnosis.

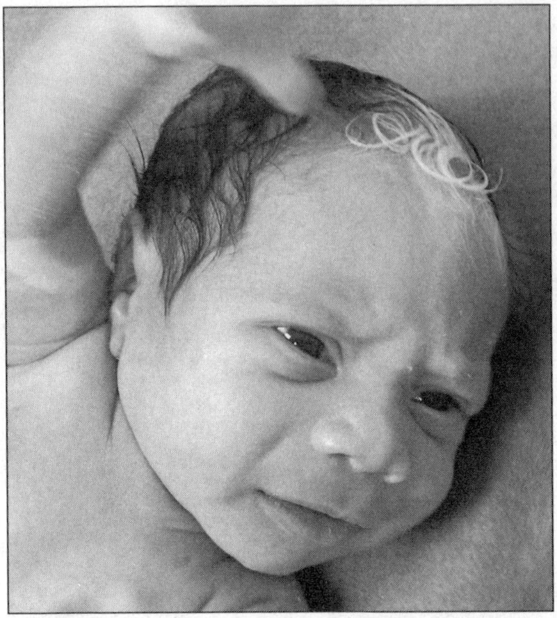

Figure 37.1. Neonate boy with prominent tuft of white hair.

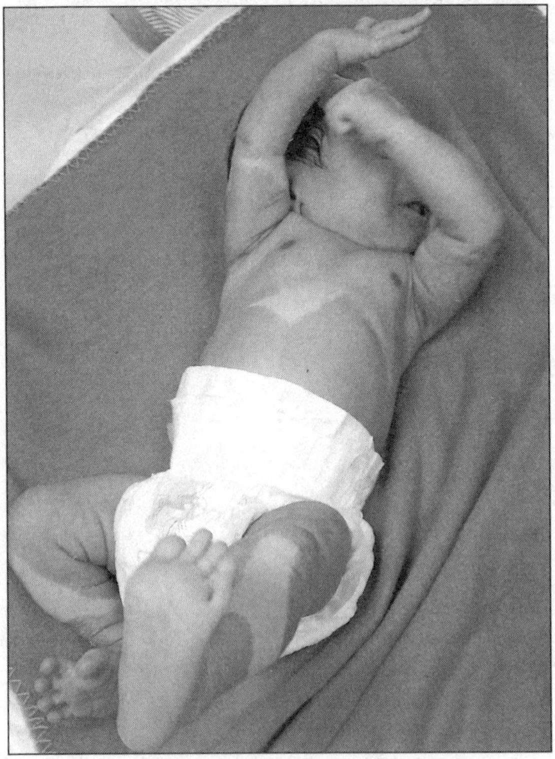

Figure 37.2. Prominent depigmented macules on torso and upper and lower extremities.

- **What is your differential diagnosis at this point?**
- **Are there any elements of history or physical examination that would help you?**
- **What additional diagnostic studies would you like performed?**

Diagnosis

On the basis of the presence of a white forelock, patches of depigmented skin, and sensorineural hearing loss, Waardenburg syndrome was diagnosed.

Discussion

Waardenburg syndrome is a rare condition characterized by congenital sensorineural hearing loss, dystopia canthorum (lateral displacement of the inner canthi), and pigmentation abnormalities of the hair, skin, and eyes. This syndrome results from a disorder of neural crest melanocyte proliferation, migration, or differentiation. Thus, the term *depigmented* is accurate, as opposed to *hypopigmented,* indicating that the skin and hair lesions are devoid of melanocytes, in contrast to a decrease in melanocyte pigment production. Waardenburg syndrome is inherited in an autosomal dominant pattern and shows no predilection for race, ethnicity, or sex. Prevalence is estimated at 1 in 42,000, and approximately 2% to 3% of deaf children have Waardenburg syndrome.

The Waardenburg Syndrome Consortium established criteria for the diagnosis of Waardenburg syndrome in 1992. Individuals born with the syndrome have either 2 major criteria or 1 major and 2 minor criteria (Table 37.1). Major criteria include congenital sensorineural hearing loss; pigment changes of the iris (irides of different color, iris bicolor, or characteristic brilliant blue irides); depigmented hair, such as a white forelock; affected first-degree relative; and dystopia canthorum with a W index (a measure of separation of the inner canthi) that exceeds 1.95 (Box 37.1).[1]

Table 37.1. Major and Minor Criteria for Waardenburg Syndrome

Major Criteria	Minor Criteria
Sensorineural hearing loss	Skin depigmentation
Pigmented changes of iris	Synophrys
Hair depigmentation	Broad high nasal root
Affected first-degree relative	Nostril hypoplasia
Dystopia canthorum (W index >1.95)	Premature graying hair

Box 37.1

W index ≥2.07 = dystopia. W index >1.87 but <2.07 = moderate dystopia. W index ≤1.87 = no dystopia.
Calculation of W index is as follows:

1. Measure (in millimeters): a = inner canthal distance, b = interpupillary distance, c = outer canthal distance.
2. Calculate $X = (2a - [0.2119c + 3.909])/c$. Calculate $Y = (2a - [0.2479b + 3.909])/b$.
3. W index = $X + Y + a/b$.

Minor criteria include depigmented skin lesions, synophrys (single eyebrow), broad high nasal root, hypoplasia of the nostrils, and premature graying hair, typically by 30 years of age.

Waardenburg syndrome is divided into 4 types. Individuals with Waardenburg syndrome type 1 must have dystopia canthorum, whereas those with Waardenburg syndrome type 2 do not. Types 3 and 4 are rare variants of the syndrome. Individuals with Waardenburg syndrome type 3, also known as Klein-Waardenburg syndrome, have hypoplasia of muscles and bones in the upper extremities, flexion contractures, and syndactyly in addition to meeting criteria for type 1. Individuals with Waardenburg syndrome type 4, also known as Waardenburg-Shah syndrome, have the type 2 phenotype associated with Hirschsprung disease. Other peripheral associations of Waardenburg syndrome include cleft lip or palate, neural tube defects, and upward scapular displacement (Table 37.2).

Most cases of Waardenburg types 1 and 3 are caused by mutations in the *PAX3* (paired box 3) gene. The *PAX3* gene is located on chromosome 2q35-37 and controls certain aspects of facial and inner ear development. Mutation of the *MITF* (microphthalmia-associated transcription factor) gene causes Waardenburg type 2. The *MITF* gene is found on chromosome 3p14.2-p14.1 and also controls some development of the ear. Both *PAX3* and *MITF* mutations are inherited in an autosomal dominant pattern. On occasion, they can be a result of de novo mutation. Type 4 has been shown to be caused by a variety of genes, including endothelin 3 at 20q13.2-q13.3, endothelin receptor type B at 13q22, *SRY* box 10 transcription factor at 22q13.1, and snail homolog 2 at 8q11, and can be inherited in either an autosomal recessive or autosomal dominant pattern. Genetic counseling is often helpful to families with a history of Waardenburg syndrome.

Congenital sensorineural hearing loss is the most serious feature of Waardenburg syndrome. Deafness generally occurs in 25% of type 1 cases and 50% of type 2 cases but has been reported to be as high as 60% and 90%. Otopathology in a subject with

Table 37.2. Types of Waardenburg Syndrome

Type	Description
1	Waardenburg Syndrome Consortium criteria with dystopia canthorum
2	Type 1 phenotype without dystopia canthorum
3 (Klein-Waardenburg)	Type 1 phenotype with upper extremity contractures
4 (Waardenburg-Shah)	Type 2 phenotype with Hirschsprung disease

Waardenburg type 1 has been reported to show partial malformations of the cochlea with absence of melanocytes, absence of stria vascularis, missing hair cells, abnormal tectorial membrane, and lack of peripheral processes of the spiral ganglion cells. These findings support a hypothesis that defective melanocyte migration or defective melanocyte function results in defective development of the inner ear structures, thus causing sensorineural hearing loss.

Deficits are generally not progressive except in type 2 cases. There are varying degrees of hearing loss within types and even within families. Hearing loss can be bilateral, asymmetric (hearing loss unequal in each side), or unilateral and can range from mild to profound. Formal audiological evaluation should be performed on all children suspected of having Waardenburg syndrome because hearing loss may not be clinically apparent in the patient or family members. These children should be referred as candidates for cochlear implants early in life.

There are few differential diagnoses to consider. Tietze syndrome, caused by mutation at a different region of the *MITF* gene, is a fully penetrant autosomal dominant disease characterized by deafness and depigmentation. In contrast to the patchy depigmented lesions of Waardenburg syndrome, patients with Tietze syndrome have frank albinism. Piebaldism is another autosomal dominant disorder in which patients present with white forelock and depigmented skin lesions only. There is no hearing loss. Vitiligo, although extremely rare in a neonate or infant, is another possible diagnosis.

Patient Course

Further history reveals that the mother and maternal grandmother have similar skin findings and white forelock. The mother dyes her forelock to match her normally black hair color. The mother also reports that she has always been hard of hearing, but her condition is not bad enough to bring to medical attention. The neonate has an otherwise uncomplicated hospital course and is discharged on day 3 of life with the preliminary diagnosis of Waardenburg syndrome type 2. He is scheduled for a comprehensive diagnostic auditory brainstem response test and appropriate follow-up appointments with a geneticist and a primary care pediatrician.

Reference

1. Reynolds JE, Marazita ML, Meyer JM, et al. Major-locus contributions to variability of the craniofacial feature dystopia canthorum in Waardenburg syndrome. *Am J Hum Genet.* 1996;58(2):384–392

Summary

- Waardenburg syndrome is an autosomal dominant disease characterized by congenital sensorineural hearing loss, dystopia canthorum, and depigmentation abnormalities of the hair, skin, and eyes.
- Rarer forms of this disease can be associated with limb contractures and Hirschsprung disease.
- Hearing loss can range from mild to profound and is not generally progressive. Affected patients should receive acoustic testing, genetic counseling, and follow-up with an otolaryngologist for the potential benefit of cochlear implants. Cognition is generally normal, and with appropriate acoustic intervention, the developmental prognosis is good.

Joshua Wong, MD, Advocate, Hope Children's Hospital, Oak Lawn, IL

CHAPTER 38

Infant With Growth Failure, Body Asymmetry, and Dysmorphic Features (Visual Diagnosis)

Presentation

A 5-month-old girl is admitted to the hospital by her pediatrician for evaluation of failure to thrive. The mother reports that her daughter has always been small and that she feels her daughter is not gaining weight as expected despite feeding her 24 oz of a 22-cal/oz premature formula each day (135 kcal/kg/d). The mother also expresses concern that her daughter has a large head, developmental delays, and a right leg that is growing longer than the left. Evaluation by an orthopedic surgeon found no evidence of hip dysplasia.

The infant's past medical history reveals an uncomplicated premature birth at 35 weeks' gestation via vaginal delivery. Her birthweight was 1.3 kg (<2 standard deviations [SD] from mean), which plotted as small for gestational age. She was hospitalized for 3 weeks for feeding and growth monitoring.

Review of systems is negative for vomiting, diarrhea, swallowing difficulties, or weight loss. She is not on any medications, and her immunizations are up to date. She is an only child and there is no history of consanguinity. Family history is unremarkable.

Physical examination reveals an alert, active, thin infant whose vital signs are normal for age. Her weight is 3.9 kg (<−3 SD from mean, according to World Health Organization Growth charts), length is 53.34 cm (<−3 SD from mean), head circumference is 40.64 cm (between 0 and −1 SD). Her head appears large in relation to the rest of her body, and she has a prominent forehead (Figure 38.1). Her right leg has larger girth and is 2.54 cm longer than the left leg (Figure 38.2). Further examination of her extremities reveals clinodactyly of her fifth fingers (Figure 38.3). She has poor head control and mild generalized hypotonia. The remainder of her physical findings are normal.

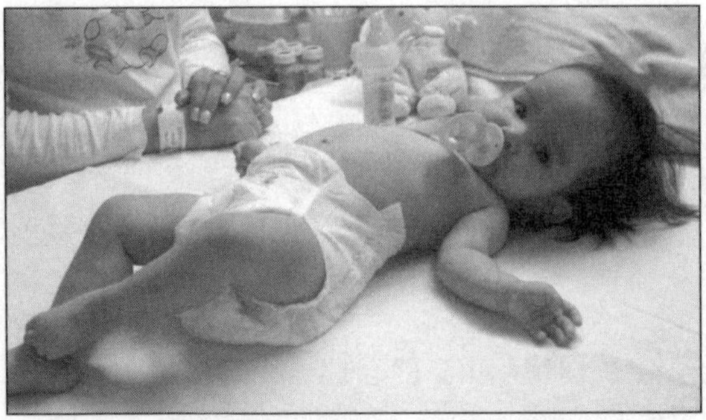

Figure 38.1. Relative macrocephaly, with prominent forehead.

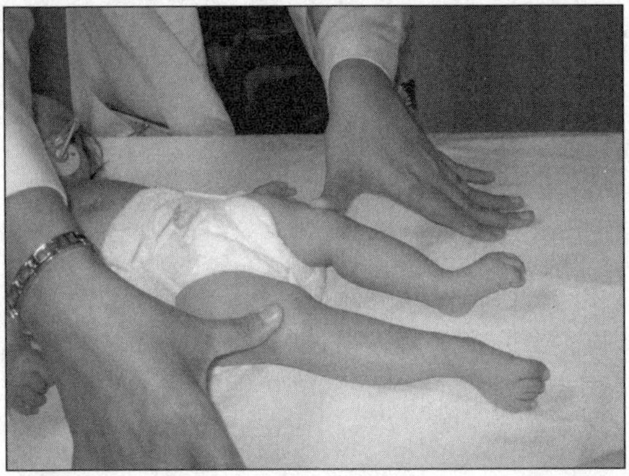

Figure 38.2. Right leg has greater girth and length than the left leg.

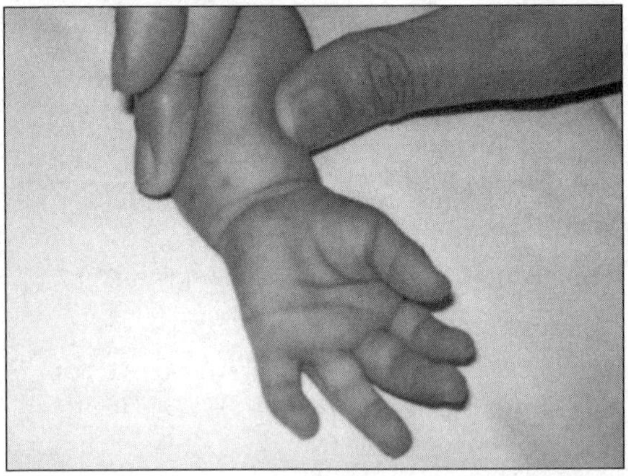

Figure 38.3. Clinodactyly of the fifth finger.

Because of the constellation of dysmorphic features described above, an underlying genetic syndrome is considered as the cause of her failure to thrive. A chromosomal analysis is normal (46,XX).

- **What is your differential diagnosis at this point?**
- **Are there any elements of history or physical examination that would help you?**
- **What additional diagnostic studies would you like performed?**

Diagnosis

The patient has Russell–Silver syndrome (RSS), a diagnosis based on the characteristic clinical features of prenatal growth restriction, failure of postnatal catch-up growth, body asymmetry, preservation of head circumference, characteristic facies, and clinodactyly.

Discussion

Russell-Silver syndrome was named after Henry Silver and Alexander Russell. This syndrome is also known as Silver-Russell syndrome and Russell-Silver dwarfism.

Epidemiology

Most cases of RSS are sporadic rather than familial. The reported incidence varies widely from 1 in 3,000 to 1 in 100,000 people, depending on the researcher because there are no well-established diagnostic guidelines. More than 400 cases have been reported so far. There is a slight male predominance and no racial predilection.

Etiology

Most cases are sporadic, but a few familial cases have been reported with autosomal recessive, autosomal dominant, and X-linked patterns of inheritance. The recurrence risk in siblings is low since most cases represent a mitotic change (somatic mutation or epimutation); for the same reason, there is likely to be a low incidence of recurrence in the offspring of probands, although that effect is not as well proven. Genetic and epigenetic mutations can be detected in about 50% of the patients. Hypomethylation of the imprinting center 1 in 11p15.5 can be detected in 40%; duplications, in 1% to 2%; and submicroscopic chromosomal aberration, in 1%. Maternal uniparental disomy of chromosome 7 is implicated in about 7% to 10% of cases. Approximately 50% of RSS cases are idiopathic in origin.

Clinical Features

In 1999, Price et al described the following clinical features considered critical for diagnosing RSS[1]:

- Intrauterine growth retardation (IUGR)
- Postnatal growth retardation
- Normal head circumference but often having the appearance of an abnormally large head in relation to the body
- Classic facial phenotype
- Limb length asymmetry

The most striking feature of this syndrome is prenatal growth restriction with failure to establish catch-up growth postnatally. This effect may be due to the high association of gastrointestinal problems seen in these infants and children. Anderson et al reported that 77% of children who have RSS also experience gastrointestinal problems, which include reflux (34%), food aversion (32%), esophagitis (25%), and failure to thrive (63%), meaning that weight for height is low even in the face of short stature.[2]

Growth velocity is normal. Patients with RSS reach a mean adult height of 151.2 ±7.8 cm in men and 139.9 ±9.0 cm in women. Growth charts designed specifically for RSS patients are available at the MAGIC Foundation Web site (www.magicfoundation.org).

Other features that help in the diagnosis are listed in Box 38.1.

Diagnosis

The diagnosis of RSS is difficult because of clinical and genetic heterogeneity. Diagnosis is essentially clinical (Box 38.1) and based on the presence of characteristic features listed above. In suspected cases, genetic evaluation includes methylation studies of imprinting center 1 at 11p15.5 and uniparental disomy of chromosome 7 studies to support the accuracy of clinical diagnosis. Molecular karyotyping may be helpful in detecting submicroscopic deletions and duplications and in excluding other diagnoses.

Box 38.1. Clinical Features of Russell-Silver Syndrome

Craniofacial Features

- Triangular face (79%), small chin, broad and bossed forehead
- Wide, thin mouth with turned-down corners of the mouth (46%)
- Large head in relation to the body (64%)
- High-arched palate
- Small, crowded teeth (28%)
- Micrognathia

Skeletal Abnormalities

- Body asymmetry (51%)
- Fifth finger clinodactyly (68%)
- Syndactyly of second and third toes (19%)
- Late closure of anterior fontanelle
- Delayed bone age
- Scoliosis

Growth

- Intrauterine growth retardation
- Low birthweight (ie, <3rd percentile) (94%)
- Failure to thrive
- Short stature (99%)

Neurologic

- Attention-deficit/hyperactivity syndrome and specific learning disorders
- Motor, speech, or cognitive delays (37%)
- Hypotonia (45%)

Skin

Café au lait spots (19%)

Other

- Blue sclerae
- Hypoglycemia
- Early puberty (13%)

Differential Diagnosis

Other diagnoses to consider in an infant with prenatal growth restriction, short stature, and dysmorphic features are listed below.

Dubowitz Syndrome

This condition is a rare, autosomal recessive disorder characterized by prenatal growth restriction, short stature, poor feeding, and mild to moderate mental retardation. Features that differentiate Dubowitz syndrome from RSS are eczema, high-pitched voice, and characteristic craniofacial features of microcephaly, high-sloping forehead, sparse hair, broad nose, micrognathia, palate abnormalities, and dysplastic ears.

SHORT Syndrome

Patients born with SHORT syndrome (**s**hort stature, **h**yperextensibility, hernia, **o**cular depression, **R**ieger anomaly, and **t**eething delay) have features very similar to RSS, such as IUGR, poor weight gain, triangular face, prominent forehead, and clinodactyly. Features that differentiate this syndrome from RSS are hyperextensibility of joints, small hands and feet, lipodystrophy, Rieger anomaly (deformity of the anterior chamber of the eye), congenital glaucoma, delayed teething, anteverted ears, and ocular depression. SHORT syndrome is extremely rare, and the genetics is uncertain.

Floating-Harbor Syndrome

This disorder is characterized by IUGR, short stature, delayed bone age, triangular face, and clinodactyly. Other features, such as speech delay and facial characteristics that include broad nasal bridge, smooth philtrum, and thin lips, can differentiate Floating-Harbor syndrome from RSS. Diagnosis is based on clinical phenotype, and the etiology remains unclear.

3-M Syndrome

3-M syndrome is a rare autosomal recessive disorder caused by mutations in the *CUL7* gene. Patients have several physical findings similar to those found in RSS, including prenatal growth restriction, short stature, triangular face, frontal bossing, relative macrocephaly, body asymmetry, and clinodactyly. Facial features include midfacial hypoplasia, upturned nose, long philtrum, and prominent mouth. These patients also have short necks, broad chests, and square shoulders, as well as hyperlordosis, long slender bones, prominent heels, and flexible joints, which differentiate this syndrome from RSS.

Mulibrey Nanism

Mulibrey nanism is an autosomal recessive disorder caused by mutations in *TRIM37*. The disorder is characterized by prenatal growth restriction, short stature, relative macrocephaly, skeletal asymmetry, triangular face, and broad forehead. Features that differentiate this syndrome from RSS include high-pitched voice, yellowish dots in the ocular fundi, hepatomegaly, cutaneous nevi flammei, and thin extremities, as well as fibrous dysplasia of the long bones, narrow shoulders, and large hands and feet.

Fetal Alcohol Syndrome

Fetal alcohol syndrome is characterized by failure to thrive and developmental delay. Features that distinguish this syndrome from RSS are microcephaly, short palpebral fissures, congenital heart disease, flat philtrum, thin upper lip, and developmental delays. Fetal alcohol syndrome results from in utero exposure to alcohol.

Bloom Syndrome

Bloom syndrome is an autosomal recessive condition caused by mutations in *BLM*. It is characterized by short stature, café au lait spots, and micrognathia, which are similar to RSS, but these infants and children have distinct facial features, such as a long and narrow face, prominent nose, butterfly rash on the cheeks, and increased susceptibility to cancer.

Turner Syndrome

Turner syndrome can be differentiated from RSS by the presence of a webbed neck, widely spaced nipples, low set ears, small fingernails, heart defects, and sterility.

Management

The main goals of treatment of RSS are to optimize nutrition and to improve both stature and developmental outcome. These goals are achieved best by a multidisciplinary approach involving orthopedics, nutrition, gastroeneterology, and endocrinology specialties, as well as early intervention, to improve the quality of life. Specific issues to manage are as follows:

Skeletal Abnormalities

Surgical lengthening can be beneficial for lower extremity discrepancies of 4.0 cm or greater. Shoe lifts are prescribed for patients with minor discrepancies. Russell-Silver syndrome is rarely associated with hip dysplasia, yet it is important to do careful hip examinations during the neonatal period and refer to an orthopedic surgeon if hip dysplasia is suspected.

Gastrointestinal Problems

Nutritional supplementation with a high-calorie diet and frequent feedings are essential in maintaining adequate nutrition in these patients. Nasogastric feeding may be necessary in some cases.

Gastroesophageal reflux may be treated with reflux precautions such as positioning, thickened feeds, and acid-blocking medications if necessary. Surgical management with fundoplication is reserved for severe cases. Feeding aversion behaviors can be corrected with speech therapy and occupational therapy.

Growth

Some studies have shown beneficial effects with the use of growth hormone in patients with RSS. However, this agent is not recommended routinely unless there is coexisting growth hormone deficiency. Although the US Food and Drug Administration has not approved the use of growth hormone specifically for treating RSS, this therapy is indicated for infants and children who experience IUGR, are small for gestational age, and fail to demonstrate catch-up growth. Growth hormone therapy in children with RSS has been shown to increase mean height velocity during the first year and sustain the increase during the first few years, but most studies have shown no significant change in the final adult height.

Neurodevelopment

Early intervention programs provide physical therapy for patients with hypotonia, and they provide speech, language, and special education courses for older children with learning disorders. Early referral and timely intervention may help improve the developmental outcome in infants and children with RSS. Psychological counseling can provide support to the child and family.

Patient Course

The infant had an unremarkable course in the hospital. Nutrition service was consulted, daily weights were obtained, and a strict calorie count was done. She did not have feeding aversion and did not require speech therapy or nasogastric feeding. She had no vomiting and gradually gained weight. The mother was made aware that low weight and short stature are part of this syndrome. The infant's length was above the 50th percentile when plotted on a RSS growth chart. The infant was discharged after 3 days, and follow-up was arranged with a gastroenterologist, geneticist, endocrinologist, orthopedist, and nutritionist. She was also enrolled into an early intervention program.

References

1. Price SM, Stanhope R, Garrett C, Preece MA, Trembath RC. The spectrum of Silver-Russell syndrome: a clinical and molecular genetic study and new diagnostic criteria. *J Med Genet.* 1999;36(11):837–842
2. Anderson J, Viskochil D, O'Gorman M, Gonzales C. Gastrointestinal complications of Russell-Silver syndrome: a pilot study. *Am J Med Genet.* 2002;113(1):15–19

Summary

- Russell-Silver Syndrome is clinically and genetically heterogeneous, which makes it difficult for physicians to diagnose this condition.
- Russell-Silver syndrome should be suspected in patients with prenatal growth restriction, postnatal growth failure, and characteristic features such as triangular facies, relative macrocephaly, and limb abnormalities (body asymmetry and clinodactyly).
- Genetic testing is available but conclusive in only about one-half of cases.
- Early recognition and appropriate intervention may play a role in improving the outcome of these patients.
- There are several support groups and organizations, such as MAGIC Foundation and the Russell-Silver Support Organization, that can provide resources for families and clinicians.

Deepa Prasad, MD, Chief Resident, and Valerie Navarrete, MD, Pediatric Resident, Department of Pediatrics, Jersey Shore University Medical Center, Neptune, NJ

Srividya Naganathan, MD, FAAP, Assistant Professor of Pediatrics, UMDNJ, and Pediatric Clerkship Site Director, Jersey Shore University Medical Center, Neptune, NJ

CHAPTER 39

Large Stature in 13-Year-Old Boy

Presentation

A 13-year-old boy is seen for evaluation of his large stature. His mother reports that he has always been bigger than other children and adolescents. His birthweight was 5.3 kg, and length was 61 cm. His mother was unable to carry him after 6 months of age because he was so heavy. She is 175.3 cm tall, and his father's height is 182.3 cm. He has 2 siblings who are of normal stature. The boy is in special classes at school.

On physical examination, his height is 193 cm, weight is 112.5 kg, and head circumference is 66 cm, all measurements well above the 95th percentile for age. His arm span is normal. His blood pressure is 110/70 mm Hg, and pulse is 68 beats/min. He has normal neurologic and funduscopic findings. His hands and feet appear very large. Some mild acanthosis is noted around his neck. His genitalia are at Sexual Maturity Rating stage 4, with normal phallus and testicular size. Scant axillary hair and mild acne are noted.

The boy's bone age is 17 years, and his epiphyses are closed. The insulinlike growth factor-1 level is normal for bone age at 400 ng/mL (52.4 nmol/L). The free tetraiodothyronine concentration is normal at 0.72 ng/dL (9.3 pmol/L), and the thyroid-stimulating hormone level is normal at 1.36 mcIU/mL. The lipid profile shows a total cholesterol level of 201 mg/dL (5.2 mmol/L), with triglycerides of 165 mg/dL (1.9 mmol/L). Results of the urinalysis and blood chemistry profile are within reference range (glucose, 93 mg/dL [5.2 mmol/L]). The insulin level is 21 mcIU/mL (146 pmol/L). Magnetic resonance imaging of the adolescent's head yields normal findings.

Further evaluation offers clues to the most likely cause of this adolescent's large stature.

- **What is your differential diagnosis at this point?**
- **Are there any elements of history or physical examination that would help you?**
- **What additional diagnostic studies would you like performed?**

Discussion

A karyotype study, analysis for fragile X chromosome, and growth hormone (GH) stimulation test gave normal results. Learning testing showed a full-scale IQ of 60. Further history revealed delayed motor milestones and febrile seizures as an infant. In view of the classic findings on history and physical examination, normal results of laboratory studies, and advanced bone age, Sotos syndrome was diagnosed.

The Condition

Sotos syndrome is characterized by excessive growth, large head size, advanced bone age, and mental retardation. Affected children and adolescents have rapid growth in utero and are likely to have a birth length at about the 97th percentile, although 85% have a birthweight below the 97th percentile. The mean of birth length in children who have Sotos syndrome is +3.2 standard deviations (SDs), with the mean of birth head circumference being +1.8 SD and the mean of birthweight being +1.0 SD.

A period of excessive growth during the first 3 years of life is common and usually striking, although growth failure may be seen in the first months after birth due to feeding problems that might mask the diagnosis in the first year of life. Adult height is variable but usually exceeds the 75th percentile and is often greater than would be expected based on the heights of family members. Bone age commonly exceeds chronologic age by 2 to 4 years, and puberty occurs early but in the reference age range.

The distinctive shape and large size of the head are important factors in making the diagnosis. Head circumference is almost always greater than the 98th percentile. The skull is typically long and narrow. A prominent forehead with a "receding hairline" and wide-set, down-slanting eyes are frequently present.

Motor, speech, and social development are often delayed. Mental retardation is common, with an average IQ of 70. However, some patients have an IQ in the reference range. Infants may have hypotonia, and older children may be described as uncoordinated. Behavior problems are frequent.

A variety of medical complications in patients who have Sotos syndrome has been described. Glucose intolerance is common. An increased incidence of malignant tumors has been described, although more recent studies indicate that early estimates may have been high, with only 2% of patients who have Sotos syndrome actually developing such tumors. Skeletal problems include scoliosis and flat feet. Seizures may occur, especially with fever.

Diagnosis and Pathogenesis

No specific laboratory test exists and no definitive cause has been found for Sotos syndrome, which is believed to have a genetic cause as yet unidentified. The diagnosis is made on the basis of 4 cardinal features: rapid early growth, both prenatally and postnatally; advanced bone age; developmental delay; and characteristic facial features. An enlarged head is another characteristic. Other identifiable disorders should be excluded. An autosomal dominant inheritance has been implicated in some families. An endocrine cause for Sotos syndrome has been sought without success. Examination typically involves evaluation for GH, insulinlike growth factor, and thyroid abnormalities. Testicular, ovarian, and adrenal functioning appear normal.

Cranial imaging might be helpful in making the diagnosis. One study of patients who had Sotos syndrome showed ventricular abnormalities, with a prominence of the trigone in 90%, prominent occipital horns in 75%, and ventriculomegaly in 63%. The finding of midline defects was common, and absence or hypoplasia of the corpus callosum was noted in almost all cases. These findings can allow differentiation of Sotos syndrome from other disorders that include macrocephaly and developmental delay. Chromosomal analyses are frequently performed as part of a thorough evaluation but are usually unrevealing, although recent work may have defined a gene that is linked with Sotos syndrome.

Differential Diagnosis

The differential diagnosis of pathologic overgrowth includes a variety of hormonal, genetic, and chromosomal conditions. Specific characteristics of each individual presentation should aid in narrowing the differential diagnosis. Clues to the diagnosis in this case were symmetric overgrowth beginning in utero, mental retardation, macrocephaly, and early puberty.

Precocious puberty, regardless of the cause, is a frequent cause of excessive growth velocity in childhood. Prepubertal secretion of the androgens or estrogen from the gonads or adrenal glands accelerates linear growth and sexual development. However, final adult height is normal or somewhat decreased.

Growth hormone excess can result in excessive height in the form of either pituitary gigantism with normal proportions or acromegaly, characterized by coarse facial features and disproportional enlargement of hands, feet, jaw, and supraorbital rim. Acromegaly results when growth hormone excess occurs in adolescence. Most cases result from primary pituitary adenomas or hyperplasia. A GH stimulation test as well as measurement of insulinlike growth factor levels aid in the diagnosis.

Hyperthyroidism should be considered in patients who grow faster than expected. Accelerated linear growth may occur with a hyperthyroid state but should return to normal after treatment.

Fragile X syndrome also deserves consideration in this case, given the tall stature, mental retardation, and large facial features. Fragile X is characterized by large ears, characteristic facies, macro-orchidism, and mental retardation. The diagnosis is made by analysis of the fragile X chromosomal site for trinucleotide repeats.

Infants of diabetic mothers and patients who have Beckwith-Wiedemann syndrome (BWS) can experience prenatal overgrowth. Postnatal rapid growth may continue with BWS. The cardinal features of BWS include large birth size, macroglossia, and abdominal wall defects. Patients are at increased risk of hypoglycemia, hemihypertrophy, and various types of tumors. The inheritance is complex. Genetic abnormalities have been mapped to region 11p15.

Macrocephaly can occur alone or, as in Sotos syndrome, in conjunction with signs and symptoms of other disease processes. Other entities to be considered include hydrocephalus, tumor, subdural effusions or hematomas, cranial skeletal dysplasias, neurocutaneous disorders, storage diseases, and BWS. Macrocephaly may also be familial, possibly with autosomal dominant inheritance, although other growth parameters should be normal.

The term *pituitary gigantism* has been used to describe conditions of pronounced growth due to isolated GH excess, usually caused by a pituitary tumor or by a high level of GH-releasing factor produced by a peripheral tumor. *Cerebral gigantism* is a name given to the condition of macrocephaly that involves no obvious pituitary abnormalities and is sometimes used as a synonym for Sotos syndrome. Today, it is thought that GH and pituitary function might play a role in the pathogenesis of Sotos syndrome, but the linkage is not clear.

Treatment

There is no specific treatment for Sotos syndrome. Early intervention for mental retardation and hypotonia is aimed at stimulation through occupational, physical, and speech therapy. Psychological counseling may be indicated for social and behavioral issues. Monitoring for glucose intolerance as well as aggressive treatment of fever are important in the primary care setting.

Robin P. Stanfield, MD, University of South Carolina, Columbia, SC

CHAPTER 40

Prolonged Generalized Seizure and Progressive Lethargy in a 15-Year-Old Boy

Presentation

A 15-year-old boy is admitted to the hospital because of a prolonged generalized seizure after having become progressively lethargic over the past 24 hours. He has a 1-week history of malaise, anorexia, and headaches. His Glasgow Coma Scale score is 8/15. Despite termination of abnormal movements following administration of intravenous anticonvulsants, his level of consciousness remains depressed, and endotracheal intubation is performed. He is admitted to the intensive care unit. A computed tomography scan of his head shows no focal abnormalities.

He has a mild global developmental delay of unknown cause. He had 3 febrile convulsions at age 3 years and one generalized seizure when 9 years of age. He takes no medication, is fully immunized, and has no family history of similar illness.

The boy fails to waken after sedative medications are stopped. On physical examination, he remains comatose and has a Glasgow Coma Scale score of 4/15. His temperature is 100.8°F (38.2°C), pulse is 98 beats/min, and blood pressure is 127/68 mm Hg. Abnormal muscle tone and intermittent extensor posturing are noted. Pupils are equal in size and reactive. No neck stiffness or rash is noted. All other physical findings are normal.

His hemoglobin concentration is 12.3 g/dL (123.0 g/L), white blood cell count is 8.0×10^3/mcL (8.0×10^9/L), and platelet count is 257.0×10^3/mcL (257.0×10^9/L). Serum electrolyte levels, C-reactive protein level, urea nitrogen concentration, creatinine concentration, and results of coagulation studies are within reference range. All culture results remain negative. An electroencephalogram shows diffuse, severe, nonspecific encephalopathy, but no epileptiform discharges. An additional test result reveals the underlying cause of his illness.

- **What is your differential diagnosis at this point?**
- **Are there any elements of history or physical examination that would help you?**
- **What additional diagnostic studies would you like performed?**

Discussion

A metabolic screening was performed and revealed severe hyperammonemia (serum ammonia concentration of 456 mcmol/L; reference range is <40 mcmol/L). A urea cycle disorder (UCD) was suspected, and additional laboratory investigations were ordered to confirm the diagnosis and identify the specific enzyme deficiency. Concentrations of citrulline and argininosuccinic acid were elevated, which suggested the condition argininosuccinate lyase deficiency, a diagnosis confirmed on red blood cell enzyme analysis.

Continuous high-flow venovenous hemofiltration was performed, and within 4 hours, the boy's serum ammonia concentration fell to the reference range. Concurrent therapy consisted of suspending protein intake, providing calories by intravenous administration of lipids and glucose, administering the nitrogen scavengers sodium benzoate and sodium phenylbutyrate, and providing supplemental arginine. Neurologically, the patient improved to a preadmission mental state within 7 days.

Two months after admission, his ammonia values remain within the reference range on a low-protein diet (approximately 1 g/kg/d) with sodium phenylbutyrate and arginine supplementation. He is back in mainstream school with special educational support.

Differential Diagnosis

Acute encephalopathy has a broad differential diagnosis that includes primary structural brain disease (eg, tumor, hemorrhage), trauma, infection (eg, meningoencephalitis), seizures, intoxication, and metabolic disorders. The differential diagnosis can be narrowed by considering age, presentation, relevant history, and physical findings. Cranial ultrasonography in neonates or computed tomography scans in older patients should be performed to rule out structural causes of encephalopathy. The electroencephalogram can both confirm global cerebral dysfunction and exclude subclinical seizures, as demonstrated in this patient.

No lumbar puncture was performed in this adolescent because of the possibility of raised intracranial pressure, but he was given antimicrobial therapy because of the potential for meningoencephalitis.

Intoxication is an important diagnostic consideration, and toxicological screening is mandatory in all patients presenting with acute encephalopathy.

The Family of Disorders

Metabolic disorders must be considered in the patient who has encephalopathy. In addition to encephalopathy, other manifestations of inborn errors of metabolism (IEM) include chronic vomiting, developmental delay, psychomotor abnormalities, seizures, failure to thrive, and psychiatric illness. Patients tend to prefer low-protein vegetarian diets. Metabolic disorders may also present as a pattern of episodic acute decompensation triggered by changes in dietary intake, fasting, intercurrent illness, trauma, or childbirth. The specific signs and symptoms depend on the condition and its severity.

Neonates who have an IEM typically appear well after birth and may become symptomatic after feeding has started because milk provides protein and carbohydrate loading. In the neonate, typical presentations include poor feeding, vomiting, lethargy, seizures, and shock. Sepsis is usually suspected initially in a neonate who shows these signs, but a metabolic disorder should always be considered if results of the septic evaluation remain negative. Other conditions that can cause a neonate to become acutely ill after a period of stability include duct-dependent heart disease, drug withdrawal, congenital viral infection, and congenital adrenal hyperplasia. Basic laboratory findings suggestive of IEM include hyperammonemia, hypoglycemia, and unexplained acid-base disorders.

Detecting IEM requires a high degree of suspicion, and these disorders can present at any time, even in adulthood. An understanding of the broad clinical manifestations of IEM provides the basis for knowing when to screen for these diseases.

Diagnostic Steps

A history and physical examination are essential and should be tailored to the age of presentation. Specific laboratory studies should be undertaken in all patients who have a suggestive history, physical findings, or initial laboratory results. Metabolic samples should be obtained while the patient is symptomatic because values can be normal when the patient is well.

Initial evaluation of suspected IEM includes the tests listed in Box 40.1. Specimens for specialized testing, as listed in Box 40.2, should be collected and stored in the acute phase and processed when indicated by the initial results and after metabolic specialist input is obtained.

Box 40.1. Initial Laboratory Tests for Suspected Inborn Errors of Metabolism

- Complete blood cell count with differential
- Arterial blood gas analysis
- Anion gap
- Glucose
- Lactate, pyruvate
- Ammonia
- Electrolyte panel, urea nitrogen, creatinine, uric acid
- Liver function tests: aminotransferase, bilirubin, prothrombin time
- Urinalysis (glucose, ketones, reducing substances)

Box 40.2. Additional Laboratory Tests for Suspected Inborn Errors of Metabolism

- Quantitative plasma and urine amino acid analysis
- Qualitative urine organic acids
- Cerebrospinal fluid amino and organic acids
- Urine orotic acid
- Acylcarnitine profile
- Very long–chain fatty acids

The Specific Condition

The urea cycle is a metabolic pathway that transforms nitrogen derived from protein metabolism to water-soluble urea, which is excreted in the urine. Urea cycle disorders are IEM characterized by episodic, life-threatening hyperammonemia resulting from partial or complete inactivity of enzymes responsible for eliminating nitrogen waste.

Deficiencies in the first 4 enzymes of the urea cycle (carbamyl phosphate synthetase I, ornithine transcarbamylase, argininosuccinate synthetase, or argininosuccinate lyase) result in accumulation of ammonia and the precursor metabolites (Figure 40.1). Metabolic decompensation resulting in hyperammonemia causes neurologic injury because free ammonia is highly toxic to the central nervous system.

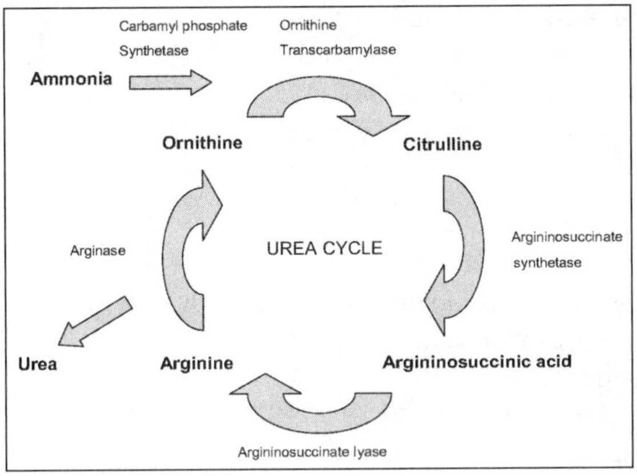

Figure 40.1. The urea cycle.

Plasma quantitative amino acid analysis identifies which precursor metabolite levels are elevated and can be used to differentiate among the UCDs. The specific UCD, however, must be confirmed by enzyme analysis of tissue samples.

Argininosuccinic aciduria is an autosomal recessive deficiency of the enzyme argininosuccinate lyase. This enzyme catalyzes the conversion of argininosuccinic acid to arginine and fumaric acid (see Figure 40.1). A deficiency in this enzyme leads to accumulation of argininosuccinic acid and the precursor metabolites citrulline and ammonia as well as a deficiency in arginine, as demonstrated in this case.

The clinical phenotype of UCDs is extremely variable and depends, in part, on the amount of protein intake. The classic presentation in neonates is similar to that of other IEM and includes poor feeding, vomiting, lethargy, and coma due to hyperammonemia.

Patients who have partial enzyme deficiencies may present outside the neonatal period. Recurrent vomiting, developmental delay, learning difficulties, seizures, brittle hair in infancy (trichorrhexis nodosa), and protein intolerance are common manifestations, and all were present in this patient on additional inquiry. Failure to thrive and psychomotor delay may warrant suspicion of a UCD. It is of interest that this boy had poor growth as a toddler but now is growing in the reference range, although he is slim. Less severe forms of enzyme deficiency may present in older patients with subtle neurologic abnormalities or psychiatric abnormalities.

Precipitants of acute hyperammonemic encephalopathy include catabolic states due to infection, trauma, or fasting. Medications affecting protein catabolism such as glucocorticoids can induce a metabolic decompensation and should be avoided in patients known to have UCD.

On further questioning, this patient's mother reported that her son had a "dairy and egg allergy" diagnosed at 2 years of age. Interestingly, the patient had self-selected a low-protein diet; he had refused to eat any meat from a young age and avoided any high-protein food. When he was less able to control his protein intake, as when eating out, he had recurrent episodes of vomiting. Furthermore, he has had brittle hair from infancy and failure to thrive, both typical features of a UCD.

General principles for managing hyperammonemic encephalopathy due to decompensation in patients who have UCDs include removing ammonia with hemodialysis or hemofiltration and nitrogen scavengers, decreasing the protein load, minimizing catabolism, and supplementing essential amino acids.

Lessons for the Physician

- A metabolic disorder should be included in the differential diagnosis of every patient who has encephalopathy of unknown cause regardless of the patient's age. Inherited metabolic disease can present at any age and requires a high degree of suspicion. This case illustrates the importance of obtaining a past medical history; this patient's history showed multiple clues of metabolic disease. Early recognition and treatment might have prevented some of his neurologic handicap.
- This adolescent's refusal to eat protein is an example of the unconscious decision-making that can occur without understanding how or why the choice was made. Patients may make such instinctive and effective adjustments to compensate for their own vulnerabilities and, in turn, minimize the manifestations of their diseases.

Nicole L. Mettauer, MD; Christine M. Pierce, MB; and Mark J. Peters, MB, PhD, Great Ormond Street Hospital, London, United Kingdom

COMMENTARY BY DR ROBERT CONWAY, METABOLIC DISORDER SPECIALIST, CHILDREN'S HOSPITAL OF MICHIGAN

Urine amino acid analysis is not routinely performed if a plasma amino acid analysis is obtained. Urine amino acid analyses are frequently nonspecifically abnormal and not helpful for most situations in which a plasma amino acid analysis would not otherwise reveal biochemical abnormalities to suggest a diagnosis in a more specific fashion. Urine amino acid analysis could be informative to identify a generalized aminoaciduria or a Fanconi-like picture of renal disease that, if present, may itself be a clinical feature of certain inborn errors of metabolism (IEM). It is also specifically helpful in the diagnosis of certain inborn errors that involve amino acid transporter proteins, as mutations in these proteins lead to specific patterns of loss of amino acids in the urine (cystinuria, Hartnup disease, and lysinuric protein intolerance are examples).

In addition, while one can perform organic acid analysis on cerebrospinal fluid, this is not often done clinically as a first-line screening method and is more helpful in situations specific to a few "cerebral" organic acidemias. Cerebrospinal fluid lactic acid is not uncommonly measured as an adjunctive screen for mitochondrial disease. The list of IEM in Box 40.2 is generally complete for conditions that present with a metabolic catastrophe, though free and total carnitine levels are often obtained to screen for presence of primary or secondary carnitine deficiency. Additional laboratory tests are often ordered as screening modalities for suspected IEM on the basis of appropriate clinical suspicion.

In addition to the therapies discussed in the case, there is a new oral medication that is available as a nitrogen scavenger, glycerol phenylbutyrate, that could also be used in lieu of sodium phenylbutyrate (Buphenyl). Some physicians may start with glycerol phenylbutyrate as it is better tolerated but others might start with sodium phenylbutyrate and then transition to glycerol phenylbutyrate.

Part 9

Hematology and Oncology

CHAPTER 41

4-Month-Old With Severe Rash Over Face and Hands

Presentation

A 4-month-old Caucasian infant is brought to the emergency department because of a severe rash over his face and hands that has been worsening over the last 3 weeks. Born after an uncomplicated pregnancy and delivery, the infant has experienced no respiratory tract infection, fever, vomiting, or diarrhea. There have been no changes in sleep pattern or appetite. His urine output has been regular, but his diapers have occasionally been stained pink or burgundy.

Physical examination reveals a normal-appearing infant in no acute distress. He has multiple, dark-colored, bullous lesions over the malar region of his face and backs of both hands. Some bullae are crusted over, and several hyperpigmented scars are present on the face. No other rash or lesions are found on the rest of the body. The remainder of the examination yields normal findings.

A complete blood cell count reveals a hemoglobin level of 8.7 g/dL (87 g/L) and a hematocrit of 25% (0.25). White blood cell count and platelet count are normal. The reticulocyte count is 6.5% (0.065). Urinalysis shows hemoglobin in the urine. Serum electrolyte levels and erythrocyte sedimentation rate are normal.

Further testing of the urine reveals the underlying disorder.

- **What is your differential diagnosis at this point?**
- **Are there any elements of history or physical examination that would help you?**
- **What additional diagnostic studies would you like performed?**

Discussion

Chemical analysis of the child's urine revealed normal levels of aminolevulinic acid and porphobilinogen, a uroporphyrinogen I level of 1,950 mcg/24 h (male reference range, 9–44 mcg/24 h), and a coproporphyrinogen level of 2,085 mcg/24 h (male reference range, 10–109 mcg/24 h), making the diagnosis of congenital erythropoietic porphyria (CEP). This condition, also known as Günther disease, is the least common of the porphyrias. It is an autosomal recessive disorder in which uroporphyrinogen III cosynthase activity is decreased, leading to an accumulation and subsequent hyperexcretion of type I uroporphyrins.

Family

Porphyrias are a diverse group of disorders that arise from an enzymatic defect in one of the 8 steps in the biosynthetic sequence of heme production. Porphyrias can be considered hepatic or erythropoietic, depending on the primary site of action of the defective enzyme. Clinically, the porphyrias are divided into 2 groups: the cutaneous porphyrias and the acute hepatic porphyrias.

The 4 cutaneous porphyrias include CEP, porphyria cutanea tarda, hepatoerythropoietic porphyria, and erythropoietic protoporphyria. This group is characterized by severe cutaneous photosensitivity and often bullous or vesicular skin eruptions. The 4 acute hepatic porphyrias include acute intermittent porphyria (the most common porphyria), delta-aminolevulinate dehydratase deficiency porphyria, variegate porphyria, and hereditary coproporphyria. The principal clinical manifestation of these porphyrias is acute episodes of neurologic disturbances, ranging from abdominal pain or nausea to muscle hypotonia, seizures, and sensory neuropathy. Patients who have acute intermittent porphyria, for example, often develop severe abdominal pain as the initial sign of an acute attack. Occasionally, the mechanism for the abdominal pain is the accumulation of porphyrin-rich gallstones in the biliary tree or terminal ileum.

Unlike most other porphyrias, the primary site of the deficient enzyme in CEP is the bone marrow rather than the liver, which accounts for the widespread distribution of porphyrin accumulation throughout the bodies of affected patients. The pigment accumulates in nearly all tissues but most frequently in the urine, feces, teeth, and other skeletal structures.

Numerous mutations have been identified in the uroporphyrinogen III cosynthase gene, all localized to chromosome 10. Congenital erythropoietic porphyria seems to occur in equal frequency in males and females and is more common in northern European populations.

Clinical Picture

Clinically, CEP usually presents in infancy with the early onset of severe cutaneous photosensitivity exacerbated by exposure to sunlight (hydroa aestivale). These infants develop subepidermal bullae that progress rapidly to crusted erosions; secondary infections are common. The bullae contain porphyrin-rich fluid that often leaves hyperpigmented scars and can lead to epidermal atrophy. Erythrodontia (reddish brown pigmentation of the teeth) that appears under UV light is virtually pathognomonic of CEP.

Because of the excessive levels of porphyrins in their urine, infants who have CEP frequently have discolored urine, ranging from pink to dark brown, that stains their diapers. In older children, CEP can present with splenomegaly, hemolytic anemia, porphyrin-rich gallstones, and erythrodontia. Because of the bone marrow involvement of CEP, many children also have recurrent pathologic fractures or vertebral compression due to the erythroid hyperplasia.

Differential Diagnosis

The differential diagnosis for bullous eruptions during infancy and childhood is extensive and includes impetigo, acute drug reactions, linear IgA dermatosis, erythema multiforme, epidermolysis bullosa, pemphigus, Stevens-Johnson syndrome, and Lyell syndrome (toxic epidermal necrolysis), as well as the cutaneous porphyrias. In infants, however, the presence of bullae is rare. Epidermolysis bullosa simplex is a genetic defect in keratin formation that leads to significant blistering and bullae formation in neonates and infants, but these lesions are widespread throughout the body and often congregate at friction points such as the palms and soles. Linear IgA dermatosis or chronic bullous dermatosis of childhood is also common in the first postnatal year, but the areas of predilection for the bullae are the genitals and buttocks. The pattern of eruptions on the sun-exposed areas of skin as well as the appearance of these bullae within the first 6 months after birth should steer the physician toward the cutaneous porphyrias as a probable cause.

Laboratory Findings

Congenital erythropoietic porphyria is diagnosed by measuring urine porphyrin levels. The most characteristic metabolic abnormality is a significantly increased urinary excretion of uroporphyrin I and coproporphyrin I. Often, levels of uroporphyrin III and coproporphyrin III are elevated as well.

Other laboratory findings in infants and children who have CEP include a normocytic, normochromic hemolytic anemia. Poikilocytes, anisocytes, or nucleated red blood cells are seen commonly in the peripheral blood smear. When CEP is suspected, UV light can demonstrate intense red fluorescence of the urine, feces, bone marrow normoblasts, and immature circulating red blood cells, as well as the teeth and other skeletal structures.

Therapy

Therapy for CEP centers on prevention. The avoidance of sunlight, trauma to the skin, and infections are the most important measures. Most affected infants and children should wear special protective clothing, gloves, and broad-brimmed hats. The use of sunscreens and oral beta carotene are useful in minimizing cutaneous reactivity.

Splenectomy has been performed frequently to relieve the hemolytic anemia and reduce the degree of porphyrinuria. Chronic transfusions with iron chelation therapy and bone marrow transplantation have also been used successfully. Other therapies include hematin therapy, administration of oral charcoal, and administration of hydroxyurea after hypertransfusion. The efficacy of these methods requires further evaluation.

Lessons for the Physician

Physicians should suspect porphyria in an infant who has a bullous eruption, especially if the bullae are prevalent in areas exposed to the sun. Unusual staining of the diaper should also raise the suspicion of porphyria.

Rui G. Rodrigues, MD, Penn State Children's Hospital, Hershey, PA

COMMENTARY BY BULENT OZGONENEL, MD, PEDIATRIC HEMATOLOGIST/ONCOLOGIST, CHILDREN'S HOSPITAL OF MICHIGAN

Patients with congenital erythropoietic porphyria can develop extensive scarring that can lead to disfigurement in exposed areas such as the face and hands, with loss of fingernails and digits. Neonates with jaundice and congenital erythropoietic porphyria should not be treated with phototherapy because of their photosensitivity. Allogeneic hematopoietic stem cell transplantation has been successful in providing a cure for some patients.

CHAPTER 42

Fever, Rash, and Decreased Oral Intake in a 10-Month-Old Boy

Presentation

A 10-month-old boy is referred to the emergency department for fever, rash, and decreased oral intake. He has asthma, eczema, and a milk-protein allergy. One week ago, he developed a mild cough and rhinorrhea. Three days later, he developed temperatures up to 103.8°F (39.9°C) but has been afebrile for the past 24 hours. Two days ago, erythematous eczematous patches appeared on his feet. The rash subsequently became vesiculopustular and spread up his legs and to his arms, chest, abdomen, back, and groin. His oral intake and urine output have decreased over the past 24 hours. He has had no diarrhea or vomiting. He has a dog at home, attends child care, and has no travel history. His only medication is occasional levalbuterol.

On physical examination, the boy is afebrile and has normal vital signs. He has enlarged tonsils (2+) with yellow ulcerations; clusters of crusted lesions on the dorsum of his feet and on all 4 extremities; and scattered vesicopustules on the dorsum of his hands, toes, back, and groin. All the lesions have surrounding erythema (Figures 42.1 and 42.2). The rest of the physical examination findings are normal.

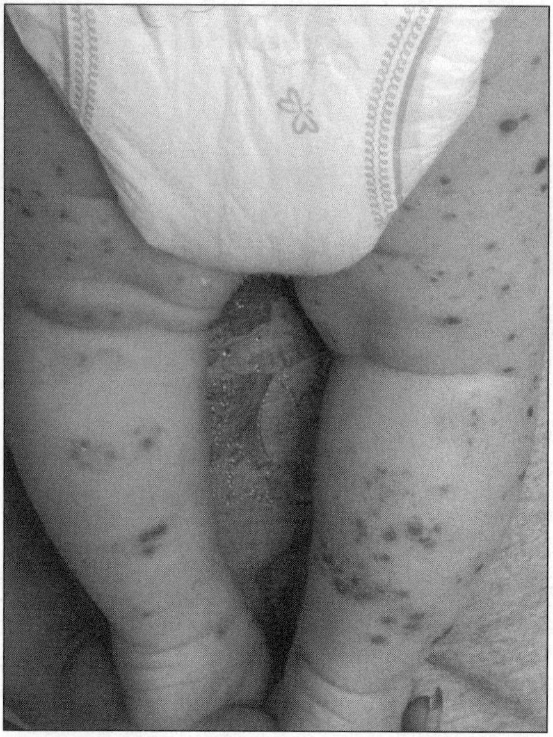

Figure 42.1. Clusters of crusted lesions on lower extremities.

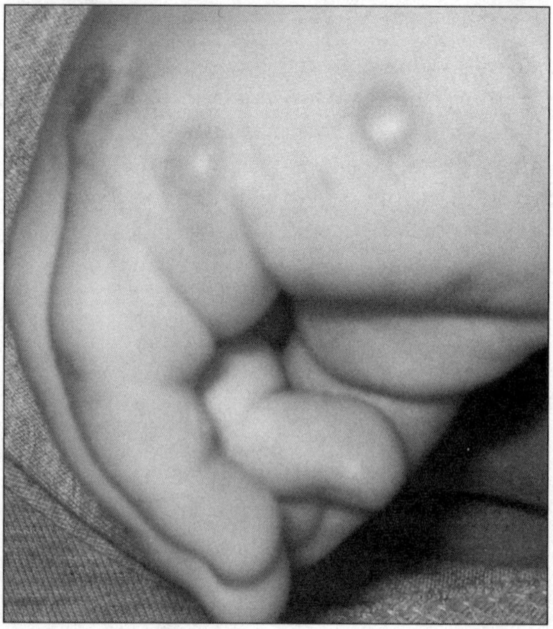

Figure 42.2. Vesiculopustular lesions with surrounding erythema on hand.

Polymerase chain reaction (PCR) testing for herpes simplex virus (HSV) and varicella-zoster virus from the base of a freshly unroofed vesicle is ordered, as well as bacterial cultures of the pustular fluid and crusted lesions. The infant is admitted and started on intravenous (IV) acyclovir and clindamycin. An additional test reveals his diagnosis.

- **What is your differential diagnosis at this point?**
- **Are there any elements of history or physical examination that would help you?**
- **What additional diagnostic studies would you like performed?**

Discussion

Polymerase chain reaction testing for enterovirus from the fluid and base of a freshly unroofed vesicle was positive, establishing the diagnosis of Kaposi varicelliform eruption (KVE). The PCR test results for HSV and varicella-zoster virus were negative, and acyclovir was discontinued. The bacterial culture was positive for *Staphylococcus aureus,* and the patient remained on IV clindamycin. Over the course of several days, his lesions crusted over and his oral intake improved; he was discharged from the hospital on a 7-day course of oral clindamycin.

The Condition

Kaposi varicelliform eruption and *eczema herpeticum* are terms often used interchangeably. Both refer to a vesiculopustular eruption in patients who have predisposing skin conditions affecting the integrity of the stratum corneum. Eczema herpeticum refers specifically to HSV infection in patients who have atopic dermatitis. *Kaposi varicelliform eruption* is a more inclusive term referring to a viral infection (eg, HSV-1 or -2, coxsackievirus A16, or vaccinia) in patients who have various skin conditions, such as atopic dermatitis, congenital ichthyosiform erythroderma, seborrheic dermatitis, Darier disease, pemphigus, Wiskott-Aldrich syndrome, pityriasis rubra pilaris, irritant contact dermatitis, psoriasis, and skin burns. The true incidence of KVE is unknown, but it is more common in infants and children than in adults.

Kaposi varicelliform eruption can occur during a primary viral infection or by autoinoculation following reactivation of HSV infection. The disrupted skin barrier allows for easy entry of viral particles. Decreased cell-mediated immunity and decreased cytokine secretion in affected skin play roles in disease pathogenesis. Patients who have atopic dermatitis have decreased expression of cathelicidins and beta-defensins, endogenous antimicrobial peptides that are first-line host defenses on the epithelium. Patients who have high serum IgE concentrations and those who have experienced the onset of atopic dermatitis at an early age are at increased risk for developing KVE.

Kaposi varicelliform eruption begins with clusters of dome-shaped vesicles that can progress to pustules, hemorrhagic crusted lesions, and punched-out erosions. The lesions are predominantly in areas affected by the predisposing skin condition and have a predilection for the head and neck. Within 2 weeks, the blisters usually become crusted and by 2 to 6 weeks are completely healed. The skin manifestations may be accompanied by systemic symptoms such as flulike illness, fever, and malaise. Viremia can result in multiorgan involvement such as hepatitis or disseminated intravascular coagulation.

Differential Diagnosis

Other vesicular and pustular eruptions should be considered in the diagnosis. Varicella presents with a similar vesicular rash along with malaise and fever. Varicella typically presents on the scalp, face, or trunk, subsequently spreading to the extremities. The vesicular eruption of herpes zoster could be confused with KVE but is typically limited to a dermatomal distribution, and patients tend to be older and have a prior history of varicella. Herpes zoster is often preceded by burning pain prior to the appearance of skin lesions. Contact dermatitis can have a blistering component, but the condition is limited to a localized area. Blistering skin disorders such as pemphigus vulgaris or bullous pemphigoid should be considered but typically produce large bullae, which are not characteristic of KVE. Bacterial superinfection of atopic areas has a similar presentation to that of KVE, with pustules, yellow crust, erythema, or induration being the prominent findings. It is important to note that bacterial superinfection can occur concurrently with KVE.

Diagnosis

Kaposi varicelliform eruption can be diagnosed clinically by the appearance of the characteristic lesions in a patient who has a predisposing skin condition, but several laboratory tests are useful and can guide treatment. A Tzanck test obtained from vigorously swabbing the base of a freshly unroofed vesicle shows multinucleated giant cells indicative of viral infection but is not sensitive or specific for HSV. Direct fluorescent antibody staining can be useful as a rapid screen for HSV-1 or -2. Polymerase chain reaction testing for HSV-1, HSV-2, or enteroviruses obtained by scraping the base of a previously intact vesicle is sensitive and specific. The diagnosis of enterovirus infection can also be established by PCR testing on serum or urine early in the course of the illness when the patient is more likely to be viremic. Viral cultures are less useful because results are not available for more than 48 hours and are often negative if taken from a crusted lesion. Complete blood cell count, serum electrolyte panel, and serum liver enzyme panel are recommended procedures to evaluate for other organ involvement. Affected skin is at risk for bacterial superinfection, and bacterial cultures should be obtained by swabbing the affected skin or obtaining fluid from a vesicle or pustule.

Treatment

Concern for KVE should prompt consideration of initiating antiviral medication. Acyclovir is effective against HSV-1 and HSV-2, especially when started within the first 72 hours of the illness. Pediatric patients are typically admitted to the hospital for IV acyclovir, pain control, and monitoring for systemic complications. If bacterial superinfection is suspected, antibiotic therapy against staphylococcal species as well as group A beta-hemolytic *Streptococcus* is warranted. Topical antibiotic preparations such as silver sulfadiazine are recommended as prophylaxis in the absence of active bacterial infection. Periocular lesions or the presence of ocular symptoms should prompt an ophthalmologic evaluation for keratoconjunctivitis, which is an ophthalmologic emergency. The role of corticosteroids and topical immunosuppressants in treating KVE is controversial. Because of a theoretical risk of immunosuppression, oral and topical corticosteroids, as well as topical calcineurin inhibitors used for treating atopic dermatitis, often are withheld until lesions are crusted.

Lessons for the Physician

- Although herpes simplex virus (HSV)-1 and HSV-2 are the most common causes of Kaposi varicelliform eruption, other viruses must be considered, especially if direct fluorescent antibody staining or polymerase chain reaction testing for HSV yields negative results.
- Polymerase chain reaction testing for enteroviruses can detect coxsackievirus that, if positive, allows discontinuation of acyclovir and can perhaps lead to fewer medication adverse effects and a shorter hospital stay.

Tashveen Kaur, MD, and Deborah Whitney, MD, The Children's Hospital of Philadelphia, Philadelphia, PA

CHAPTER 43

Acute Urinary Retention in a 13-Month-Old Boy

Presentation

A 13-month-old Caucasian boy presents to the emergency department with sudden onset of abdominal discomfort and lethargy. There is no history of fevers, vomiting, or diarrhea. He was born at 39 weeks' gestation by spontaneous vaginal delivery. He has had no surgery, and he does not take any medications. His immunizations are up to date and he is developmentally appropriate. Some older family members have had gastric, uterine, and cervical cancers.

Physical examination reveals a crying but consolable child. He is afebrile with a heart rate of 123 beats/min, blood pressure of 107/60 mm Hg, respiratory rate of 37 breaths/min, and oxygen saturation of 97% on room air. His abdomen is soft and nontender, with mild guarding; there are no masses or hepatosplenomegaly. Neurologic examination reveals normal strength and deep tendon reflexes. A rectal examination is deferred because of parental request.

His laboratory results reveal a serum sodium level of 134 mmol/L (134 mmol/L), potassium of 4.4 mmol/L (4.4 mmol/L), chloride of 105 mmol/L (105 mmol/L), bicarbonate of 13 mmol/L (13 mmol/L), urea nitrogen of 83 mg/dL (29.6 mmol/L), creatinine of 5.4 mg/dL (477 mcmol/L), glucose of 98 mg/dL (5.4 mmol/L), calcium of 8.6 mg/dL (2.15 mmol/L), and lipase of 24 U/L (0.4 mckat/L). The complete blood cell count is normal for age, and urinalysis on a catheterized specimen shows moderate occult blood but is negative for protein, white blood cell esterase, or nitrites. He receives intravenous fluids to correct his prerenal failure. Subsequently, he develops urinary retention that requires frequent urinary catheterizations. Renal ultrasonography shows bilateral hydronephrosis, and a voiding cystourethrogram shows 2 small bladder diverticula and the absence of spontaneous emptying of the bladder. An advanced imaging study reveals the diagnosis.

- **What is your differential diagnosis at this point?**
- **Are there any elements of history or physical examination that would help you?**
- **What additional diagnostic studies would you like performed?**

Discussion

Despite a normal neurologic examination, the voiding cystourethrogram results raised concern for a neurogenic bladder. Therefore, magnetic resonance imaging (MRI) of the thoracic, lumbar, and sacral spine was performed and was completely normal, thus ruling out demyelinating lesions, transverse myelitis, spinal cord injury or hematoma, spinal dysraphism, spina bifida occulta, tethered cord, and epidural abscess.

Posterior urethral valves might have been considered, but the history was not suggestive. A pelvic mass obstructing the urinary tract should potentially have been seen in the imaging studies performed earlier. Urinary tract infection is a possibility, but both bacterial and viral urine cultures were negative.

The decision was made to perform cystoscopy. During cystoscopy, a firm nodular prostate gland was noted and prostatic biopsies were obtained. Pelvic MRI revealed a 5.0 × 4.2 × 3.5–cm mass involving the prostate. The mass seemed to be invading the bladder. The pelvic and inguinal lymph nodes were also prominent (Figure 43.1). On further review of the original spinal MRI, some images appeared to suggest an enlarged prostate.

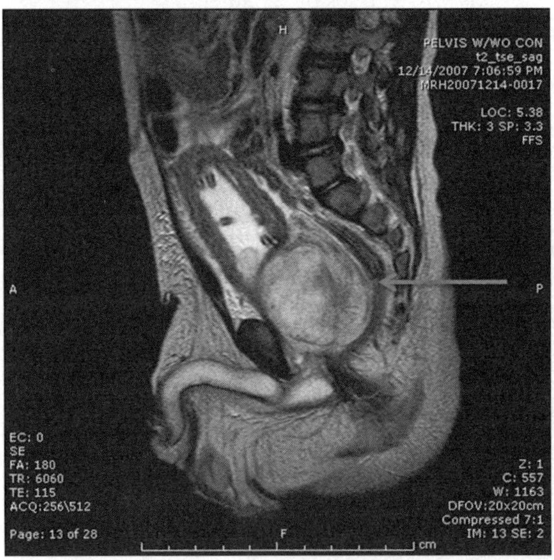

Figure 43.1. Pelvic magnetic resonance imaging showing a mass involving the prostate.

Histopathology was positive for spindle cell tumor. The histologic and immunophenotypic features were consistent with embryonal rhabdomyosarcoma of the prostate. Metastatic evaluation, including bone marrow aspirate and biopsy, bone scan, and computed tomography of the chest, abdomen, and pelvis, was negative for metastases.

The Condition

Rhabdomyosarcoma is the most common soft-tissue sarcoma in children. The frequency in children and adolescents younger than 15 years is 6 cases per 1 million per year. Approximately 250 new cases of rhabdomyosarcoma are diagnosed in the United States per year. Genitourinary rhabdomyosarcomas account for 15% to 30% of all rhabdomyosarcoma cases in children. This percentage equates to an incidence of genitourinary rhabdomyosarcoma of approximately 1 case per million children per year. The specific incidence of isolated prostate rhabdomyosarcoma in pediatrics is even less than 1 per million per year. Rhabdomyosarcoma, in general, ranks fourth in frequency among childhood malignancies, behind central nervous system tumors, neuroblastoma, and Wilms tumor.

Typical presenting signs of prostatic rhabdomyosarcoma include dysuria, hematuria, and hesitancy. Progressive disease leads to symptoms of bladder outlet obstruction, abdominal pain, or rectal compression.

Prognosis

Localized genitourinary rhabdomyosarcoma has a 5-year survival rate of 65% to 80% with treatment by surgery, radiation, and chemotherapy. Metastatic disease has a 5-year survival of less than 30%.

Management

The management of genitourinary rhabdomyosarcoma requires a multidisciplinary approach involving an oncologist, radiation oncologist, and urologist. This patient underwent 1 year of chemotherapy consisting of vincristine, actinomycin D, and cyclophosphamide. He then underwent radiation therapy and a subsequent prostate resection. It has been nearly 2.5 years since his diagnosis and he is doing well.

Lessons for the Physician

- Imaging studies that are focused on one aspect of anatomy (in this case the spine) can be suboptimal for viewing other locations in close proximity (such as the pelvis).
- In the pediatric population, more attention should be paid to rectal examination and even prostate evaluations in children who present with signs of urinary outlet obstruction.
- Rhabdomyosarcoma is an uncommon malignancy in children and has a good prognosis when the disease is localized, before the tumor metastasizes.

Sameer Pathare, MD, Pediatric Hospitalist, CHOC Children's Hospital, University of California, Irvine, Orange, CA

CHAPTER 44

4-Year-Old Girl With Intermittent Abdominal Pain for 3 Months, Difficulty Passing Stools for 2 Weeks, and Intermittent Vomiting for 2 Days

Presentation

A 4-year-old girl has experienced intermittent abdominal pain for 3 months, difficulty passing stools for 2 weeks, and intermittent vomiting for 2 days. The pain is mild, dull, and located in the left side of her abdomen. No aggravating or relieving factors can be identified. Mild abdominal distension has been noted for 3 weeks, ascribed by her parents to gaseous distension. Before this 2-week period of passing hard stools with difficulty, the child had experienced intermittent constipation. There is no history of weight loss, dietary changes, medication use, or fever. Her pediatrician prescribed symptomatic measures for constipation. For a few days she had softer, more frequent stools but then resumed difficulty in defecating.

Physical examination reveals a well-developed, comfortable child. Her temperature is 99°F (37.2°C), pulse is 108 beats/min, blood pressure is 100/62 mm Hg, and respiratory rate is 20 breaths/min. Her abdomen is mildly distended, more on the left side, and a somewhat firm, nontender, nonmobile mass that has rounded margins is palpable in the left lower quadrant and left lumbar regions. No guarding, rigidity, tenderness, fluid wave, or shifting dullness is noted. Bowel sounds are audible. Rectal examination reveals no tenderness or masses and an empty rectal vault.

The child's complete blood cell count and serum urea nitrogen, creatinine, glucose, and electrolyte levels are within reference range. Urinalysis shows 1+ protein and 2 to 5 white blood cells per high-power field. Radiography of the abdomen reveals a hazy mass in the left flank that gives the impression of hardened stools. More vigorous measures to combat the constipation are prescribed, and her stool pattern improves, but the characteristics of the mass do not change, prompting further testing.

- **What is your differential diagnosis at this point?**
- **Are there any elements of history or physical examination that would help you?**
- **What additional diagnostic studies would you like performed?**

Discussion

In this child, who had a history of and clinical picture consistent with constipation, the physicians were concerned that some improvement in her bowel pattern did not bring relief. They could not convince themselves that the left-sided mass was stool and suspected that an obstructive phenomenon on her left side was interfering with the free passage of stool.

The child underwent abdominal ultrasonography that revealed a minimally vascular renal mass on the left side, and contrast-enhanced computed tomography (CT) of her abdomen and pelvis showed a mass arising from the upper pole of the left kidney and occupying the left lumbar and left upper quadrant regions. There was tumor extension through the left renal vein into the inferior vena cava and right atrium. The inferior vena cava was obstructed, and numerous collateral vessels were present. The child was referred for biopsy, which established the diagnosis of Wilms tumor.

The Condition

Wilms tumor accounts for the highest number of pediatric renal tumors and occurs with almost the same frequency in both sexes and all races. The median age at the time of diagnosis is 3 years. The physical sign noted most commonly is an abdominal mass, detected by parents while bathing or clothing the child or by a physician during a routine examination. The mass often is asymptomatic and varies in size at the time of presentation (average of 11 cm in one study). About 50% of affected children have abdominal pain, vomiting, or both. Abdominal pain is more likely when hemorrhage occurs in the tumor (8% of cases). Hypertension has been noted in as many as 60% of cases, possibly from renal ischemia due to pressure on the renal artery. About 25% of patients have hypertension at the time of presentation. Constipation occurs in 4% of patients.

An important feature of Wilms tumor is its association with congenital anomalies in a small number of cases (genitourinary abnormalities, hemihypertrophy, and sporadic aniridia). It may be a component of rare syndromes such as WAGR syndrome (**W**ilms tumor, **a**niridia, **g**enitourinary abnormalities, mental **r**etardation), Denys-Drash syndrome (Wilms tumor, genitourinary abnormalities, nephropathy), and Beckwith-Wiedemann syndrome (multiple embryonal tumors, visceromegaly, macroglossia).

Diagnosis

Wilms tumor must be suspected in any young child who has an abdominal mass. Microscopic hematuria is suggestive of a renal tumor and is detectable at presentation in 10% to 25% of children who have these tumors. Many physicians consider renal ultrasonography to be the appropriate initial imaging procedure. Ultrasonography can usually differentiate intrarenal from extrarenal masses and cystic from solid lesions. Wilms tumors tend to invade vascular spaces, and ultrasonography can access vessels for flow and tumor thrombosis.

An abdominal CT scan offers several advantages in the evaluation of a possible Wilms tumor, such as confirmation of the intrarenal origin of the tumor (usually ruling out neuroblastoma), detection of multiple masses, determination of the extent of tumor, and evaluation of the opposite kidney. Slight tumor enhancement may occur after injection of contrast medium.

Hematogenous metastases are recognized in 10% to 15% of cases at the time of diagnosis (85% lung, 7% liver, 8% lung and liver). Most metastatic lung disease presents with multiple bilateral lung lesions seen on 2-view chest radiographs. A CT scan of the chest may be useful in evaluating the lung bases below the domes of diaphragm and in following the response to therapy. Controversy exists over whether to perform chest CT in patients who present with negative findings on chest radiograph. Additional lesions are rarely identified by CT scanning of children who have negative findings on chest radiographs, and the prognosis is very good for children who have lesions detectable only by CT scan and are treated appropriately.

Evaluation of the bone and bone marrow should be considered only if the patient has persistent bone pain or in cases of clear cell sarcoma of the kidney and rhabdoid tumor of the kidney. Some rare paraneoplastic syndromes may be associated with Wilms tumor. The tumor may produce erythropoietin, leading to polycythemia.

In addition to imaging, evaluation of a child who has an abdominal mass should include a complete blood cell count, urinalysis, liver and renal function tests, and a serum calcium level. Calcium may be elevated in patients who have mesoblastic nephroma or rhabdoid tumor of the kidney.

Differential Diagnosis

The differential diagnosis of a renal mass in a young child should include hydronephrosis, renal cysts, mesoblastic nephroma (most common in neonates in whom Wilms tumor does not occur), and other renal malignancies, such as renal cell carcinoma, soft-tissue sarcoma, and lymphoma. Intrarenal location of the tumor, noncrossing of the midline, and less obvious illness in the child at presentation favor the likelihood of Wilms tumor and may differentiate it from neuroblastoma, which must be considered in the differential diagnosis.

Treatment

The immediate treatment for unilateral tumors is surgical removal of the affected kidney through a wide flank incision or transabdominal approach, even if pulmonary metastases are present. Surgery also facilitates proper staging of the tumor. The contralateral kidney should be inspected carefully to assess the possibility of bilateral tumor before nephrectomy is performed, and the liver and intra-abdominal contents should be palpated for metastasis. In the absence of bilateral disease, the tumor-involved kidney and a generous segment of the ureter should be removed en bloc.

The renal vein stump, other renal vessels, and retroperitoneal lymph nodes should be examined. Although radical lymph node dissection is not recommended, adequate lymph node sampling is necessary because about 15% of patients have regional lymph node involvement at the time of diagnosis. Examination of the wall above the renal vein and artery for evidence of invasion or thrombosis also is necessary.

Every possible attempt should be made to avoid spillage of the tumor during surgery. Because postoperative radiotherapy and chemotherapy effectively destroy residual tumor, complete resection should not be attempted if it poses serious risks.

Routine postoperative radiation therapy is not necessary for patients who have stage I disease and favorable histology or anaplasia or stage II disease with favorable histology if postnephrectomy chemotherapy includes both vincristine and actinomycin D. Patients who have stage III disease and a favorable histology benefit from the addition of doxorubicin as well as intra-abdominal radiation. Those who have stage IV disease and favorable histology should receive the 3 chemotherapeutic agents plus abdominal and whole lung radiation. Patients who have stage II to IV disease and diffuse anaplasia may benefit from the regimen of cyclophosphamide, etoposide, vincristine, actinomycin D, and abdominal irradiation. Preoperative therapy is generally not recommended for unilateral disease, but it is indicated in bilateral disease to allow later renal salvage procedures. Treatment of children who have bilateral disease aims at eradicating all tumor while preserving as much normal renal tissue as possible and must be individualized.

The patient's prognosis depends on the disease stage (Table 44.1). Recurrence carries a poor prognosis, although the addition of newer agents may improve the outcome in a small group of these patients.

Table 44.1. National Wilms Tumor Study Group Classification and Survival Rates

Stage	Description	2-Year Survival Rate (%)	4-Year Survival Rate (%)
FH I	Limited to the kidney and can be excised completely with intact capsular surface	98	97
FH II	Extends beyond the kidney but can be excised completely	96	94
FH III	Postsurgical residual nonhematogenous extension confined to the abdomen	91	88
FH IV	Hematogenous metastasis that most frequently involves the lung	88	82
V	Bilateral involvement of kidneys	Variable	Variable
UFH I	(Focal or Diffuse Anaplasia) Stage I	89	89
UFH II–IV	(Focal or Diffuse Anaplasia) Stage II–IV	56	54

Abbreviations: FH, favorable histology; UFH, unfavorable histology.

Lessons for the Physician

Many children present with the complaint of constipation in everyday clinical practice. Although the diagnosis of simple constipation is very common and frequently correct, other sinister abdominal conditions, such as abdominal tumors, should not be overlooked. In this case, the patient's continued symptoms, despite some relief of the constipation, and palpation of a mass on careful examination and reexamination led to the procedures that made the diagnosis.

Muhammad A. Khan, MD, Lincoln Medical Center, Bronx, NY

COMMENTARY BY MAXIM YANKELEVICH, MD, PEDIATRIC HEMATOLOGIST/ONCOLOGIST, CHILDREN'S HOSPITAL OF MICHIGAN

The risk of developing a Wilms tumor (WT) is somewhat higher in African American children and lower in Asian children. Patients with subcapsular hemorrhage can present with rapid abdominal enlargement, anemia, hypertension, and fever. Hematuria is observed in 12% to 25% of patients. Once a WT is suspected, abdominal palpations should be done carefully, without excessive pressure, to avoid capsular rupture and tumor spillage, which changes the tumor local stage to III and results in more intensive chemotherapy and addition of radiation therapy. An abdominal magnetic resonance image is, in general, diagnostically equal to computed tomography not associated with radiation exposure and may provide somewhat better details of a tumor capsule; however, it requires significantly longer sedation times. Coagulation studies may be considered because approximately 8% of patients with WT have acquired von Willebrand disease at diagnosis.

Current survival rates of approximately 90% in WT patients were achieved through stepwise advances made by several cooperative clinical trials in North America and Europe. Subsets of patients with unfavorable features like anaplastic histology still have survival rates well below 90% and require more intensive therapy. All recent improvements in outcomes for children with WT have been achieved mostly through better stratification of patients into risk groups and delivery of risk-directed therapy based on the clinical and biological prognostic markers. For example, the most recent National WT Study # 5 confirmed that loss of heterozygosity for chromosomes 1p and 16q is a significant negative prognostic factor in patients with favorable histology WT. Additional risk factors used in the current stratification system include stage, histology, patient age, tumor weight, and rapidity of lung nodule response. Preoperative chemotherapy is generally not recommended for unilateral disease except when tumor thrombus is above the level of the hepatic vein, resection may require removal of contiguous structures other than adrenal gland, or a surgeon judges that immediate nephrectomy would result in significant morbidity or tumor spillage.

CHAPTER 45

Fever and Multiple Ruptured Bullae in a 6-Year-Old Boy (Visual Diagnosis)

Presentation

A 6-year-old previously healthy boy presents to an urgent care clinic with the complaint of fever and several tender, erythematous, circular lesions on his skin. The child had been doing well until 2 days ago, when he developed the abrupt onset of subjective fever, frontal headache, nausea, and vomiting. Yesterday, he began complaining of pain over his left elbow. The skin over the elbow became progressively erythematous, with a small papule appearing that increased in size and started to blister. Overnight, the lesion ruptured and the parents noted several similar lesions starting to appear, one on the right shoulder and 2 others on the left chest. These lesions progressed similarly, all having ruptured by the time of presentation to the clinic.

Review of systems reveals decreased activity and mild fatigue. His appetite has been normal, with good intake of food and liquids. His urine output has not decreased, and his stool pattern has not changed. The rest of the review of systems is negative.

The boy's past medical history is unremarkable. He was born at term following an uncomplicated pregnancy. He had had no prior hospitalizations or surgeries, and apart from some occasional doses of acetaminophen during this febrile illness, he took no medications. His immunizations are up to date. The family history reveals no significant medical problems. No similar symptoms are present in family or social contacts. He has not traveled recently and has no exposure to animals.

Physical examination reveals a pleasant boy who is alert and cooperative but minimizes movement of his left arm. Vital signs include a temperature of 102.2°F (39.0°C), heart rate of 139 beats/min, respiratory rate of 20 breaths/min, and blood pressure of 95/45 mm Hg. There is an approximately 2-cm, well-circumscribed, circular lesion on the distal posterolateral aspect of his left elbow that appears to be a ruptured bulla with a thin, flat, hemorrhagic ring surrounding the lesion that is surrounded further by mild erythema (Figure 45.1). The region is tender to palpation, and passive range of motion of the elbow is mildly painful. He has a similar lesion on his right anterior upper extremity, approximately 1 cm in diameter (Figure 45.2), another 1-cm lesion adjacent to his left areola, and a fourth 1-cm lesion on his left chest (Figure 45.3).

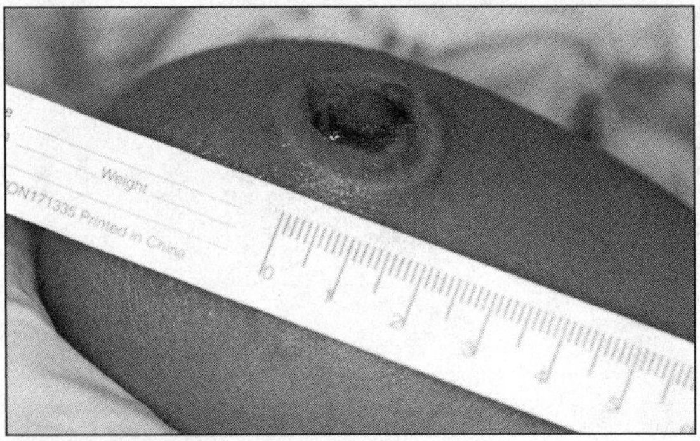

Figure 45.1. Initial skin lesion distal to the left elbow with a thin halo of erythema.

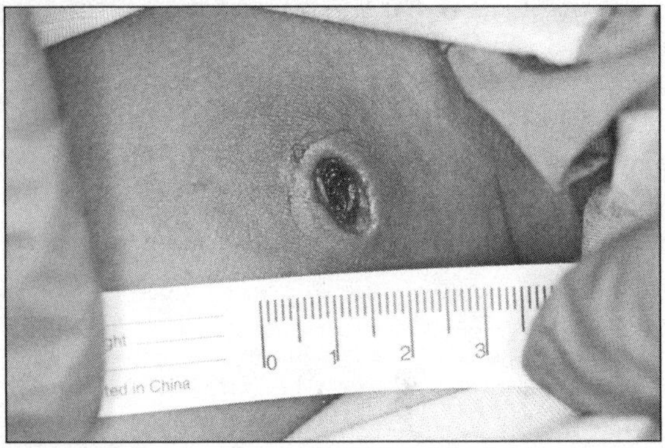

Figure 45.2. Lesion on right upper extremity 4 days after presentation (note deep gray-black eschar).

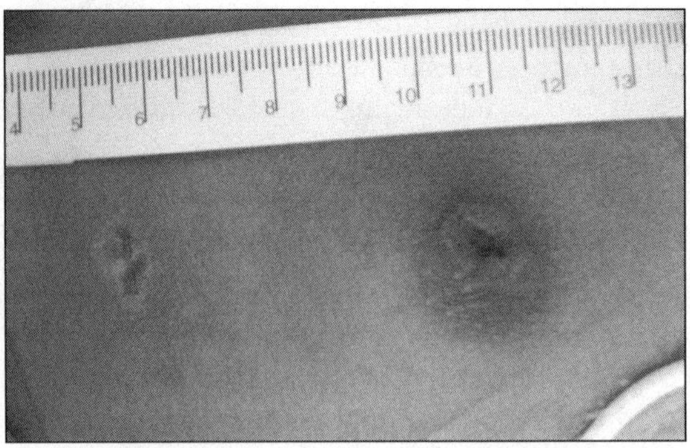

Figure 45.3. Left chest lesions.

All of the lesions are well circumscribed and appear to be ruptured bullae with demonstrable tenderness of the surrounding skin. Eye examination shows multiple conjunctival hemorrhages. Cardiac examination reveals a grade 2/6 systolic ejection murmur at the left sternal border without radiation to the axillae. Respiratory and abdominal examinations yield unremarkable findings. No significant cervical, axillary, or inguinal lymphadenopathy is appreciated. The remainder of his physical examination findings are within reference range.

The white blood cell count is 8.5×10^3/mcL (8.5×10^9/L) with 95% lymphocytes, 1% bands, 2% neutrophils, 1% monocytes, and 1% eosinophils. The hemoglobin measures 4.8 g/dL (48 g/L), and the platelet count is 39×10^3/mcL (39×10^9/L). A blood culture is obtained and broad-spectrum antibiotic therapy, initiated. Packed red blood cells are typed and cross-matched for transfusion, and the patient is admitted with a presumptive diagnosis of acute lymphocytic leukemia.

A clinical diagnosis for the skin lesions is presumed.

- **What is your differential diagnosis at this point?**
- **Are there any elements of history or physical examination that would help you?**
- **What additional diagnostic studies would you like performed?**

Diagnosis

The clinical presentation and skin findings appeared consistent with a diagnosis of ecthyma gangrenosum (EG). Flow cytometry and bone marrow biopsy confirmed the working diagnosis of acute lymphocytic leukemia. Culture of material from a skin swab of the primary lesion grew *Pseudomonas aeruginosa,* confirming the presumptive diagnosis of EG. Empiric antibiotic therapy (vancomycin and piperacillin-tazobactam) for neutropenic fever was initiated. Blood and urine cultures showed no growth.

Ecthyma gangrenosum is a distinct skin lesion that typically begins as an erythematous macule that indurates, frequently becoming papular. Although often painless initially, EG also may present as a painful macule. The macule or papule subsequently progresses to a hemorrhagic, bullous lesion. Over a short time, often 12 to 24 hours, the skin sloughs off and forms a deep, gangrenous ulcer that has a gray-black eschar (see Figure 45.2). The surrounding skin forms an erythematous halo, and localized cellulitis may occur beyond the halo.

Ecthyma gangrenosum lesions may occur singly or at multiple sites. Although lesions may arise anywhere, the most common sites are the gluteal or perineal region (57%), extremities (30%), trunk (6%), and face (6%). Associated symptoms can include fever, myalgias, and localized pain and tenderness. The hematogenously disseminated form of EG presents with signs of sepsis such as tachycardia, tachypnea, and hypotension.

Classically associated with and for a time pathognomonic of *Pseudomonas* infection, EG has been reported to arise from multiple infectious causes (Box 45.1). Lesions are caused by bacterial or fungal multiplication within vessel walls, leading to arterial and venous thrombosis–induced dermal necrosis. Lesions may occur at a primary site on the skin due to direct inoculation without concomitant bacteremia or because of septic seeding to the skin by an infectious organism. Mortality in the septic form is high; even without bacteremia, mortality is approximately 15%.

Pseudomonas species are found ubiquitously in the environment and have become a significant health care–associated infection. They tend to have low virulence, typically not causing invasive or severe infections in immunocompetent patients. However, *Pseudomonas* species can cause skin infections in otherwise healthy hosts, particularly if the skin is moist. *Pseudomonal folliculitis,* in particular, is well known to occur following exposure to *P aeruginosa*–contaminated hot tubs, whirlpools, and swimming pools.

Skin lesions may accompany *P aeruginosa* sepsis in up to 39% of patients. Other than EG, skin manifestations of *P aeruginosa* sepsis include localized vesicles or bullae; a gangrenous cellulitis that often begins as a well-demarcated, painless, necrotic lesion; and macular, papular, or nodular lesions that are typically small, oval, and painless and usually located on the trunk.

Like *Pseudomonas* in general, EG occurs predominately in children who have impaired host cellular or humoral immunity. Neutropenia, in particular, seems to place patients at higher risk for mortality. Other underlying impairments in host

Box 45.1. Pathogens Associated With Ecthyma Gangrenosum

- *Pseudomonas aeruginosa*
- *Staphylococcus aureus*
- *Streptococcus pyogenes*
- *Serratia marcescens*
- *Klebsiella*
- *Escherichia coli*
- *Enterobacter*
- *Proteus*
- *Citrobacter freundii*
- *Burkholderia cepacia*
- *Neisseria meningitidis*
- *Aeromonas hydrophila*
- *Xanthomonas maltophilia*
- *Stenotrophomonas maltophilia*
- *Chromobacterium violaceum*
- *Aspergillus*
- *Candida*
- *Fusarium*
- *Rhizopus*

immunity that have been reported with EG include malignancy (nonleukemic), intrinsic immunodeficiencies such as chronic granulomatous disease or hypogammaglobulinemia, immunosuppressive medications, malnutrition, and diabetes. Ecthyma gangrenosum may also occur in patients who have extensive burns or those who have undergone protracted courses of antibiotic therapy, particularly with penicillin. Although multiple pediatric and adult cases of EG without obvious underlying immunodeficiency have been reported, evaluation for immunodeficiency should be considered when EG develops in children. These cases typically occur in the setting of a disruption of the mechanical barrier of skin or mucosa, but many children who have this presentation are found to have an occult immunodeficiency.[1]

Differential Diagnosis

Although it has a relatively unique appearance, EG must be distinguished from other similar skin disorders. Two of the most important similar disorders are necrotic arachnidism (the necrotic spider bite) and cutaneous anthrax. Most patients and physicians attribute brown recluse spider (*Loxosceles reclusa*) bites to otherwise unexplained hemorrhagic or necrotic lesions. Most bites are initially painless, and unless the brown recluse spider is seen and caught, the diagnosis is speculative at best. The brown recluse spider bite typically becomes painful several hours after the bite, with the development of erythema, local cyanosis, and edema. Necrosis at the site of the bite to the point of requiring skin grafting may occur. Cutaneous anthrax, spread by spores of *Bacillus anthracis,* is of particular concern because of the underlying possibility of bioterrorism. Isolated cases of anthrax may occur in endemic areas, but a history of livestock exposure is often present. Cutaneous anthrax characteristically begins as a painless or pruritic papule that becomes necrotic.

Other possible diagnoses include drug eruptions, which occasionally cause bullous and hemorrhagic lesions; necrotic vasculitis; cryoglobulinemia; polyarteritis nodosa; pyoderma gangrenosum; hyperviscosity syndrome; leukemic infiltrates; and skin infections such as ecthyma or ecthyma contagiosum. Ecthyma is a streptococcal infection that presents as ulcers covered by yellowish crusts extending into the dermis and surrounded by a raised purplish border (Figure 45.4). Ecthyma contagiosum, also known as orf, is a disease typically found in patients who have been exposed to infected sheep or goats. Caused by a parapoxvirus, ecthyma contagiosum begins as a small, firm papule that develops into a hemorrhagic pustule or bulla and forms a crust due to weeping fluid. Other infectious causes to consider are ulceroglandular tularemia, plague, and cutaneous tuberculosis.

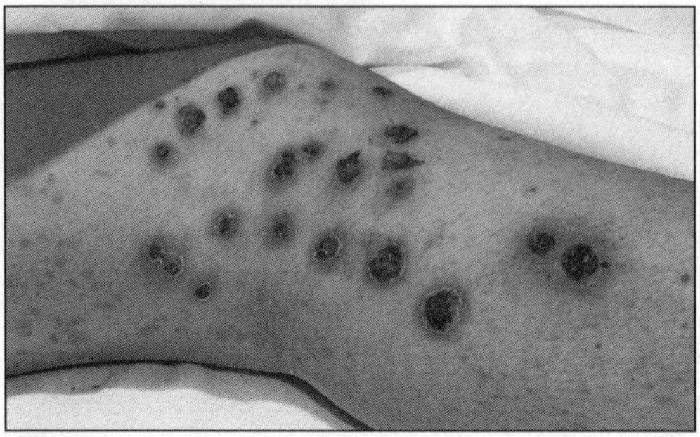

Figure 45.4. Ecthyma due to streptococcal skin infection characterized by ulcers with yellowish crusts extending into the dermis and surrounded by raised purplish borders.

Diagnosis

Ecthyma gangrenosum has a characteristic appearance, but the diagnosis should be confirmed by microbiological or histopathologic analysis. Needle aspiration of intact lesions or Gram stain and culture of a skin swab of tissue beneath a ruptured bulla may provide rapid identification. If these procedures are not diagnostic, skin biopsy for culture and histopathologic analysis with special bacterial stains may help. Histopathologic analysis typically reveals a necrotizing, hemorrhagic vasculitis.

Blood cultures obtained on initial presentation and during fever spikes may help identify the causative organism.

Treatment

Following collection of culture specimens, broad-spectrum antibiotic therapy that includes coverage for *P aeruginosa* should be initiated. Because of its significant mortality, timely identification of EG and initiation of antibiotic medications are crucial. Combination therapy consists of β-lactam and aminoglycoside antibiotics. Following several weeks of intravenous antibiotics, treatment may be changed to oral fluoroquinolone therapy. For localized infection, topical therapy such as wet compresses with silver nitrate or acetic acid or applications of silver sulfadiazine cream may be sufficient but should be instituted only after ruling out invasive disease. In cases of severe necrosis, surgical debridement and skin grafting may be necessary.

Patient Course

Intravenous vancomycin and piperacillin-tazobactam therapy for neutropenic fever was initiated for this boy. Following culture susceptibility results, the therapy was changed to piperacillin-tazobactam and gentamicin. The skin lesions turned black during the hospitalization, consistent with the typical course of EG (Figure 45.5). The patient tolerated induction chemotherapy well and was discharged from the hospital to complete a full 3-week course of antibiotic therapy and to continue chemotherapy. Factors that predisposed this patient to EG included neutropenia and hematologic malignancy.

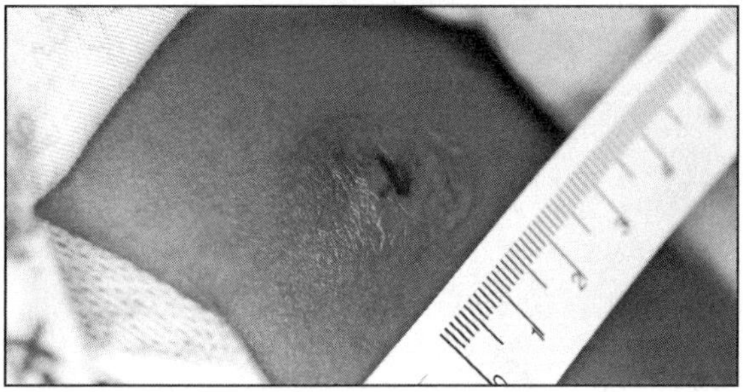

Figure 45.5. Blackening of an ecthyma gangrenosum lesion during hospitalization.

Reference

1. Zomorrodi A, Wald ER. Ecthyma gangrenosum: considerations in a previously healthy child. *Pediatr Infect Dis J.* 2002;21(12):1161–1164

Summary

Ecthyma gangrenosum is a serious infection that requires timely identification and institution of antimicrobial therapy that includes coverage for *Pseudomonas*. Although the appearance of ecthyma gangrenosum is distinct, suspected cases should be confirmed by bacterial culture or skin biopsy. Ecthyma gangrenosum in a previously healthy child should prompt an evaluation for an underlying immunologic impairment. Rapid diagnosis and treatment may help prevent the significant morbidity and mortality associated with this rare disease.

Nathan D. Tofteland, MD, Fourth-Year Medical-Pediatrics Resident, and Robert R. Wittler, MD, Professor, Department of Pediatrics, Pediatric Infectious Disease, University of Kansas School of Medicine-Wichita, Wichita, KS

CHAPTER 46

Bilateral Hip and Lower Back Pain in a 9-Year-Old Girl

Presentation

A 9-year-old girl is admitted to the hospital on the orthopedic service because of bilateral hip and lower back pain of 1 month's duration that has worsened over the last week. She describes the pain as constant with moderate intensity, nonradiating, worse with walking, and slightly relieved by lying on her side. The child denies any recent infections, rashes, cough, fever, or vomiting. She had oral surgery 5 years ago. Her family history is unremarkable.

Physical examination reveals an obese child who is alert but uncomfortable. Her temperature is 97.8°F (36.6°C), respirations are 18 breaths/min, heart rate is 84 beats/min, and blood pressure is 143/77 mm Hg. Her height is 144 cm (96th percentile), weight is 72.2 kg (significantly higher than the 97th percentile), and body mass index is 36 kg/m^2 (significantly higher than the 97th percentile). Extension of both hips causes pain, but no pain is elicited on flexion. There is decreased range of motion of her hip joints, but she is able to bear weight. There are no tender points over her spine, and no pain is elicited by moving her knees. When asked to point to her pain, she indicates both hips. There is mild tenderness on palpation of the lower abdomen but no hepatosplenomegaly or palpable masses. The remainder of the physical findings are normal.

Her white blood cell count is 15.6 × 10^3 mcL (15.6 × 10^9/L), erythrocyte sedimentation rate (ESR) is 55 mm/h, and C-reactive protein (CRP) level is 113.0 mg/L (1,076.2 nmol/L). Radiographs of the lumbosacral spine, hips, and knees yield normal findings.

- **What is your differential diagnosis at this point?**
- **Are there any elements of history or physical examination that would help you?**
- **What additional diagnostic studies would you like performed?**

Discussion

Differential Diagnosis

Causes of persistent hip and lower back pain of 1 month's duration include musculoskeletal disorders (slipped capital femoral epiphysis, diskitis, toxic synovitis, juvenile rheumatoid arthritis, vertebral osteomyelitis, stress fractures, sprains of the pelvis or spine, various bone tumors, herniated intervertebral disc, osteitis pubis, spondylosis), renal disease (urinary tract infection, hydronephrosis), gastrointestinal conditions (bowel spasms, dietary intolerance, infections of the gastrointestinal tract, hernias), and genital disorders (ovarian cyst, genital tract malformation or infection). A persistently elevated ESR or CRP value may indicate an ongoing inflammatory process (chronic pelvic inflammatory disease, pelvic serositis, inflammatory bowel disease, spondylitis, tumors of the pelvis and lower spine, appendicitis, abdominal abscess).

An Unlikely Finding

A bone scan and magnetic resonance imaging failed to reveal any hip or lumbosacral disease. Blood work revealed an ongoing inflammatory process, with the ESR and CRP values increasing on the second hospital day to 82 mm/h and 135.0 mg/L (1,285.7 nmol/L), respectively. Other tests gave normal results, including urinalysis, rheumatoid factor, antinuclear antibody, C3 and C4 complement levels, antistreptolysin O titer, and Lyme titer. Blood and urine culture results were negative.

On the second day of admission, the patient's pain continued in her lower abdomen and bilateral inguinal region as well as her hips. The pain was severe, and the surgical team was consulted to evaluate the patient's abdomen. She complained of diffuse tenderness when her abdomen was palpated, but it was soft. The physical findings did not match the patient's pain level, and computed tomography of the abdomen was performed.

Computed tomography revealed a very large, complex, cystic mass involving the abdomen and pelvis and measuring 35 × 20 × 10 cm. Multiple separations were seen within the mass. The mass extended into the cul-de-sac, displacing the bladder anteriorly. The large size of the mass obscured the origin, but potential causes included ovarian cystadenoma, lymphangioma, mesothelioma, cystadenocarcinoma, and hydrometrocolpos. The patient underwent surgery to remove the mass.

During surgery, the mass was found to be retroperitoneal, behind the uterus, and not attached to the ovaries, fallopian tubes, mesentery, or bowel. The tumor was excised, and because there was some attachment to the appendix, an appendectomy was performed.

The Lesion

The tumor was described as a hemorrhagic, multiloculated cystic mass, weighing 0.31 kg and measuring 14 × 10 × 6 cm. Histologic examination revealed it to be a benign cystic mesothelioma. Immunohistochemistry testing confirmed that the cells lining the cysts were positive for vimentin and monoclonal mouse anti-human keratin (*SLC4A1* and *SLC4A3* [formerly *AE1* and *AE3*]), findings consistent with a mesothelial origin.

Benign cystic mesothelioma (an adenomatoid tumor) is a rare lesion of the peritoneum characterized by the formation of multiple multilocular cysts. Although cases of childhood lesions in both girls and boys have been reported, the tumor is extremely rare in the pediatric age group, occurring predominantly in young to middle-aged women, and is frequently associated with previous abdominal surgery, pelvic inflammatory disease, and leiomyoma of the uterus. Most patients are females of reproductive age, suggesting a key role for female sex hormones in the tumor's pathogenesis.

This tumor tends to be located in the pelvis, with some reports of involvement of the upper abdomen and retroperitoneum. The process spreads superficially over peritoneal surfaces without significant organ invasion. The most common presenting symptom is lower abdominal pain, although back pain and asymptomatic lesions have been noted. This patient's bilateral hip pain is an unusual initial presentation.

Therapy

Current management of mesothelioma includes resection of the mass. However, despite resection, the lesion tends to recur. Recurrence has been documented in 27% to 75% of patients within 3 months to 22 years of the initial resection. Although this tumor is currently described as benign, there have been reports of malignant transformation.[1,2] The long-term outcome for patients who have this tumor is not yet known.[3]

References

1. Mohamed F, Sethna K, Elias D, Sugarbaker PH. Challenging and unusual cases: case 3. Peritoneal cystic mesothelioma. *J Clin Oncol.* 2003;21(7):1419–1420
2. Gonzalez-Moreno S, Yen H, Alcorn KW, et al. Malignant transformation of "benign" cystic mesothelioma of the peritoneum. *J Surg Oncol.* 2002;79(4):243–251
3. McCullagh M, Keen C, Dykes E. Cystic mesothelioma of the peritoneum: a rare cause of "ascites" in children. *J Pediatr Surg.* 1994;29(9):1205–1207

Lessons for the Physician

Often in teaching medicine we use the adage "When you hear hoof beats, think horses, not zebras!" Yet, a careful, methodical approach to a diagnosis can often be rewarding and lead to finding a "zebra," as in this case. This obese 9-year-old was admitted initially to the orthopedic service for what was likely a slipped capital femoral epiphysis, given her weight, age, and presentation. By following her clinical course over several hospital days, listening closely to the history, and performing follow-up physical examinations, the physicians were able to gallop into the underlying diagnosis.

Thomas Foley, MS IV, Mary Fury, DO, and Sam Adler, MD, Monmouth Medical Center, Long Branch, NJ

CHAPTER 47

Epistaxis and Melena in a 9-Year-Old Boy

Presentation

A 9-year-old boy presents to the emergency department with a 4-day history of epistaxis and melena. There has been no trauma except for nose picking. Physical examination reveals a pale but well-nourished boy. His heart rate is 140 beats/min, blood pressure is 110/85 mm Hg, respiratory rate is 25 breaths/min, and temperature is 99°F (37.2°C). Blood is visible in both nares. He is treated with topical silver nitrate and electrocautery.

Radiographs of the sinuses yield normal results. The hemoglobin level is 7 g/dL (70 g/L), mean corpuscular volume is 82 mcm^3 (82 fL), and platelet count is 300 × 10^3/mcL (300 × 10^9/L). Coagulation studies reveal a prothrombin time (PT) of more than 212 seconds (reference range, 10–12.9 seconds) and activated partial thromboplastin time (APTT) of more than 212 seconds (reference range, 26–36 seconds). Both values correct with 1:1 mixing with normal serum. Fibrinogen level is 0.25 g/dL 7.4 mcmol/L) (reference range, 0.19–0.39 g/dL [5.6–11.5 mcmol/L]). Clotting factor quantification is as follows: factor II activity, 4% (0.4) (reference range, 83%–117% [0.83–1.17]); factor V activity, 107% (1.07) (reference range, 50%–150% [0.5–1.5]); factor VII activity, less than 2% (0.2) (reference range, 65%–135% [0.65–1.35]); and factor X activity, 4% (0.4) (reference range, 45%–155% [0.45–1.55]). The serum warfarin level is below limits for detection (<1 mcg/mL [3.24 mcmol/L]).

Fresh frozen plasma (FFP) and intravenous vitamin K are administered, and the bleeding ceases. By the next morning, however, the nasal packing and drip pad are saturated. An additional test reveals the diagnosis.

- **What is your differential diagnosis at this point?**
- **Are there any elements of history or physical examination that would help you?**
- **What additional diagnostic studies would you like performed?**

Discussion

Causes for prolonged bleeding within the setting of a prolonged PT and APTT include vascular malformations with inherent consumptive coagulopathy, liver disease with decreased hepatic synthetic function, and vitamin K deficiency. Although vascular malformations can present as epistaxis, severe or prolonged bleeding within this setting is most often due to disseminated intravascular coagulation and platelet consumption. This condition seemed unlikely, given this patient's normal platelet count and fibrinogen level. Although platelet function defects and bleeding have also been observed in liver disease, a hallmark of liver disease is decreased synthesis of factors V, VII, and fibrinogen. Given the boy's normal factor V and fibrinogen findings, liver disease also seemed an unlikely cause.

Vitamin K deficiency should be suspected in any instance of acquired bleeding tendency that involves prolonged PT and APTT and a normal platelet count. Vitamin K deficiency often results from a malabsorption syndrome. Frequently, there are physical clues to this disorder, such as delayed growth, skin findings, or a history of loose stools. Vitamin K deficiency also occurs in association with antibiotic, salicylate, and anticonvulsant therapy. Treatment with parenteral vitamin K usually results in normalization of the PT within 4 to 8 hours and concomitant resolution of the bleeding, adding an important diagnostic clue. This patient's markedly decreased vitamin K–dependent clotting factors, which normalized on 1:1 mixing with normal serum, strongly supported the diagnosis of vitamin K deficiency.

The persistent nature of this boy's epistaxis, despite treatment with FFP and parenteral vitamin K, suggested an ongoing depletion of vitamin K stores or disruption of activation of vitamin K–dependent clotting factors (factors II, VII, IX, and X), effects that suggest warfarin exposure. Although a thorough search of the patient's environment failed to discover warfarin, the boy's serum tested positive for brodifacoum.

The boy later admitted to eating rat poison surreptitiously over a number of weeks that he had found in the basement of his home. The boy's incredulous mother attributed the rat poison ingestion to the boy's longstanding diagnosis of conduct disorder.

The Condition

Brodifacoum is a long-acting anticoagulant commonly found in mouse and rat poisons, with thousands of ingestions being reported to United States poison control centers each year. Although asymptomatic ingestions by children represent most exposures, repeated, large, or prolonged exposures to brodifacoum can result in major morbidity and death. Brodifacoum, like warfarin, exerts its anticoagulant effect by inhibiting the enzyme 2,3-epoxide reductase. Brodifacoum is much more potent than warfarin, is highly soluble in lipids, and is eliminated from the body slowly. Vitamin K_1 stores decline rapidly, resulting in decreased gamma-carboxylation and decreased activation of the vitamin K–dependent clotting factors. Because the half-life of brodifacoum is very long (at least 24.2 days), vitamin K deficiency and the abnormal PT may persist or recur following initial therapy.

Treatment and Prognosis

It is uncommon for a single unintentional ingestion of brodifacoum by a child to result in coagulopathy and bleeding, suggesting that most children ingesting the poison once can be monitored for signs of bleeding as outpatients and without laboratory evaluation. Fresh frozen plasma and parenteral vitamin K are the mainstays of treatment when bleeding occurs. With cessation of bleeding and normalization of the PT, oral vitamin K therapy can be substituted for parenteral vitamin K. The length of treatment can vary from days to months. Factor VII has the shortest half-life of the vitamin K–dependent factors (3–5 hours), making it a useful parameter to monitor when determining how long vitamin K administration is necessary.

Lessons for the Physician

Vitamin K deficiency is a common cause of coagulopathy and should be considered in children who present with bleeding. The diagnosis of vitamin K deficiency is usually not difficult to establish, but identification and treatment of the underlying cause may be challenging. For vitamin K–deficient children who present with bleeding, administration of fresh frozen plasma and parenteral vitamin K usually corrects the coagulopathy and stops the bleeding within a few hours. For those who do not respond, the physician must consider unusual causes of vitamin K deficiency, including exposure to long-acting anticoagulants.

MaryEllen Cavalier, MD, James Whitcomb, Riley Hospital for Children, Indianapolis, IN

CHAPTER 48

Fever and Changes in Mental Status in a 12-Year-Old Girl

Presentation

A 12-year-old girl is brought to the emergency department because of changes in mental status and fever. She was well until 4 days ago, when she complained of general malaise and had tactile fever. Last night, her condition worsened; she became lethargic and disoriented. The patient was having her menstrual period, which was expected.

On physical examination, the patient is lethargic, disoriented, and combative. She is extremely obese, weighing 175 kg, with a height of 155 cm, a temperature of 103.9°F (39.9°C), blood pressure of 90/60 mm Hg, and pulse of 110 beats/min. There are no skin rashes. Her fundi are normal, there are no meningeal signs, and respiratory and cardiovascular examinations reveal no abnormalities. Pelvic evaluation shows only minor bleeding.

Laboratory studies show hemoglobin, 7.0 g/dL (70 g/L); platelet count, 20×10^3/mcL (20×10^9/L), and reticulocyte count, 4.0% (0.040). The urea nitrogen level is 80 mg/dL (28.6 mmol/L), and the serum creatinine level is 3.0 mg/dL (265.2 mcmol/L). Both a direct Coombs test and antinuclear antibody determination give negative results. Findings on chest radiography and abdominal ultrasonography are normal. The results of additional blood tests lead to the diagnosis.

- **What is your differential diagnosis at this point?**
- **Are there any elements of history or physical examination that would help you?**
- **What additional diagnostic studies would you like performed?**

Discussion

A serum lactate dehydrogenase level was 700 U/L (11.7 mckat/L). A peripheral blood smear showed schistocytes, helmet cells, and a few spherocytes. These findings established the diagnosis of thrombotic thrombocytopenic purpura (TTP).

The Condition

Thrombotic thrombocytopenic purpura is a rare syndrome (3.7 cases/1,000,000 population) characterized by the pentad of thrombocytopenia, microangiopathic hemolytic anemia, fever, renal dysfunction, and neurologic abnormalities. All of these clinical features may not be noted at the time of presentation. Thrombotic thrombocytopenic purpura occurs most commonly in individuals between the ages of 10 and 40 years, with a peak occurrence during the second decade of life. Single-episode and intermittent TTP are seen most commonly in adults; chronic TTP is seen in children, but the incidence is extremely low.

Pathophysiology

Thrombotic thrombocytopenic purpura appears to be related to a deficiency of a metalloproteinase enzyme responsible for cleaving to von Willebrand factor (vWf). In normal plasma, the enzyme cleaves the peptide bond between tyrosine and methionine in positions 842 and 843, respectively, creating monomeric subunits of vWf, hence degrading large vWf multimers. During acute TTP episodes, patients have little or no vWf-cleaving metalloproteinase activity. Because one of the functions of vWf is to allow platelet aggregation, inadequate degradation of vWf leads to the major problem of platelet aggregation. Chronic TTP is believed to be caused by congenital deficiency of the vWf metalloproteinase; intermittent or single-episode TTP results from the action of autoantibodies against the enzyme that are present intermittently or transiently in affected patients.

Although TTP has been reported to occur in association with systemic lupus erythematosus, rheumatoid arthritis, polyarteritis, Sjögren syndrome, pregnancy, and carcinoma after chemotherapy, the disorder occurs in the absence of any other systemic disease.

Differential Diagnosis

The diagnosis of TTP is supported by microangiopathic findings (schistocytes, spherocytes, helmet cells) on the peripheral blood smear, elevation of the reticulocyte count and serum lactate dehydrogenase level, and the absence of laboratory evidence of a consumptive coagulopathy, as is seen in disseminated intravascular coagulopathy (prolonged prothrombin time and partial thromboplastin time, elevation of fibrin split product levels and fibrin time, hypofibrinogenemia, decreased factors V and VIII levels, fast fibrinogen turnover). Disseminated intravascular coagulopathy may accompany TTP, complicating the picture.

Hemolytic uremic syndrome is a closely related disorder that involves a microangiopathic hemolytic anemia along with renal failure, which is the predominant manifestation. Most cases are associated with diarrhea, often caused by an enterohemorrhagic strain of *Escherichia coli* (O157:H7). The bacterium elaborates a verotoxin (a cytotoxin that injures the endothelium and is so named because it affects Vero kidney cell cultures). Neurologic involvement is not a consistent feature, as it is in TTP, but seizures occur in some patients. Evans syndrome and malignant hypertension may also present with renal failure, microangiopathy, and encephalopathy. A distinction among these conditions must be made. Evans syndrome is the simultaneous or sequential occurrence of direct Coombs test–positive autoimmune hemolytic anemia and idiopathic thrombocytopenia. Significant elevation in the arterial blood pressure is the primary presenting feature of malignant hypertension.

Reticulocytosis and elevated, indirect bilirubin level are seen in most patients who have TTP. The reticulocyte count of 4.0% (0.040) in this patient seems low for a person who has a hemoglobin level of 7.0 g/dL (70 g/L), but it was recorded early in the course and might be ascending. Also, an antecedent viral infection can depress the marrow response. The markedly elevated serum lactate dehydrogenase level may be used as an indicator for therapy. The platelet count has a wide range, but invariably it is low in affected patients. Anemia is always present, and microangiopathic changes can be seen in the peripheral blood smear. The demonstration of characteristic microvascular occlusions in biopsies of skin, gingiva, or other tissues lends further support but is not required to make a presumptive diagnosis and initiate therapy. The direct Coombs test is rarely positive, and the prothrombin time and partial thromboplastin time usually are normal or prolonged only slightly. The use of an assay of vWf-cleaving protease may help in making the diagnosis.

Therapy

Thrombotic thrombocytopenic purpura should be considered a medical emergency, and therapy should be instituted promptly because of the high mortality associated with the condition. Treatment is largely empiric. The cornerstone is administration of fresh frozen plasma (FFP). Plasmapheresis that uses FFP as replacement fluid for total plasma exchange is performed daily. If plasmapheresis is not available, FFP should be administered intravenously every 6 to 8 hours. The extent to which administration of plasma can be repeated is limited by the protein load, expansion of intravascular volume, and heart failure. Plasma therapy should continue until neurologic restoration and normalization of serum lactate dehydrogenase and platelet count occur.

Treatment of the anemia requires transfusions of packed red blood cells. Platelet transfusion should be avoided, unless it is essential to control bleeding, because it may accelerate thrombosis. Adding antiplatelet medications (eg, aspirin, dipyridamole) and steroids (eg, prednisone, methylprednisolone) has been reported to be useful. Relapses are common and may occur even years after the initial presentation. Relapsing and refractory cases may benefit from the use of immunoglobulin for 5 days, vincristine once a week, or "cryopoor" plasma (plasma from which cryoprecipitate has been removed) as the replacement fluid for plasmapheresis. Splenectomy is controversial and should be considered only as a last resort.

The patient in this case was treated initially with FFP, followed by daily plasmapheresis until her neurologic symptoms improved and the lactate dehydrogenase level decreased. She was discharged from the hospital on antiplatelet medications.

Edwin Rodríguez-Cruz, MD; Rosa M. Cintrón-Maldonado, MD; and Elizabeth Contreras, MD, Henry Ford Hospital, Detroit, MI

PEDIATRICS IN REVIEW EDITOR'S NOTE

Thrombotic thrombocytopenic purpura and hemolytic uremic syndrome (HUS) share so many clinical features that some authors discuss them as thrombotic thrombocytopenic purpura-HUS syndrome. Thrombotic thrombocytopenic purpura usually affects older individuals and has more consistent neurologic involvement than HUS. Microangiopathic hemolytic anemia occurs when conditions in capillaries, including endothelial damage and the presence of fibrin strands, lead to shearing and destruction of red blood cells. Schistocytes, burr cells, and helmet cells are examples of the damaged cells. Because mechanical erythrocyte damage can occur in larger vessels, as when there is an exposed portion of a synthetic heart valve, some authors prefer to use the more inclusive terms of *fragmentation* or *vascular hemolytic anemia.*—LFN

COMMENTARY BY DR MICHAEL CALLAGHAN, HEMATOLOGIST/ONCOLOGIST, CHILDREN'S HOSPITAL OF MICHIGAN

At the time this case was published, the pathophysiology of thrombotic thrombocytopenic purpura (TTP) was coming into greater focus. The case report describes a metalloproteinase enzyme responsible for cleavage of von Willebrand factor multimers. Our current understanding of the thrombotic microangiopathies has benefited from an understanding of the role of this protein, now called ADAMTS-13, in the development of microangiopathy. Upshaw and Schulman independently described patients with congenital TTP which have subsequently been determined to result from autosomal recessive deficiency of ADAMTS-13. Other thrombotic microangiopathies have been described in the setting of congenital or acquired deficiencies of complement proteins (CFH, CFI, CFB, C3, and CD46) as well as deficiencies of thrombomodulin and mutations in diacylglycerol kinase, epsilon (*DKGE*), or methylmalonic aciduria and homocystinuria type cblC (*MMACHC*) genes. These have in common uncontrolled activity of complement, vascular injury, or uncontrolled von Willebrand factor activity. In the time since this case was reported this new understanding of the pathophysiology of thrombotic microangiopathies has lead to diagnostic and clinical tools that have improved our ability to accurately diagnose and treat these disorders. Importantly for the case described, measurement of ADAMTS-13 levels assist in accurate diagnosis of TTP and anti-ADAMTS-13 antibody testing correctly categorizes congenital versus acquired TTP. Acquired TTP should be managed initially with plasmapheresis to remove these antibodies and replenish ADAMTS-13 by plasma infusion. This is done in parallel with immunosuppression to stop formation of new antibodies. First-line immunosuppression is most often accomplished with corticosteroids with anti-CD20 humanized monoclonal antibodies added for refractory cases, although many physicians choose to use anti-CD20 therapy up front.

CHAPTER 49

13-Year-Old Boy With a Lump on His Back

Presentation

A 13-year-old boy was noted to have a lump on his back when his father was hugging him 2 weeks ago. The lump is about the size of a small fist, is located below the right scapula, and has caused no pain. It has been enlarging slowly. The boy feels well and denies fever, weight loss, other lumps, or trauma to the area.

On physical examination, the boy is awake, alert, and in no distress. His vital signs are within reference range. There is a poorly defined, fixed mass, measuring 8 × 10 cm, without induration or erythema, at the level of the eighth rib on the right side of his back. His lungs are clear bilaterally. No lymphadenopathy is noted. Normal laboratory results are reported for complete blood cell count, basic chemistry panel (including calcium), erythrocyte sedimentation rate, lactic acid dehydrogenase, uric acid, and liver function tests. Radiography of the chest confirms the presence of a mass. An additional study reveals the diagnosis.

- **What is your differential diagnosis at this point?**
- **Are there any elements of history or physical examination that would help you?**
- **What additional diagnostic studies would you like performed?**

Discussion

The rapidly enlarging mass on this boy's back raised concern for a neoplastic lesion of bone or soft tissue. The differential diagnosis included neuroblastoma, non–Hodgkin lymphoma, osteosarcoma, Ewing sarcoma, rhabdomyosarcoma, lipoma, malignant fibrous histiocytoma, osteomyelitis, and benign tumors of bone.

Computed tomography of the chest revealed the mass to be emerging from, or infiltrating, the right eighth rib (Figure 49.1).

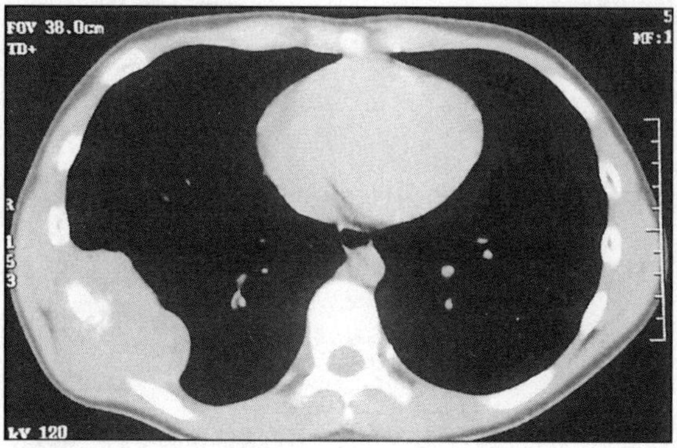

Figure 49.1. Computed tomography scan showing a mass that is emerging from, or infiltrating, the right eighth rib.

Biopsy of the lesion and a bone marrow aspirate were performed. Pathologic analysis revealed a tumor of the "small, round, blue cell" group, a group of disorders that includes rhabdomyosarcoma, neuroblastoma, Ewing sarcoma, and primitive neuroectodermal tumor (PNET). Further studies indicated a PNET, a tumor classified as part of the Ewing sarcoma family. Both PNETs and Ewing tumors are believed to be of neural crest origin and typically demonstrate the t(11;22) translocation. This patient's tumor also stained positively for CD99 (MIC2) and neuron-specific enolase. These results were consistent with the diagnosis of PNET. A thoracopulmonary PNET is called an Askin tumor.

The boy underwent a bone scan and bone marrow biopsy. These evaluations, in addition to computed tomography, failed to reveal metastases to the lungs or bone marrow. He began systemic chemotherapy to reduce the size of the tumor, and a cardiothoracic surgeon was consulted to discuss surgical resection.

Epidemiology

Tumors of the bone are relatively rare in children and adolescents. Approximately 50% of these tumors are malignant. Malignant bone tumors in children comprise approximately 6% of childhood cancers. Of bone tumors in children and adolescents, 90% are either osteosarcomas or tumors in the Ewing sarcoma family.

Osteosarcomas are about equally prevalent in African American and Caucasian patients, but Ewing sarcomas are very rare in African Americans. The incidence of bone tumors peaks during adolescence, somewhat earlier in girls than in boys. This timing is most likely associated with the adolescent growth spurt.

Clinical Features

Osteosarcomas represent the most common childhood bone tumors. They typically arise from the metaphyses of the long bones, especially those of the lower extremities. Patients may present with chronic or intermittent pain in the affected knee, leg, or arm. The affected area is often edematous and tender. The classic sunburst pattern on radiography suggests this tumor. The serum alkaline phosphatase level may be elevated.

In contrast to osteosarcomas, tumors of the Ewing family most commonly arise in the bones of the central axis, as in this case. Primitive neuroectodermal tumors represent close relatives of Ewing sarcomas, distinguished by only the degree of cellular differentiation. Ewing sarcomas typically arise in bony structures; PNETs generally arise in soft tissues such as central nervous system tissue, although either tumor may emerge from either tissue.

This patient's presentation was somewhat unusual in that he had no pain, despite having a palpable mass. Patients with Ewing sarcoma or PNET typically present with palpable, painful masses. The PNET tumor may occur in the vertebrae, ribs, or surrounding soft tissues. Pathologic fractures may occur. Metastatic disease may cause systemic symptoms such as fever, weight loss, focal pulmonary findings, or leukemialike symptoms if the bone marrow is involved. Neurologic impairment may reflect involvement of spinal nerves.

Therapy and Prognosis

Therapy for patients who have bone tumors typically involves a multifaceted approach, including radiotherapy, surgery, and systemic chemotherapy. Bone tumors involving a limb historically required amputation, but today most patients undergo a limb-sparing procedure, usually with insertion of a stabilizing rod. Radiotherapy or chemotherapy may be performed prior to surgery to reduce tumor burden and possibly prevent metastasis.

Ongoing evaluation of patients who have bone tumors includes close radiographic surveillance for recurrence of the tumor or metastases while the patient is receiving chemotherapy. Bone marrow support and management of fever, neutropenia, or drug toxicity are critical.

The patient's prognosis depends on a number of factors, including the presence or absence of metastatic disease, age (younger patients have a better prognosis), and sex (females generally fare better than males). Five-year survival rates for patients having osteosarcomas and tumors of the Ewing family in one recent series were 63% and 58%, respectively.

Lessons for the Physician

A rapidly enlarging mass can be a neoplastic lesion, regardless of its location. Tenderness or erythema in the region of the knee or long bones, especially in a young adolescent, suggests the possibility of osteosarcoma and should prompt at least a radiograph. Similar findings in the chest or back may indicate Ewing sarcoma or primitive neuroectodermal tumor and are especially concerning in the presence of systemic or neurologic symptoms or signs. Prompt diagnosis is critical because metastatic disease may affect the prognosis adversely and profoundly.

David I. Rappaport, MD, and Jay Greenberg, MD, INOVA Fairfax Hospital for Children, Falls Church, VA

COMMENTARY BY JOANNE WANG, MD, CHILDREN'S HOSPITAL OF MICHIGAN

Peripheral primitive neuroectodermal tumor and Ewing sarcoma (EWS) share molecular and morphologic features and are now regarded as essentially the same entity and referred to simply as Ewing sarcoma. Progress has been made in the diagnosis and treatment of Ewing sarcoma over last decade. It is known that the chromosomal translocation involving the EWS, which is readily detected by conventional cytogenetic methods or fluorescent in situ hybridization techniques, is essential for oncogenesis. Fluorodeoxyglucose positron emission tomography-computed tomography has now been widely used in staging and assessing response to initial chemotherapy, which has been shown to be the most important prognostic factor. Treatment still includes chemotherapy to help shrink the tumor followed by local control with surgical resection or radiotherapy if a negative margin cannot be achieved. In addition, administering the chemotherapy at a shorter interval has further improved the outcome for patients with nonmetastatic Ewing sarcoma, with an expected survival rate greater than 70%. However, no more than 30% of patients with metastatic Ewing sarcoma are long-term survivors. Many new targeting agents, such as antibodies targeting the insulinlike growth factor receptor-1, are being tested in clinical trials, which may prove to be effective in the treatment of EWS.

CHAPTER 50

Epistaxis in a 15-Year-Old Boy

Presentation

A 15-year-old boy is seen because of a "massive nosebleed" that occurred earlier today but has stopped. He has had a runny nose for months, with green discharge at times, and for 1 month has experienced headaches and orbital pain. Five days ago, at another institution, facial radiographs were obtained and sinusitis was diagnosed, for which he was given amoxicillin. There is no history of trauma, blood dyscrasia, allergic rhinitis, or use of nasal sprays.

The boy's blood pressure is 105/74 mm Hg, and the rest of his vital signs also are within reference range. There is tenderness on deep palpation of the right infraorbital area. Examination of the nasal passages reveals blood clots on the right side but no prominent vessels in the anterior septum. The septum is deviated mildly to the left. Cranial nerve function is intact. No cervical masses or adenopathy are noted. The remainder of his physical findings are normal. Continuation of the antibiotic course is recommended.

Eight days later, the boy experiences right-sided epistaxis during sleep. In the emergency department, a posterior pack is placed. The procedure is painful for the patient and extremely difficult and time consuming for the physician. Complete blood cell count, prothrombin time, and partial thromboplastin time are normal. An otorhinolaryngologist is consulted, who notes a posterior nasal mass. A radiologic study provides the diagnosis.

- **What is your differential diagnosis at this point?**
- **Are there any elements of history or physical examination that would help you?**
- **What additional diagnostic studies would you like performed?**

Discussion

Computed tomography showed a mass filling the right nasopharynx, causing destruction of the right cribriform plate and extending into the right ethmoid and sphenoid sinuses; the floor of the sphenoid sinus was destroyed as well. Sinusitis was also identified in the left maxillary and right frontal sinuses. Angiography revealed a tumor blush in the right nasopharynx in an area supplied by the internal maxillary artery. No further tumor blush was identified after embolization was performed. A few days later, the patient underwent resection of the mass, which was found to be a nasopharyngeal angiofibroma.

A Variety of Causes

Bleeding from the nose is a common occurrence in childhood and adolescence, emanating more than 90% of the time from the anterior inferior septal region (Kiesselbach area). The terminal arterioles in the plexus under the mucous membrane bleed easily after being traumatized by nasal or facial trauma, nose picking, excessive drying, sneezing, blowing of the nose, upper respiratory tract infection, allergic rhinitis, or chemical irritation.

The diagnosis is usually made easily by inspection of the anterior nasal septum, which reveals prominent blood vessels. Posterior epistaxis cannot be seen on a thorough anterior examination; the bleeding comes from the larger nasal branches of the internal maxillary artery or from the ethmoidal arteries.

Epistaxis has been reported to occur in systemic illnesses such as sickle cell anemia, leukemia, hemorrhagic disorders (only 3% of patients who have epistaxis), and hypertension. Various infectious disorders have been associated with epistaxis, including sinusitis, nasal diphtheria, and infectious mononucleosis. Epistaxis has occurred in patients who have rheumatic fever. Use of anticoagulant medications such as aspirin can be a cause. Hemangioma should be considered, especially in the young infant. Rendu-Osler-Weber syndrome (hereditary hemorrhagic telangiectasia) should be suspected in the presence of small telangiectasias throughout the nasal mucosa, oral mucosa, and face.

A foreign body should be sought, especially in chronic or recurrent epistaxis. An ulcer or perforated septum may cause chronic nasal bleeding. Such a condition should raise the suspicion of cocaine use.

Bleeding caused by a nasal fracture can begin at any site, but most often it is seen in the nasal roof, coming from the ethmoidal vessels. Fractures may be responsible for persistent bleeding.

Tumors are rare causes of epistaxis. Polyps may cause bleeding and lead to a diagnosis of cystic fibrosis. An olfactory neuroepithelial tumor causes recurrent epistaxis, nasal congestion, and olfactory dysfunction. Nasopharyngeal lymphoepithelioma causes trismus, torticollis, and unilateral tender cervical lymphadenopathy in addition to epistaxis. Lymphoma, rhabdomyosarcoma, and sarcomas of the bone can cause nasal bleeding if they invade and destroy the nasal vault.

Juvenile nasopharyngeal angiofibroma develops almost exclusively in pubertal boys and is an androgen hormone–dependent tumor. It causes progressive nasal obstruction, nasal discharge, and recurrent copious epistaxis due to its marked vascularity. This histologically benign growth arises from the fibrocartilaginous tissue overlying the upper cervical vertebrae and the area around the sphenopalatine foramen. It manifests clinically as a reddish brown, smooth mass that invades the nose, temporalis region, or cheek. The tumor is usually not seen in the anterior nasal passages, but it can become visible in the posterior nasal cavity as a result of its growth from the nasopharynx. Bulging of the soft palate may be felt on the ipsilateral side. The compression of cranial nerves may result in neurologic symptoms, the most typical being facial pain or numbness due to trigeminal injury.

Treatment

Because most epistaxes are anterior and located in the Kiesselbach area, they stop after adequate nasal compression. Moistening agents such as petroleum jelly or cautery with silver nitrate can be used. If control is not gained or if recurrence is a problem, an anterior pack is inserted. Traumatizing agents such as nasal sprays should be discontinued.

In posttraumatic epistaxis, bleeding usually stops spontaneously within several minutes. When resolution occurs and there is no cosmetic deformity, no immediate treatment is indicated, but the patient should be reexamined in a few days to be sure the airway is adequate and to rule out the development of a septal hematoma. Nasal fractures that cause no cosmetic damage may be responsible for persistent epistaxis; impacted nasal bones may need to be disimpacted to stop the bleeding.

Persistent posterior epistaxis requires the placement of a posterior pack; a referral usually is indicated for this purpose.

When present, any underlying hemorrhagic, infectious, vascular, or neoplastic disorder should be managed appropriately.

The treatment of juvenile nasopharyngeal angiofibroma is surgical resection after embolization of the tumor to control bleeding. Embolization is accomplished by using a catheter that is introduced into the femoral artery and advanced as near as possible to the vessels that supply the angiofibroma. A contrast agent is injected to identify the appropriate vessels, following which an embolizing material is injected. In this case, the agent used was polyvinyl alcohol, a spongy substance made of microparticulate material. Contrast and embolizing material are injected alternately to guide the procedure and to indicate when the desired obliteration has occurred.

Lessons for the Physician

- Although epistaxis is extremely common and unlikely to portend a serious disorder, the nasal passages should be examined carefully in every case of epistaxis, especially in an adolescent boy. When the results of the examination do not reveal a cause and the bleeding is recurrent or profuse, as in this case, the posterior portion of the nose should be inspected carefully by a specialist.
- The presence of an angiofibroma should be suspected when there is a history of nasal obstruction and profuse epistaxis in combination with a neurologic sign that could be due to tumor invasion, such as facial pain or numbness. This adolescent had intact cranial nerve function, and his facial pain was attributed initially to his sinusitis. This situation reminds us again that 2 conditions can exist simultaneously.
- In general, if a child or adolescent who has not sustained a fracture and has no other obvious cause for the epistaxis requires a posterior pack, the physician must consider unusual causes. If the bleeding is profuse, juvenile nasopharyngeal angiofibroma is at the top of the list in this age group. This boy required placement of a posterior nasal pack. Although this procedure always is hard to perform and uncomfortable for the patient, its extreme difficulty in this case made the emergency department physician suspect that the nasal passage might be obstructed. The possibility of nasal obstruction in association with normal results on an anterior examination, profuse posterior bleeding, and a neurologic symptom should prompt consultation with an otorhinolaryngologist.

N. Zvi Avigdor, MD, St. Vincent's Catholic Medical Centers, Brooklyn, NY

CHAPTER 51

Acute Shortness of Breath and Coughing Up Blood in a 16-Year-Old Girl

Presentation

A 16-year-old girl comes to the emergency department because of acute shortness of breath and "coughing up a cup of blood." She has been diagnosed as having asthma and uses bronchodilators as needed. Over the past 7 months, her cough and wheezing episodes have increased, and she has produced blood-streaked sputum but has not sought care. She denies any fevers, weight loss, lethargy, decreased appetite, unusual travel, or major illness.

On physical examination, she is uncomfortable and is breathing at 35 breaths/min but without respiratory distress. Her temperature is 98.5°F (36.9°C), heart rate is 96 beats/min, blood pressure is 129/66 mm Hg, and oxygen saturation is 95% by pulse oximetry. Breath sounds over the right hemithorax are diminished, but no retractions, wheezing, or crackles are noted. The remaining physical findings are normal.

Her hemoglobin concentration is 14.1 g/dL (141 g/L), white blood cell count is 14.6×10^3/mcL (14.6×10^9/L) (90% neutrophils, 5% lymphocytes, 5% monocytes), and platelet count is 183×10^3/mcL (183×10^9/L). Coagulation study results, serum electrolyte measurements, and liver enzyme values are normal. A chest radiograph reveals complete opacification of the right lung and the presence of a convex density in the right mainstem bronchus. A computed tomography scan of the chest demonstrates a mass in the right mainstem bronchus resulting in extensive atelectasis. A tuberculin test is applied and sputum, obtained for cell count, Gram stain, and culture. Ceftriaxone therapy is initiated.

Bronchoscopy is performed, and tissue specimens from the mass reveal the diagnosis.

- **What is your differential diagnosis at this point?**
- **Are there any elements of history or physical examination that would help you?**
- **What additional diagnostic studies would you like performed?**

Discussion

This girl had a bronchial carcinoid tumor presenting with hemoptysis and collapse of her right lung.

The Sign

Hemoptysis—the spitting of blood—is a rare sign in children and adolescents and can range from a small amount of blood-streaked sputum to a fatal hemorrhage causing asphyxiation. It is difficult to ascertain whether the blood is produced in the lungs, bronchi, upper airway, pharynx, or other areas of the gastrointestinal tract.

The differential diagnosis of hemoptysis is extensive and includes infectious causes, foreign bodies, congenital defects, congenital heart disease, vasculitis, cystic fibrosis, pulmonary embolus, coagulopathy, arteriovenous malformations, and autoimmune diseases. On rare occasions, the production of blood can be factitious. For neonates up to 30 days after birth, likely causes are hemorrhagic disorder, sepsis, cardiopulmonary malformations, and bacterial pneumonia. Infants between the ages of 1 and 12 months may have pulmonary hemosiderosis, pneumonia, cardiopulmonary malformations such as bronchogenic cyst and arteriovenous malformation, and tumors.

The initial evaluation of hemoptysis should include a thorough history and physical examination. It is important to inquire about the possibility of aspiration because foreign bodies (especially vegetable matter) or caustic agents may lead to pulmonary or esophageal bleeding. The history may reveal a previous bleeding diathesis. Hemoptysis with no other findings than intermittent respiratory symptoms is seen in the pulmonary hemorrhage syndromes and in children and adolescents who have unrecognized vascular malformations.

Dyspnea and cough are common in patients who have hemoptysis caused by lower respiratory tract bleeding. Pulmonary hemorrhage may lead to altered air exchange and crackles (coarse or fine), often with wheezing in the affected areas. Signs and symptoms of infection should be sought because infectious processes can cause pulmonary bleeding.

Radiography of the chest may localize the disease, and a computed tomography scan may define bronchiectasis or malformations. Bronchoscopy is useful for localizing the bleeding and sampling the lower airway for blood and blood products. In very rare cases, thoracotomy and open lung biopsy may be the only methods to diagnose the cause of bleeding. Urinalysis and measurements of serum creatinine and urea nitrogen can reveal signs of renal involvement.

Many of the more common causes of hemoptysis could be excluded by the duration of symptoms experienced by this patient. Her long-standing history of cough and hemoptysis and the absence of additional symptoms suggested an uncommon cause. The presence of an opacity in the right mainstem bronchus suggested a pulmonary tumor in the airway as the source of bleeding.

The Underlying Condition

Pulmonary tumors are a rare cause of hemoptysis in the pediatric and adolescent population. Primary benign and malignant tumors are unusual, with most malignant tumors being metastases. Bronchial carcinoid tumors are the most common primary malignant lung tumor in children and tend to arise in the perihilar region.

Carcinoid tumors are rare neuroendocrine tumors, occurring most often in the gastrointestinal tract, particularly the appendix. In the lung, they arise from the basal layer of the bronchial epithelium and usually present in the fifth decade of life but have been described in pediatric patients. These tumors can be associated with systemic symptoms due to the release of a variety of hormones such as insulin, gastrin, serotonin, vasoactive intestinal peptide, or histamine. The release of serotonin into the systemic circulation is thought to cause the carcinoid syndrome, which consists of episodic flushing, wheezing, and diarrhea. This constellation of signs and symptoms suggests a carcinoid tumor. This patient had elevated urinary levels of 5-hydroxyindoleacetic acid, a metabolite of serotonin, but did not experience symptoms associated with elevated serotonin levels.

Clinical Features

Patients who have pulmonary carcinoid tumors may present with recurrent pneumonia, cough, hemoptysis, wheezing, asthma, or chest pain. This patient experienced several of these symptoms, including those associated with an acute lung collapse. Carcinoid syndrome is noted in less than 1% of patients who have carcinoid tumors and was not present in this patient.

Diagnosis

Once a carcinoid tumor is diagnosed on the basis of histologic features, it is important to determine the extent of tumor spread. When metastasis occurs, it usually develops in mediastinal lymph nodes, liver, bone, or skin. An octreotide scan in this patient revealed focal uptake in the right mainstem area without metastasis. Octreotide is a somatostatin analog that binds somatostatin receptors. These receptors are present in some malignancies, including most bronchial carcinoids.

Treatment and Prognosis

Conservative resection is the preferred treatment for localized pulmonary carcinoid tumors. Survival rates of greater than 90% are achieved by patients who have focal disease and typical histologic features of carcinoid tumor. No lymph node involvement was noted on microscopic examination of surgical specimens in this patient, and the carcinoid tumor appeared to be localized to the right mainstem bronchus. She did well immediately following a right pneumonectomy and has had an uneventful postoperative course.

Lessons for the Physician

True hemoptysis is encountered infrequently in children and adolescents and warrants further evaluation of the lower respiratory tract. Pulmonary tumors, although rare, should be considered in the evaluation of hemoptysis because a delay in diagnosis and treatment can influence the prognosis.

Mark Puczynski, MD; Rama Jasty, MD; and Nizar Kheralla, MD, Medical College of Ohio, Toledo, OH

CHAPTER 52

Abdominal Pain in a 16-Year-Old Girl

Presentation

A 16-year-old girl is seen in the emergency department because of abdominal pain of 4 days' duration. An abdominal radiograph obtained by her physician on the first day had revealed stool throughout the colon, and she was instructed to increase fluid and fiber intake.

The pain has worsened and is constant and cramping, with radiation to the pelvis. She has no other symptoms, and her past history is significant only for taking oral contraceptive pills (OCPs) for 3 months. Her last menstrual period was 2 weeks ago. A pelvic examination performed 3 months ago yielded normal results, including negative cervical cultures for *Chlamydia* and *Gonococcus.* She is sexually active in a monogamous relationship. The family history is significant for colon cancer in a grandmother.

Physical examination reveals tenderness to palpation in the left lower quadrant and suprapubic regions of the abdomen. No other abnormalities are appreciated. In the radiology suite, awaiting pelvic ultrasonography, the patient is noted to have swelling of her left thigh area, and she comments, "My thigh is even bigger and redder than earlier!" Additional studies are performed.

- **What is your differential diagnosis at this point?**
- **Are there any elements of history or physical examination that would help you?**
- **What additional diagnostic studies would you like performed?**

Discussion

In addition to pelvic ultrasonography, which showed normal findings, Doppler ultrasonography of the left lower extremity was performed. The venous sonogram revealed thrombosis of the left common femoral vein extending to the left popliteal vein. The patient was diagnosed as having a deep venous thrombosis (DVT).

Laboratory test results included a normal complete blood cell count; negative urine pregnancy test; negative antinuclear, anticardiolipin, and anti–double-stranded DNA antibodies; negative tests for lupus anticoagulant and prothrombin mutation; and normal levels of serum homocysteine, antithrombin III, factor VIII, protein S, protein C, and von Willebrand factor. Additional testing revealed a genotype for heterozygosity for factor V Leiden deficiency.

Therapy with the anticoagulant low-molecular-weight heparin (enoxaparin) was initiated. After 5 days, the patient's symptoms resolved, physical therapy was initiated, and she was discharged from the hospital on 5 additional days of enoxaparin. She was started on warfarin on the last day of hospitalization, and outpatient follow-up with a pediatric hematologist was arranged.

Differential Diagnosis

The diagnosis of acute abdominal pain in an adolescent girl can be far from simple. The list of diagnoses related to the gastrointestinal and genitourinary systems alone is extensive. In this case, the patient's pain arose from a thrombosis of a deep vein that extended to the abdomen and not from a process within the abdomen itself. The manifestations of the more distal aspects of the thrombus, which was not causing symptoms in the leg, provided the diagnosis.

The clinical features of venous thrombosis in a deep vein of the leg include leg pain, tenderness, swelling, a palpable cord, discoloration, venous distention, prominence of the superficial veins, and cyanosis. Patients who are at higher risk for developing thromboses (those who have hypercoagulability) may not exhibit the typical clinical features, and the physician must be aggressive in obtaining appropriate imaging studies to confirm the diagnosis when a thrombosis is suspected.

Pulmonary emboli typically cause pleuritic chest pain, dyspnea, and hemoptysis. They may, however, manifest as abdominal or back pain or cause no symptoms. Pulmonary emboli originate from thrombi in the proximal deep veins of the leg in 90% or more of patients. Other, less common sources of pulmonary emboli include the deep pelvic veins, the renal veins, the inferior vena cava, the right ventricle, and the axillary veins. Pulmonary embolism occurs in 50% of patients who have documented proximal leg venous thrombosis. Usually only part of the thrombus embolizes, and 50% to 70% of patients who have pulmonary emboli documented by angiography have detectable DVT of the legs at the time of initial evaluation. The clinical significance of pulmonary embolism depends on the size of the embolus and the cardiorespiratory reserve of the patient.

A number of conditions can mimic venous thrombosis of the leg and include (in approximate order of frequency) muscle strain, direct twisting injury to the leg, cellulitis, lymphangitis and lymphatic obstruction, venous reflux, muscle tear,

Baker cyst, and reflex sympathetic dystrophy. Despite diagnostic measures, however, the cause of pain, tenderness, and swelling of the leg remains uncertain in a number of individuals.

Pathogenesis

Deep venous thrombosis is a common problem that, in many cases, is preventable. Based on current knowledge, at least 30% to 50% of affected individuals harbor an inherited thrombophilic defect.

Risk factors related to thrombosis include aging, immobilization longer than 3 days, pregnancy, major surgery in the past 4 weeks, trauma, vasculitis of any cause, intravenous drug use, sepsis, use of OCPs, and genetic predisposition (heritable defects of the hemostatic mechanism).

Oral contraceptive pills can increase the incidence of DVT by a factor of 10. Initially, this effect was believed to be due to alteration of the procoagulant and fibrinolytic system. However, more recent data suggest that the increased prevalence of thrombosis is due to the individual having a genetic predisposition because of an inherited defect of the hemostatic system.

Adolescent girls who have a genetic defect have a significantly increased prevalence of DVT when they take OCPs. Of these defects, the most common of the inherited disorders is the factor V Leiden mutation, which occurs in 2% to 10% of individuals who have a European background but is found in 20% to 40% of patients who experience thrombosis. The factor V mutation predicts the replacement of arginine 506 with a glutamine residue, which results in the loss of the ability of activated protein C to neutralize ongoing activation of the factor V molecule. The factor V mutation is found predominantly in Caucasians.

The second most common genetic risk factor for thrombosis (found in 6%–8% of patients who develop thrombi) is a single mutation (*G20210A*) in the 3′ untranslated region of the prothrombin gene. The mutation does not impair prothrombin function, but is associated with slightly increased concentrations of prothrombin in plasma, leading to a threefold to fivefold increase in the risk of forming a thrombosis. Heterozygous deficiency of protein C, protein S, or antithrombin III also increases the risk of thrombosis (present in 1%–3% of patients who have thrombosis), but these deficiencies are uncommon in the general population.

The antiphospholipid syndrome (lupus anticoagulant) is an acquired risk factor for thrombosis. This condition can persist and cause both arterial and venous thrombosis. Antibodies in the plasma of affected patients are directed against a protein-lipid complex. The antiphospholipid syndrome is associated with an increased risk of pregnancy-related complications, including miscarriage.

Other conditions associated with a predisposition toward thrombosis include hyperhomocysteinemia and dysfibrinogenemia.

Diagnosis

The signs and symptoms of thrombosis in any individual are related to the degree of obstruction and whether the thrombosis is arterial or venous. In addition, vessel wall inflammation may alter the clinical manifestations of the thrombosis. The patient may be asymptomatic or a variety of signs and symptoms can be present, including swelling, local pain, edema, cyanosis, and pain with dorsiflexion of the foot as well as tenderness, warmth, or erythema of the skin. Physical findings can include unilateral edema, localized tenderness of the lower extremity, calf pain on forced dorsiflexion of the foot (Homan sign), a reddish purple hue of the overlying skin, pallor of the extremity from arterial spasm, and low-grade fever.

The formation of a DVT in a patient who has been taking OCPs for a short time suggests the presence of a defect in coagulation and mandates laboratory investigation. At present, there are no simple laboratory screening tests to uncover such defects. Therefore, in the United States it has not proven cost effective to subject the patient to extensive testing before starting OCPs unless there is a strong family history of thrombotic disorders. A congenital hypercoagulable disorder is suggested by a strong family history of DVT or pulmonary embolism.

Clinical diagnosis with Doppler flow studies is adequate for establishing the diagnosis of DVT in the leg; further laboratory studies are not needed. Concern regarding pulmonary embolism may require the use of D-dimer and radiologic investigation (serial computed tomography of the chest).

The initial laboratory investigations needed to confirm an inherited thrombophilic state are listed in Box 52.1. Additional assays, such as platelet glycoprotein assay, may be required for the rarer group of inherited defects.

Box 52.1. Tests for Detecting a Hypercoagulable State

- Activated protein C resistance assay
  - Factor V Leiden mutation
  - Factor VI or VIII mutation
- Prothrombin 20210A mutation assay
- Protein C and protein S assays (activity and antigen)
- Antithrombin III assay (activity and antigen)
- Homocysteine level
- Lupus anticoagulant and anticardiolipin assays
- Clottable fibrinogen assay

Treatment

The goals of treatment are to reduce morbidity and to prevent pulmonary emboli. The regimen of choice is anticoagulation with low-molecular-weight heparin because of its better pharmacokinetic properties compared with unfractionated heparin and because it allows better hemostatic control with a single daily subcutaneous injection. After a few days of combined treatment with heparin and warfarin, the low-molecular-weight heparin is discontinued and warfarin is continued, generally for 3 to 6 months. The risk of bleeding complications must always be weighed against the benefits of anticoagulation, especially if an anticoagulant is used for longer than 6 months, at which point the risk of recurrent thrombosis has probably declined.

Lessons for the Physician

This case illustrates several important points. When evaluating an adolescent patient, it is important to ask about specific signs and symptoms because answers to general questions may omit important information. A complete physical examination is required, even when the complaints seem to center on a specific area of the body. Pediatricians must realize that even young people can experience deep venous thrombosis, with oral contraceptive pill use being an important risk factor.

Christine A. Rothermel, MD; Ulfat Shaikh, MD, MPH; and Jack Lazerson, MD, University of Nevada School of Medicine, Las Vegas, NV

COMMENTARY BY MEERA CHITLUR, MD, CHILDREN'S HOSPITAL OF MICHIGAN

Treatment of secondary venous thromboembolism in children/adolescents

Anticoagulation is typically administered for 3 months when the venous thromboembolism has occurred in association with a clinical risk factor that has subsequently resolved. If the thrombus is still present on imaging, at the end of 3 months, anticoagulation may be continued for a total of 6 months. In the presence of a persistent risk factor, anticoagulation may be continued for as long as the risk factor persists (eg, central venous line). The presence of an inherited thrombophilia does not change the duration of therapy. Acute anticoagulation typically consists of unfractionated heparin or low-molecular-weight heparin (initiated at 1 mg/kg subcutaneously, twice a day). Ongoing treatment may be low-molecular-weight heparin in children as it is easier to titrate (not affected by dietary changes) and needs to be monitored only once every 4 weeks once therapeutic levels are attained. Switching to vitamin K antagonists like warfarin may be considered if subcutaneous administration is a concern. Prolonging the duration of treatment beyond the 6 months in those with a transient risk factor that resolved has not been found to be beneficial.

CHAPTER 53

Painless, Intermittent Vaginal Spotting in a 16-Year-Old Girl

Presentation

A 16-year-old African American girl comes to the emergency department because of 1 week of painless, intermittent vaginal spotting without nausea, vomiting, vaginal discharge, or previous bleeding. The patient is sexually active, has multiple sexual partners, and uses condoms occasionally. Her last menstrual period was 3 months ago, and a urine pregnancy test was positive 2 months ago. She underwent an abortion at age 14 years and a miscarriage at age 15 years. Her menarche was at age 11 years, and her menstrual pattern has been regular. There have been no prior medical problems, including sexually transmitted infections.

Physical examination reveals an obese girl in no distress. Her pulse is 83 beats/min, blood pressure is 100/70 mm Hg, respiratory rate is 16 breaths/min, and temperature is 98.7°F (37.1°C). The abdomen is soft, nonrigid, nontender, and free of palpable masses. The vagina shows no discharge or bleeding. A speculum examination reveals some bloody discharge but no clots or fetal parts. The cervix is closed and has no erosions. A bimanual examination shows no cervical or adnexal tenderness or fullness in the adnexal area. The uterus is large; the examiner could not get around it with his fingers. Laboratory tests lead to the diagnosis.

- **What is your differential diagnosis at this point?**
- **Are there any elements of history or physical examination that would help you?**
- **What additional diagnostic studies would you like performed?**

Discussion

The girl's serum chorionic gonadotropin (β-hCG) level was 280,000 mIU/mL (280,000 IU/L). Pelvic ultrasonography showed a thickened, heterogeneous endometrial lining ("Swiss cheese" appearance) with multiple hypoechoic spaces typical of molar pregnancy. The next day the patient underwent suction evacuation of the endometrial cavity, and histopathologic examination of the specimen confirmed the diagnosis.

The Disorder

Gestational trophoblastic diseases represent a spectrum of benign and malignant conditions derived from early embryonic tissues of conception. Gestational trophoblastic diseases are categorized into 4 distinct forms. Hydatidiform mole is defined as products of conception that lack an intact fetus and show gross cystlike swellings of the chorionic villi due to accumulation of fluid. There is disintegration and loss of blood vessels in the villous core.

Hydatidiform mole has 2 principal forms: partial and complete. Partial moles are characterized by focal hydropic villi with scalloping, focal mild to moderate trophoblastic hyperplasia, and identifiable fetal or embryonic structures. Chromosome analysis reveals a polypoid karyotype, which most frequently is triploid. Complete moles are characterized by hydropic swelling of all villi, marked hyperplasia and anaplasia of the trophoblast, and complete absence of fetal structures. The karyotype of the complete mole is 46,XX. Chromosomal banding studies show that the chromosomal material of complete hydatidiform moles is inherited completely from the paternal contribution and is not chromosome Y–related.

About 80% of complete hydatidiform moles resolve after evacuation of the uterus. The remaining patients develop malignant trophoblastic sequelae (invasive mole or choriocarcinoma), with local uterine invasion being almost 4 times as common as distant spread. In contrast, patients who have a partial molar pregnancy are much less likely to develop persistent trophoblastic disease, with a range from 0% to 6.6%.

Invasive hydatidiform mole is a locally invasive, rarely metastatic lesion characterized microscopically by trophoblastic invasion of the myometrium and identifiable villous structures. Microscopically, this lesion is characterized by hyperplasia of cytotrophoblastic and syncytial elements as well as persistence of villous structures.

Choriocarcinoma is an uncontrolled growth of the cytotrophoblast and syncytiotrophoblast without the presence of villous structures. Columns and sheets of trophoblastic tissue invade normal tissues and spread to distant sites, the most common of which are lungs, brain, liver, pelvis, vagina, spleen, intestines, and kidney. Most cases of choriocarcinoma appear to follow a recognizable gestation. About 50% of choriocarcinomas are preceded by a hydatidiform molar pregnancy, 25% follow a spontaneous abortion, 22.5% follow a normal pregnancy, and 2.5% follow ectopic pregnancy. About 1 of every 40 molar gestations is followed by choriocarcinoma.

Abnormal uterine bleeding is the most frequent clinical presentation of choriocarcinoma. Other common signs include bizarre neurologic symptoms and asymptomatic lesions on routine chest radiography. Choriocarcinoma can be divided into nonmetastatic and metastatic forms, the latter being subdivided into those having a good prognosis and those carrying a poor prognosis. Nonmetastatic choriocarcinoma is diagnosed when β-hCG titers are persistently elevated or there is a tissue diagnosis of uterine choriocarcinoma in the absence of detectable metastatic disease.

Metastatic choriocarcinoma with a good prognosis is associated with the last pregnancy having occurred fewer than 4 months previously, a low β-hCG level (<100,000 IU in a 24-hour urine specimen or <40,000 mIU/mL [40,000 IU/L] in the blood), absence of liver or brain metastases, and no prior chemotherapy. Metastatic choriocarcinoma with a poor prognosis is characterized by the last pregnancy having occurred more than 4 months previously, an elevated β-hCG level (>100,000 IU in a 24-hour urine sample or >40,000 mIU/mL [40,000 IU/L] in the blood), liver or brain metastases, prior chemotherapy, and occurrence after a term pregnancy.

Placental-site trophoblastic disease is an extremely rare tumor arising from the placental implantation site. It resembles an exaggerated form of syncytial endometritis.

In addition to its potential for developing malignancy, molar pregnancy is associated with other significant complications, including hemorrhage, infection, and toxemia. Molar pregnancy rates in population-based studies range from 0.2 to 1.2 cases per 1,000 pregnancies. The 2 clinical risk factors most associated with molar pregnancy are being at the extremes of the reproductive years and having a history of prior molar pregnancy. The mechanisms leading to molar pregnancy are not well known. A maternal locus responsible for the familial form of hydatidiform mole was mapped on chromosome 19q13.3–13.4. Recent research focusing on the molecular bases of gestational trophoblastic disease has uncovered important data concerning the roles of certain receptors, adhesion molecules, oncoproteins, and mitochondrial factors in the pathogenesis of this disease.

Diagnostic Factors

Frequent clinical manifestations of a molar pregnancy are uterine size larger than dates, hyperemesis, pregnancy-induced hypertension in the first or second trimester, vaginal bleeding or passage of vesicles, abdominal pain, and clinical hyperthyroidism. The differential diagnosis should include disorders that are associated with the presenting complaint. Currently, because of sophisticated ultrasonographic technology and the practice of obtaining ultrasonography in the first trimester, a significant proportion of patients who have molar pregnancy are diagnosed before they develop symptoms.

Management

Once a hydatidiform mole has been diagnosed, suction evacuation of the uterus should be performed, followed by curettage of the endometrium. A baseline chest radiograph should be obtained to rule out metastatic disease. Normally, the serum β-hCG level falls toward zero 10 to 12 weeks after evacuation of molar pregnancy. Declining serum levels of β-hCG may be assessed every 1 to 2 weeks until the level is negative twice and then monthly for 1 year. A physical examination, including a pelvic examination, is recommended every 2 weeks until remission and then every 3 months for 1 year. Patients must be advised to use contraception for 1 year.

Invasive mole, nonmetastatic choriocarcinoma, and metastatic good-prognosis choriocarcinoma are usually treated with single-agent chemotherapy, although hysterectomy has been performed on the occasional patient in whom preservation of reproductive function is not an issue. Single-agent chemotherapy usually employs methotrexate with leucovorin unless the patient has abnormal liver function, in which case actinomycin D is used.

Poor-prognosis metastatic choriocarcinoma and persistent, relapsing, or resistant disease require complex regimens of chemotherapy and surgery. One regimen used in patients who have high-risk disease is etoposide, methotrexate, actinomycin D, cyclophosphamide, and vincristine. Patients who have relapsing or resistant disease require surgery and cisplatin together with a combination of etoposide, platinum-etoposide, methotrexate, and actinomycin D. Hysterectomy is the treatment of choice for patients who have placental-site trophoblastic disease

Lessons for the Physician

In this case, the patient knew that she was pregnant on the basis of a positive urinary chorionic gonadotropin test. She had no prenatal care. The diagnosis could have easily been missed because of mild symptoms and the patient's obesity. Pregnancy at a young age is a high risk factor for molar pregnancy, and whenever there is a presenting complaint suggestive of abnormal progression of pregnancy, the diagnosis of gestational trophoblastic disease should be entertained. Findings on evaluation, including high levels of chorionic gonadotropin (>100,000 mIU/mL [100,000 IU/L]), raised the suspicion of molar pregnancy. Ultrasonography that showed no viable fetus and an endometrial lining with multiple hypoechoic spaces further supported the diagnosis, and the histopathology confirmed it. The current criterion standard for diagnosing molar pregnancy is confirmation by histopathologic examination.

Yasser Mansour, MD, and Gheorghe R. Ganea, MD, Albert Einstein College of Medicine, Bronx-Lebanon Hospital Center, Bronx, NY

CHAPTER 54

Left Arm Swelling and Pain in a 17-Year-Old Boy

Presentation

A 17-year-old boy presents with a 1-day history of left arm swelling and pain from the midbiceps to the forearm. He denies fever, trauma, or muscle strain but does report having lifted weights last week. He has had a port wine stain since birth and underwent laser surgery at 3 months of age where it affected his face but still has the stain on his left upper extremity. He drinks protein shakes but takes no medications, smokes one cigarette per week, and occasionally smokes marijuana, most recently 3 weeks ago. He has been sexually active since age 15 years, has had 5 lifetime partners, and uses condoms occasionally.

On physical examination, his left upper arm circumference is 36.5 cm at the midpoint compared to 29 cm for his right upper arm. He has mild tenderness at the left antecubital fossa and full range of motion of his left shoulder and wrist but mild limitation of flexion and extension at the elbow due to pain. His port wine stain is visible on his left neck, chest, upper back, and left arm to the thumb. Thus, erythema is difficult to assess, but there is no warmth.

His complete blood cell count, serum electrolyte panel, urinalysis (negative for blood), and erythrocyte sedimentation rate yield normal findings. His aspartate aminotransferase (AST), alanine aminotransferase (ALT), and creatine kinase values were initially and mildly elevated but decreased during the hospitalization.

Hypercoagulation evaluation (proteins C and S, antithrombin III, lupus anticoagulant, homocysteine, antiphospholipid antibody, factor V Leiden, and factor II mutation G2012A) is negative. A blood culture does not show any growth. Imaging studies reveal the diagnosis.

- **What is your differential diagnosis at this point?**
- **Are there any elements of history or physical examination that would help you?**
- **What additional diagnostic studies would you like performed?**

Discussion

Upper extremity Doppler ultrasonography performed at an outside hospital revealed deep venous thrombosis (DVT) of both left brachial veins. On repeat evaluation at our hospital, the clots had resolved. Contrast venography showed increased narrowing of the left subclavian vein at the thoracic outlet with left arm abduction, consistent with thoracic outlet syndrome. Thus, Paget-Schroetter syndrome (spontaneous thrombosis of the axillary or subclavian veins or effort thrombosis) was diagnosed.

Differential Diagnosis

The most common reason for upper extremity swelling in a young patient is a fracture. This patient's lack of trauma and the normal findings on radiographs refuted this diagnosis. The presentation could have been caused by cellulitis, but the lack of fever or warmth to touch (although erythema could not be assessed) did not support this diagnosis. The next consideration would be an upper extremity DVT, which is usually diagnosed by Doppler ultrasonography, although the clavicle and sternum can interfere with the imaging. If an upper extremity DVT is suspected clinically despite negative ultrasonographic findings, the venous anatomy must be defined by venography.

Deep venous thromboses of the upper extremity can be primary or secondary. Catheters for dialysis, chemotherapy, and parenteral nutrition and pacemakers are causes of secondary DVT. Primary DVT can be due to a hypercoagulable state (protein C, protein S, and antithrombin III deficiencies; factor V Leiden and prothrombin gene mutations; hyperhomocysteinemia; and antiphospholipid antibody syndrome) or thoracic outlet syndrome, as in this patient. Deep venous thromboses may also be idiopathic.

An unusual cause of upper extremity swelling in an adolescent or young adult is superior vena cava syndrome, usually associated with malignant tumors such as lymphoma and lung cancer. This syndrome causes severe reduction in venous return from the head, neck, and upper extremities, with resulting swelling of those structures. Eosinophilic fasciitis is a rare cause of upper extremity swelling in adults and is a sclerodermalike syndrome of unknown cause that results in inflammation and later sclerosis of the deep fascia. Patients usually have a sudden onset of symmetric extremity tenderness and swelling followed by induration, with marked early eosinophilia. Finally, lymphedema, either primary (congenital) or secondary (to previously resected cancer or infiltrative infections such as filariasis), can rarely cause swelling of the upper extremities in an adolescent.

The Condition

Paget-Schroetter syndrome is a spontaneous axillary subclavian venous thrombosis. Patients are typically young and healthy and develop a DVT in the dominant arm after repetitive, strenuous upper extremity exercise, such as weightlifting. Heavy exertion leads to microtrauma to the vessel intima and activation of the coagulation cascade, which causes thrombosis, particularly if there is external compression, usually due to thoracic outlet syndrome.

In thoracic outlet syndrome, compression of the neurovascular bundle (brachial plexus, subclavian vein, and subclavian artery) in the area delineated by the scalene muscles, clavicle, and first rib is usually caused by bony anomalies (eg, cervical rib) or hypertrophied surrounding muscles. The syndrome generally presents in the third or fourth decade of life with pain, numbness, tingling, weakness, and fatigability of the affected extremity.

On examination, the patient may have positive results to provocative tests (increase in paresthesias and decrease in radial pulse). Provocative tests include the Adson test (abduct arm and extend and rotate neck toward affected side), the Halstead test (pull shoulders back and down to depress clavicle onto first rib), the Wright test (hyperabduct shoulder to 180°), and the Roos test (abduct and externally rotate shoulders and open and close hands for 3 minutes). When the syndrome presents in childhood, it occurs in adolescence with vascular complications such as a subclavian venous thrombosis or venous or arterial impingement.

The Other Problem

This patient had elevated AST and ALT values, which are nonspecific and can be of nonhepatic origin. Aspartate aminotransferase is also found in the heart, kidney, skeletal muscle, and brain. Myocardial infarction and skeletal muscle injury are known causes of AST and ALT elevation. Because this patient also had an elevated creatine kinase value, we postulate that these elevations were from transient left arm ischemia and muscle injury, possibly due to transient arterial impingement from thoracic outlet syndrome.

Treatment

Treatment for Paget-Schroetter syndrome includes anticoagulation, initially with heparin and then warfarin for a minimum of 3 months, to prevent the thrombus from becoming a life-threatening pulmonary embolus. Acute thrombolysis with or without angioplasty and early or delayed surgical removal of any extrinsic compression by resecting part of the first rib or surrounding muscles are controversial treatments. This patient underwent immediate anticoagulation with low-molecular-weight heparin and was begun on warfarin. He underwent thoracic outlet decompression 2 months later by having a left anterior and middle scalenectomy, first rib resection, and brachial plexus neurolysis.

Lessons for the Physician

- The list of common problems causing upper extremity swelling in an adolescent or young adult is fairly short.
- In the absence of fever or trauma, an effort thrombosis or Paget-Schroetter syndrome should be considered, particularly if there is a history of repetitive exertion by the upper extremities.
- Because pulmonary embolism is a complication of a deep venous thrombosis and immediate anticoagulation is required, the proper imaging should be ordered expeditiously.

Holly D. Smith, MD, and Avni Shah, MD, The University of Texas Health Science Center at Houston, Houston, TX

CHAPTER 55

Blue Skin Discoloration, Headache, and Difficulty Breathing in an 18-Year-Old Girl

Presentation

An 18-year-old Hispanic girl presents to her obstetrician for elective termination of pregnancy. She is estimated to be 14 weeks' pregnant. The procedure includes the use of *Laminaria japonica,* a brown algae, as a dilating agent of the uterine cervical os, followed by dilatation and curettage, usually within 24 hours. The patient changes her mind regarding pregnancy termination, and the *Laminaria* seed is removed. She receives a prescription for topical vaginal benzocaine cream, which she applies liberally to her vaginal area. Approximately 7 days later, she presents to the emergency department because of blue skin discoloration, headache, and difficulty breathing.

Physical examination shows a well-developed young adult in no acute distress. Her temperature is 98.0°F (36.7°C), heart rate is 120 beats/min, respiratory rate is 22 breaths/min, blood pressure is 104/62 mm Hg, and oxygen saturation is 92% on room air. She has perioral and peripheral cyanosis. Her lungs are clear to auscultation, and cardiac examination yields normal results.

Laboratory analysis reveals a white blood cell count of 10.8×10^3/mcL (10.8×10^9/L) with a normal differential, hemoglobin level of 11.6 g/dL (116 g/L), hematocrit of 34.2% (0.342), mean corpuscular volume of 86.8 mcm^3 (86.8 fL), and platelet count of 176×10^3/mcL (176×10^9/L). Results of hepatic and renal profiles as well as urinalysis are normal. A urine pregnancy test is positive, and her chorionic gonadotropin measures 53,810 U/mL. Arterial blood gas analysis shows a pH 7.48, PCO_2 of 26.7 mm Hg, PO_2 of 294 mm Hg, bicarbonate level of 20 mmol/L, and oxygen saturation of 98.8%. Electrocardiography, chest radiography, and computed tomography angiography of the chest yield normal results. Specific laboratory findings lead to the diagnosis.

- **What is your differential diagnosis at this point?**
- **Are there any elements of history or physical examination that would help you?**
- **What additional diagnostic studies would you like performed?**

Discussion

Possible conditions that could cause blue discoloration of the skin, headache, and difficulty breathing include congenital heart disease, lung disorders, arterial or venous obstruction, anemia, methemoglobinemia, sulfhemoglobinemia, argyria, and skin contamination with blue dye. A blood co-oximetry test showed a carboxyhemoglobin concentration of 0%, methemoglobin concentration of 16.9%, oxyhemoglobin concentration of 82.4%, and oxygen saturation of 98.8%. A diagnosis of methemoglobinemia was established. The red blood cell glucose-6-phospate dehydrogenase (G6PD) value and hemoglobin electrophoresis results were normal.

After receiving 3 doses of methylene blue intravenously over 3 days, her methemoglobin value was reduced to 1.7%. She aborted spontaneously while still in the hospital. On further questioning, she reported that her older brother has "blue lips and fingers." Her parents' health status is unknown. Additional studies revealed a cytochrome-b_5 reductase (methemoglobin reductase) value of 0.1 IU/g Hg (reference range, 8.2–19.2 IU/g Hg), indicating cytochrome-b_5 reductase deficiency.

The use of benzocaine cream apparently precipitated methemoglobinemia in this patient, who was highly susceptible because of her severe deficiency of the enzyme that maintains hemoglobin iron in its normal reduced Fe^{+2} state. An intriguing and as yet unanswered question is whether the use of brown algae *L japonica* might have contributed to the methemoglobinemia and whether the chemicals called brown algae polyphenols[1] might be implicated. One report suggests that brown algae polyphenols neutralize the cancer-causing oxygen radicals that are produced by UV-B exposure and that they lower skin concentrations of cyclooxygenase and prostaglandin E_2, both indicators of cell proliferation and inflammation. Could the same mechanism be operative in the oxidation and reduction of hemoglobin and the generation of methemoglobin? The role of brown algae, thus, needs additional study regarding its possible causative role in methemoglobinemia.

The Condition

Methemoglobinemia, a condition in which hemoglobin iron is oxidized from its normal Fe^{+2} state to Fe^{+3}, is a rare cause of cyanosis in infants and children. It can be congenital, resulting from a genetic defect in hemoglobin metabolism or structure, or it can be acquired after exposure to oxidant drugs or toxins. Hereditary methemoglobinemia or cytochrome-b_5 reductase deficiency is a rare disorder that has an autosomal recessive inheritance. Hemoglobin M disease is of autosomal dominant inheritance and involves a mutation resulting in a structural alteration of α or β globin chains of hemoglobin. Symptoms usually present in infancy.

Most cases, however, are acquired due to exogenous agents that increase methemoglobin formation. One of the most common causes is topical anesthetic agents, such as benzocaine, which is used in many over-the-counter analgesic preparations. Drug absorption is enhanced if too much is used. Another cause of methemoglobinemia—perhaps the most common of all—is an acute episode of diarrhea and metabolic acidosis in infants between 2 and 6 months of age. The accompanying alterations in intestinal chemistry and permeability result in abnormal absorption of nitrites, causing severe methemoglobinemia.

Clinical Presentation

Usually, patients born with congenital methemoglobinemia are asymptomatic, but they can become symptomatic if methemoglobin concentrations increase because methemoglobin does not transport and release oxygen to the tissues effectively. The primary concern is "cyanosis," or "blue color of the skin." At methemoglobin concentrations of approximately 30% to 50% of the total hemoglobin concentration, patients may have dyspnea, dizziness, tachycardia, fatigue, and headache. At 50% to 70% methemoglobin concentrations, severe lethargy and stupor may be present, and death may occur at concentrations greater than 70%.

Diagnosis

The presence of clinical cyanosis with a normal arterial Po_2 or "chocolate brown blood" should raise the suspicion of methemoglobinemia. Pulse oximetry readings are inaccurate. One bedside diagnostic test is to oxygenate the patient's blood in vitro by placing a drop of blood on paper or cloth and waving it in the air for 30 to 60 seconds; normal blood appears bright red, but when methemoglobinemia is present, the blood remains reddish brown. Methemoglobinemia can be confirmed by blood co-oximetry, which measures the actual concentration of methemoglobin. Family history may suggest hereditary forms of methemoglobinemia, and electrophoresis and enzymatic assays can recognize specific defects.

Treatment

Therapy for methemoglobinemia involves recognition and discontinuation of the offending agents. Because methemoglobin is hemoglobin in which iron has been oxidized to the Fe^{+3} state, treatment employs reducing agents, such as methylene blue, ascorbic acid, glutathione, or riboflavin. For severe symptoms, methylene blue, which acts rapidly, can be administered at a dose of 1 to 2 mg/kg of body weight. A second dose can be provided 1 hour later if symptoms persist. The maximum dose should not exceed 7 mg/kg due to toxicities.

Failure to decrease methemoglobin concentrations with methylene blue may be a result of G6PD deficiency. Methylene blue acts as a cofactor with nicotinamide adenine dinucleotide phosphate produced by G6PD to reduce methemoglobin. Ascorbic acid, 500 mg/d, can reduce methemoglobin directly. In severe cases, hyperbaric oxygen and exchange transfusion may be needed.

Reference

1. Hwang H, Chen T, Nines RG, Shin HC, Stoner GD. Photochemoprevention of UVB-induced skin carcinogenesis in SKH-1 mice by brown algae polyphenols. *Int J Cancer.* 2006;119(12):2742–2749

Lessons for the Physician

Methemoglobinemia, although an uncommon cause of cyanosis, should be considered in the differential diagnosis. The hallmark is cyanosis unresponsive to oxygen in the absence of cardiac or pulmonary disorders. Caution should also be used against the indiscriminate use of topical anesthetics such as benzocaine without first asking the patient specifically about a history of cyanosis, blue nail beds, blue lips, or any other symptoms suggestive of methemoglobinemia.

Madhuri Penugonda, MD; Dominick Sabatino, MD; Saumya Sharma, MD; Peter Ciminera, MD; Sujatha Kosuri, MD; and Jacob J. Rosenberg, MD, Nassau University Medical Center, East Meadow, NY

Part 10

Infectious Diseases

CHAPTER 56

2-Week-Old Has a Red, Peeling Rash (Visual Diagnosis)

Presentation

A 2-week-old term neonate presents to the emergency department with a history of an abrupt, generalized red rash with peeling of the skin. Her mother reports that she first noticed the skin peeling around her daughter's umbilicus 3 days ago, about the same time the umbilical cord stump fell off. She also noted some brownish discharge from the umbilicus at that time. Twenty-four hours earlier, the infant had developed irritability and a generalized red rash over her body, with areas of peeling skin. There is no history of fever, cold, hypothermia, cough, or eye discharge. Up to this point, the neonate has been feeding and stooling well.

The neonate was born term via a normal spontaneous vaginal delivery without complications. Birthweight was 2.7 kg, and Apgar scores were 9 and 9 at 1 and 5 minutes, respectively. However, the maternal group B *Streptococcus* status was unknown; the mother received 2 doses of intravenous penicillin 4 hours before delivery.

On physical examination, the patient's vital signs are appropriate for age, and there is no fever. The neonate reacts to touch as if it hurts. Examination of the skin reveals erythroderma (scaling erythematous dermatitis) and large, thin sheets of peeling skin with underlying shallow, bright red erosions around the face (Figure 56.1), lower abdomen, axillae and antecubital fossae (Figure 56.2), and both ankles and feet (Figure 56.3). There are no vesicles or bullae. There is no increased erythema around, or oozing or crusting from, the periumbilical area. The mucous membranes of the mouth and anus are unaffected. The rest of the physical examination findings are normal for age. A clinical diagnosis is made.

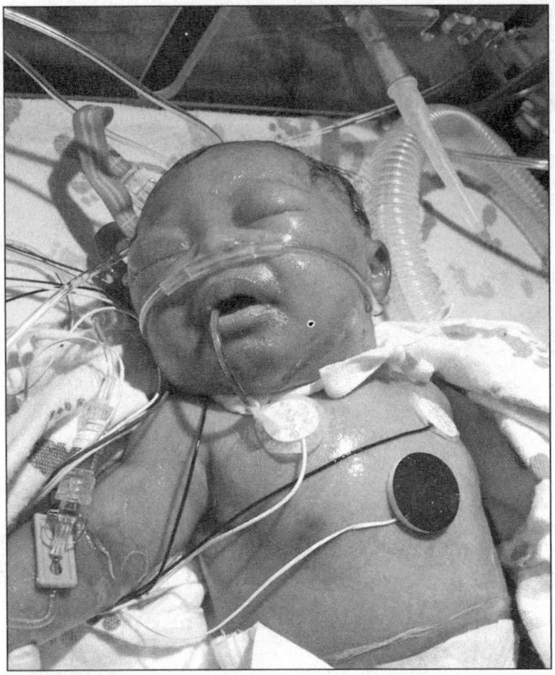

Figure 56.1. Bright red face with thin sheets of peeling skin and underlying shallow erosions.

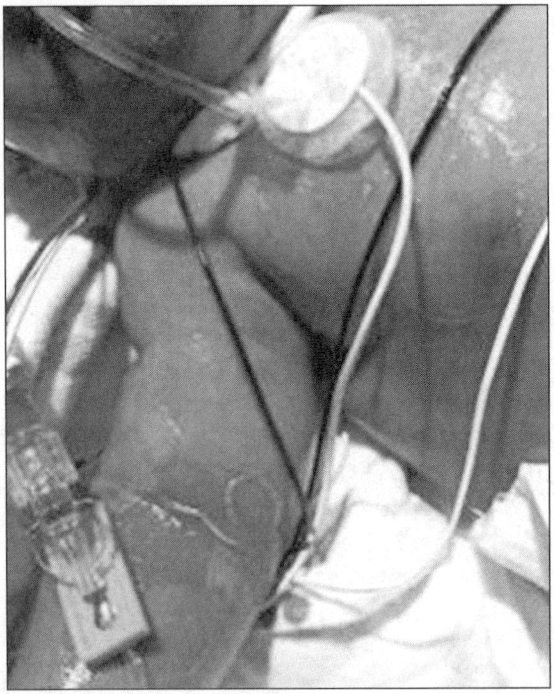

Figure 56.2. Thin sheet of peeling skin with underlying shallow, bright red erosion in antecubital fossa.

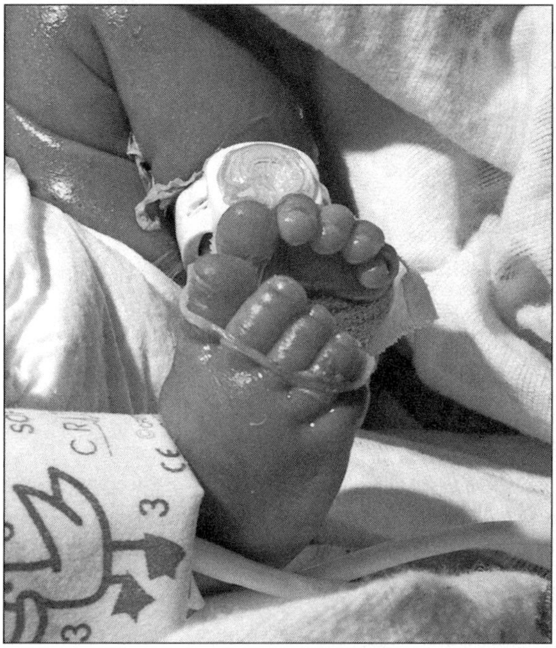

Figure 56.3. Erythroderma (scaling erythematous dermatitis) of the feet.

- **What is your differential diagnosis at this point?**
- **Are there any elements of history or physical examination that would help you?**
- **What additional diagnostic studies would you like performed?**

Diagnosis

The diagnosis of staphylococcal scalded skin syndrome (SSSS) was based on the classic clinical presentation of a generalized, faint, orange-red, macular erythema with cutaneous tenderness and a positive Nikolsky sign (the separation of superficial skin from the deeper skin layers after application of light pressure).

Discussion

Other names for forms of SSSS are Ritter disease and impetigo neonatorum in neonates. Staphylococcal scalded skin syndrome is a toxin-mediated exfoliative dermatitis caused by toxigenic strains of *Staphylococcus aureus* that usually belong to phage group 2 (types 3A, 3B, 3C, 55, or 71). The exfoliative toxins (ET) usually involved are A (ETA) and B (ETB), with ETA occurring more commonly (89% of cases) than ETB (4%). Exfoliative toxins cause intraepidermal splitting by destroying the protein desmoglein 1, an important cell-to-cell attachment protein found only in the superficial epidermis. This breakdown leads to bullae formation and diffuse, sheetlike desquamation. The spectrum of SSSS from localized bullous impetigo to full-blown SSSS depends on the distribution of the toxin.

Staphylococcal scalded skin syndrome is primarily a disease of children; 62% of affected children are younger than age 2 years, and 98% are younger than age 6 years. Predisposing factors for SSSS are immunocompromise and lower titers of enterotoxin-specific antibodies, which are lowest in infants and young children up to age 2 years. Most maternal antibodies transferred to infants via human milk are thought to be partially protective, but neonatal disease can still occur, possibly as a result of inadequate immunity or immature renal clearance of exotoxin.

In neonates, *Staphylococcus* commonly colonizes the skin, eyes, perineum, wound sites, circumcision wounds, and umbilical stumps. Approximately 30% of neonates are colonized by *S aureus* strains within 1 week of birth, although some studies have shown carriage rates of 60% to 90% in neonates discharged from hospitals, particularly when there are staphylococcal outbreaks and where the use of antiseptic umbilical cord care is discouraged.

Usually, SSSS begins with a local skin infection by an *S aureus* strain that produces ET, which affects the immediate area. By contrast, the generalized form of SSSS affects neonates (Ritter disease), infants, and children but rarely adults. In this form, fluid from intact bullae is generally sterile, and the infecting strain is usually recovered from distant sites, such as the throat or nose. Generalized SSSS is thought to arise from systemic ET absorption from local sites, followed by bloodstream diffusion to cutaneous targets. The incubation period from skin infection to the appearance of SSSS usually is 1 to 10 days.

Staphylococcal scalded skin syndrome typically presents clinically with the sudden appearance of diffuse tender erythroderma. Usually, there is a preceding upper respiratory tract infection, conjunctivitis, and, rarely, infection with staphylococcal superinfection as a complication of varicella or measles. Early SSSS commonly includes fever, irritability, and generalized, faint, orange-red, macular erythema with cutaneous tenderness. Within 1 to 2 days, a positive Nikolsky sign develops, and flaccid, thin-walled bullae appear. Within hours of bullae formation, the bullae spontaneously rupture, and the superficial epidermis separates in large sheets to reveal widespread areas of moist red undersurface. Within the next 1 to 3 days, these denuded areas of dry skin undergo a secondary flaky desquamation. Unless infection of the exposed dermis supervenes, the affected skin heals without scarring within 14 days of the onset of skin separation.

The definitive diagnosis of SSSS depends on culture and biopsy results. It is important to culture the skin sites in all patients who have suspected SSSS to identify the causative organism and to determine antibiotic sensitivities. Results of blood cultures are almost always negative in children who have SSSS. Skin biopsy results of affected skin in children who have SSSS reveal intraepidermal cleavage, with splitting beneath and within the stratum granulosum. The cleavage space may contain free-floating or partially attached acantholytic cells. Unaffected surrounding epidermis appears unremarkable, and the dermis contains no inflammatory cells.

Differential Diagnosis

The differential diagnosis for SSSS includes streptococcal scarlet fever, Stevens-Johnson syndrome, toxic epidermal necrolysis (TEN), toxic shock syndrome, and Kawasaki disease. Distinguishing features are severity of the disease, percentage of total body surface area affected, involvement of mucous membranes, skin biopsy findings, and systemic signs and symptoms. For example, SSSS differs from the more severe TEN by histology and absence of mucosal pathologic evidence. In SSSS, there is intradermal cleavage of the skin; in TEN, there is necrosis of the full epidermal layer. Table 56.1 presents ways to differentiate SSSS from TEN.

Table 56.1. Differentiating Staphylococcal Scalded Skin Syndrome and Toxic Epidermal Necrolysis

Features	Staphylococcal Scalded Skin Syndrome	Toxic Epidermal Necrolysis
Patients affected	Infants, young children, immunocompromised adults	Older patients
Patient history	Recent staphylococcal infection	Drug use, infections, and renal failure
Level of epidermal cleavage	Within the granular cell (outermost) layer of the epidermis as shown below 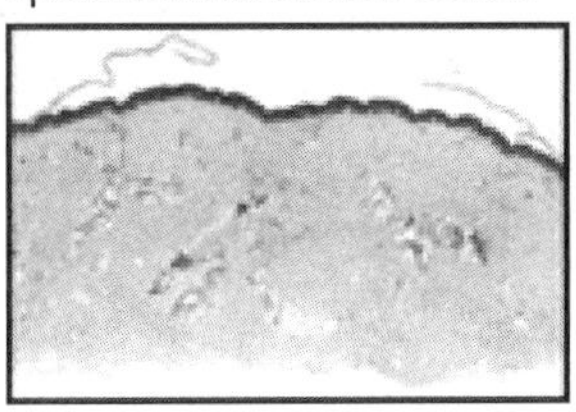	Between the epidermis and dermis or at the level of the basal cell as shown below 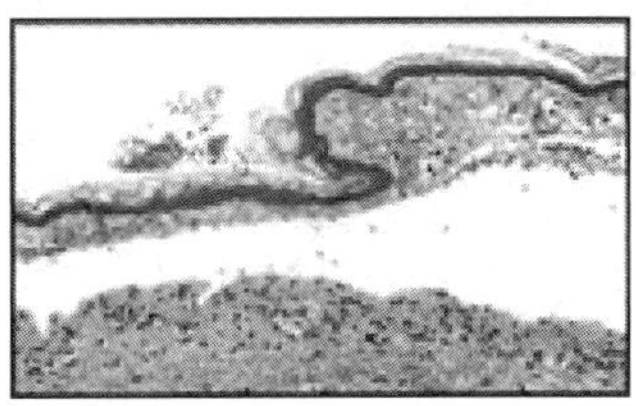
Mucous membrane involvement	Mucous membranes usually not involved	Mucous membranes involved

Management

The mainstay of therapy for SSSS is eradication of the staphylococcal focus of infection by using antibiotic medications, as well as supportive care with careful attention to hydration and monitoring of electrolyte levels due to fluid loss through the denuded skin. Fluid rehydration plays an important role if a large percentage of body surface area is affected. Management of the skin in SSSS is similar to treating severe burns. Topical wound care of denuded areas is important and includes applying a bland emollient to decrease pruritus and tenderness. In addition to the use of bland emollients on the skin, nonadherent dressings such as petrolatum-impregnated gauze can be used to cover erosions.

Staphylococcal scalded skin syndrome in neonates and infants should be treated with a parenteral β-lactam antimicrobial such as nafcillin or oxacillin or, if methicillin-resistant *S aureus* is a consideration, with intravenous vancomycin or oral clindamycin to decrease the staphylococcal bacterial load. Corticosteroids are not indicated, and topical antimicrobials are of no benefit.

Ongoing research has demonstrated that infusing anti-ET antibodies into mice can halt progression of exfoliation. However, this technique has not yet been tested in humans.

Patient Course

The patient was admitted to the pediatric intensive care unit for observation, intravenous fluid and vancomycin therapy, and burn care. Both the infectious disease and dermatology services were consulted. Skin care included applying petroleum jelly to keep the skin moist and reduce water permeability. A complete blood cell count on the peripheral blood smear revealed a normal white blood cell count of 5,200/mm^3 with 25% neutrophils, 3% bands, 52% lymphocytes, and 20% monocytes. Wound cultures from the mouth, nose, umbilicus, and skin lesions grew *Staphylococcus epidermidis,* which was most likely commensal. Pain was relieved with rectal acetaminophen. The neonate was transferred to the hospital floor in 2 days. She remained afebrile and her skin condition improved without further peeling after 7 days. The patient was discharged from the hospital on oral clindamycin to complete 14 days of therapy.

Summary

- Although staphylococcal scalded skin syndrome is relatively uncommon, usually diagnosed on clinical grounds, and readily treated with conventional antibiotics, it is important to emphasize that mortality rates are still unacceptably high and outbreaks are difficult to control.
- Staphylococcal scalded syndrome can occasionally lead to serious complications, such as pneumonia, septic arthritis, hypothermia, dehydration, and secondary infections, particularly in neonates, in whom complications may be lethal.
- Early diagnosis and appropriate treatment can prevent the morbidity and mortality associated with these complications. With appropriate management, mortality due to staphylococcal scalded skin syndrome in children remains below 5% compared to approximately 60% in adults.

Anita Gupta, MD, Neonatology Fellow, Ann & Robert H. Lurie Children's Hospital of Chicago, Chicago, IL

Norman Jacobs, MD, Attending Physician, John H. Stroger Jr. Hospital of Cook County, Chicago, IL

CHAPTER 57

Evaluation of Eosinophilia, Loose Stools, and Low-grade Fever in a 3½-Year-Old Boy

Presentation

A 3½-year-old boy, who lives in the southeastern United States, is referred for evaluation of eosinophilia that was detected on laboratory tests performed during a routine health supervision visit. A few days ago, he had loose stools, without blood or mucus, associated with low-grade fever. He has no history of significant illness, allergies, respiratory symptoms, weight loss, sick contacts, or travel. He is not taking any medications. He lives with his mother, aunt, 3 siblings, 4 cousins, and 2 dogs in a rural area that has city water and sewage. He frequently plays outside the house.

Physical findings, including vital signs, are within reference range except for some scratch marks on his trunk and extremities. His white blood cell count is 35×10^3/mcL (35×10^9/L) with 56% eosinophils (absolute eosinophil count [AEC] of 19.8 $\times 10^3$/mcL [19.8×10^9/L]). The rest of the laboratory evaluation, including a metabolic panel and a C-reactive protein assessment, yields normal results. Stool examination for ova, cysts, and parasites shows negative results. Serum concentrations of IgG, IgM, and IgA are normal, but the IgE value is elevated (1,358 IU/mL). Immunophenotyping for T and B lymphocytes and natural killer cells is within reference range. Additional laboratory evaluation leads to the diagnosis.

- **What is your differential diagnosis at this point?**
- **Are there any elements of history or physical examination that would help you?**
- **What additional diagnostic studies would you like performed?**

Discussion

The eosinophilia and elevated serum IgE value raised the suspicion for parasitic infestation. Therefore, stool studies for ova, cysts, and parasites were repeated 3 times. The third sample was reported positive for *Strongyloides stercoralis.*

The accepted upper range for normal AEC is ill defined, but a count above 0.6×10^3/mcL (0.6×10^9/L) is usually considered abnormal. Eosinophilia can be categorized as mild, with an AEC ranging from more than 0.6×10^3/mcL (0.6×10^9/L) to less than 1.5×10^3/mcL (1.5×10^9/L), moderate from greater than 1.5×10^3/mcL (1.5×10^9/L) to less than 5×10^3/mcL (5×10^9/L), and high if greater than 5×10^3/mcL (5×10^9/L). The causes of eosinophilia can be categorized as primary, secondary, and idiopathic.

Primary eosinophilia is caused by clonal expansion of eosinophils, which occurs in hematologic malignancies such as leukemia. Secondary eosinophilia can be due to infectious causes, the most common being tissue-invasive parasites, and noninfectious causes, such as allergic disorders, immunodeficiency, autoimmune disease, and endocrine disorders. Secondary eosinophilia can also be caused by toxins or medications such as aspirin or ranitidine. Idiopathic eosinophilia is diagnosed when neither primary nor secondary causes can be identified.

Usually, allergic diseases such as allergic rhinitis or asthma cause mild eosinophilia, whereas parasitic diseases, tumors, hyper-IgE syndrome, and IL-2 therapy cause moderate to high eosinophilia. For a febrile patient who has eosinophilia, noninfectious causes such as adrenal insufficiency should be suspected because most acute bacterial or viral infections cause eosinopenia but not eosinophilia.

Evaluation of patients who have eosinophilia requires a history, including allergic symptoms, environmental exposures, animal contacts, travel, medications, and constitutional symptoms. A physical examination should be performed to identify signs of allergies or malignancies. After narrowing the differential diagnosis based on the history and physical examination, laboratory evaluation should begin with testing 3 stool specimens for ova and parasites.

Some of the major parasites that should be included in the evaluation of patients who have eosinophilia are *S stercoralis, Ascaris lumbricoides,* hookworm (*Necator americanus* and *Ancylostoma duodenale*), and *Toxocara canis.* Stool examination may help diagnose all except *T canis,* which can be diagnosed by enzyme immunoassay for *Toxocara* antibody in serum. Also, unlike the other parasites, toxocariasis can present with hepatomegaly and hypergammaglobulinemia.

Strongyloidosis may be difficult to diagnose by stool examination because only a few parasites may be present in the specimen. Therefore, multiple fresh stool samples may need to be submitted to the laboratory for testing. Occasionally, serologic testing for antibodies to *Strongyloides* may be necessary. Patients who have had 3 negative stool study results may also need serologic studies to rule out tissue or blood-dwelling helminthic infections caused by *Trichinella* or *Toxocara.*

The Underlying Condition

Strongyloidosis is caused by a nematode prevalent in tropical and subtropical regions of the world and is endemic in the southeastern United States. *S stercoralis* is one of the only common nematodes that reproduces within the human host, the other being *Capillaria philippinensis.* Infective larvae are acquired from the soil through skin penetration. Poor sanitation and crowded living conditions lead to high transmission rates. Eosinophilia is a prominent feature of strongyloidosis, as seen in this patient. Infection with *Strongyloides* can persist for decades without being symptomatic. A hyperinfection syndrome can be seen in the immunocompromised host and consists of disseminated strongyloidosis. This disorder may present with abdominal pain, distention, pulmonary manifestations, and neurologic symptoms that can progress to shock; the disorder is potentially fatal.

Treatment

Treatment of strongyloidosis consists of ivermectin or thiabendazole, each of which is administered in the same dose for children and adults. Ivermectin is the preferred treatment, prescribed at a dose of 200 mcg/kg/d as a single daily dose for 2 days. Thiabendazole is an alternative, prescribed at a dose of 50 mg/kg/d (maximum 3 g/d) divided in 2 daily doses for 2 days; this dose may cause adverse effects and may need to be decreased. Because treatment failure can occur, therapeutic efficacy should be confirmed by using either stool studies or examination of duodenal contents about 2 weeks after starting treatment. Decreasing titers of antibodies to *Strongyloides* by enzyme immunoassay also supports adequacy of therapy and should be repeated at approximately 3 months. Persistent eosinophilia after many months of treatment may suggest treatment failure or a different cause for the high eosinophil counts. This patient was treated with thiabendazole but was lost to follow-up.

Lessons for the Physician

- The differential diagnosis for eosinophilia is vast but can be narrowed by a detailed history, thorough physical examination, and consideration of the degree of eosinophilia.
- To confirm the diagnosis of strongyloidosis, at least 3 stool examinations should be performed for the patient who has high eosinophilia because the initial results may be negative, as seen in this patient.
- A high degree of suspicion is required for the diagnosis of strongyloidosis, especially in an immunocompromised host.

Roshan P. George, MD, and Joseph A. Bocchini, MD, Louisiana State Health Sciences Center, Shreveport, LA

COMMENTARY BY NAHED ABDEL-HAQ, MD, INFECTIOUS DISEASES SPECIALIST, CHILDREN'S HOSPITAL OF MICHIGAN

Ivermectin remains the drug of choice for the treatment of strongyloidosis. The case report states thiabendazole as the alternative treatment for strongyloidosis. However, the current Centers for Disease Control and Prevention and *Red Book* 2015 recommend albendazole as alternative treatment rather than thiabendazole. Albendazole is an alternative agent because cure rate is lower than ivermectin. The recommended dose is 400 mg/d divided in 2 doses for 7 days. Thiabendazole in not currently available in the United States.

CHAPTER 58

Sore Throat and Difficulty Swallowing in a 9-Year-Old Boy (Visual Diagnosis)

Presentation

A 9-year-old boy presents with sore throat and difficulty swallowing of 3 days' duration. He was seen at a clinic on the first day of his illness, where the result of a rapid streptococcal antigen test was negative. He was discharged with a diagnosis of sore throat with cough and prescribed a 5-day course of azithromycin and a 3-day course of prednisolone suspension. However, his sore throat has persisted and his dysphagia has worsened. His mother is seeking further medical attention because she has noted the roof of his mouth to be red and swollen posteriorly. The boy describes a feeling that "something is stuck in my throat" but still can swallow. Dysphagia occurs with both solids and liquid foods.

On physical examination, his vital signs are within reference range; there is no fever or respiratory distress. Examination of the pharynx reveals an erythematous, swollen uvula (Figure 58.1). He has no drooling, cervical lymphadenopathy, or erythema or exudate on his pharyngeal wall. No other abnormality is noted. He has taken 3 doses of azithromycin and 2 doses of prednisolone.

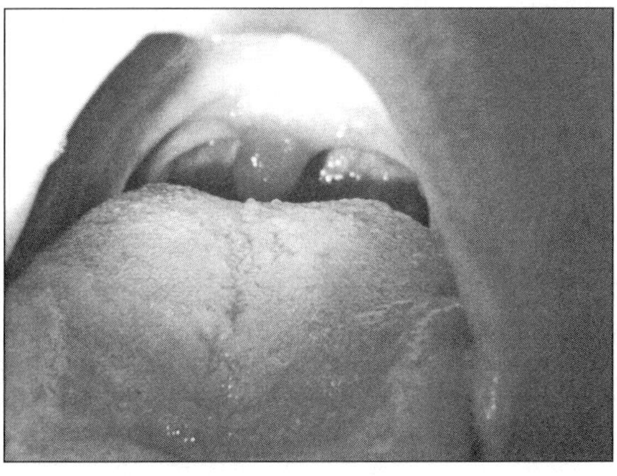

Figure 58.1. Erythematous, swollen uvula.

The boy had croup last winter, has occasional nasal symptoms due to seasonal allergies, and underwent tonsillectomy with adenoidectomy 2 years ago for repeated ear infections. His immunizations are up to date. He has had no ill contacts.

Diagnosis is made on clinical findings.

- **What is your differential diagnosis at this point?**
- **Are there any elements of history or physical examination that would help you?**
- **What additional diagnostic studies would you like performed?**

Diagnosis

The diagnosis of uvulitis is based on the complaints of a sore throat with dysphagia; the presence of a red, swollen uvula; and the absence of physical findings suggestive of other causes of sore throat and dysphagia, such as retropharyngeal abscess or peritonsillar abscess.

Discussion

Uvulitis is defined as inflammation of the uvula and typically presents with marked uvular edema and erythema.[1] The condition most commonly results from cellulitis due to infection by group A *Streptococcus* in children 5 to 15 years of age. Among unimmunized children younger than 5 years, *Haemophilus influenzae* type b is the next most common bacterial cause.[1–3] Other reported pathogens include *Fusobacterium nucleatum, Prevotella,* and *Streptococcus pneumoniae.*[4] Uvulitis can also be caused by viral infections due to coxsackievirus, herpes simplex virus, and varicella-zoster virus and by fungal infection due to *Candida albicans.* Noninfectious causes of uvulitis include trauma during instrumentation (eg, intubation), inhalation of chemical irritants (eg, cannabis), inhalation of steam, and vasculitis.[5,6]

Presentation

Uvulitis usually presents with fever, sore throat, dysphagia, drooling, and respiratory distress. Significant respiratory distress is uncommon unless there is an associated epiglottitis or if the uvulitis is due to a noninfectious cause such as a chemical irritant. Diagnosis is based on clinical characteristics alone in the absence of other findings. However, if respiratory distress is present or if an adequate examination of the oropharynx cannot be performed, imaging is essential to rule out epiglottitis or retropharyngeal abscess.[2] Blood and throat cultures may help identify an infectious cause.

Differential Diagnosis

The most common differential diagnosis for uvulitis is streptococcal pharyngitis, which presents with pharyngeal edema and erythema with tonsillar exudates and palatal petechiae. Other potential diagnoses include retropharyngeal and peritonsillar abscesses and epiglottitis. Retropharyngeal abscesses present with swelling of the pharyngeal wall; peritonsillar abscesses manifest with tonsillar swelling and deviation of the uvula. Both may present with signs of upper airway obstruction and limited ability to open the mouth adequately for examination. Epiglottitis presents with fever, drooling, stridor, anxiety, and rapid progression of upper airway obstruction.

Management

Treatment should be decided on a case-by-case basis and directed at the most likely pathogens that cause age-associated symptoms (pharyngitis or epiglottitis) and local antimicrobial susceptibility data. Many children can be treated as outpatients. If group A *Streptococcus* is isolated or suspected on the basis of associated pharyngitis, oral therapy with penicillin or amoxicillin is appropriate. The initial treatment of isolated uvulitis without evidence of pharyngitis or epiglottitis or uvulitis with epiglottitis consists of empiric antimicrobial treatment, such as a third-generation cephalosporin (eg, ceftriaxone) to provide coverage for typical pathogens such as *Haemophilus influenzae* type b and *S pneumoniae,* which may produce β-lactamase or be resistant to penicillin, respectively. Once blood cultures are negative, changing to an oral antibiotic such as amoxicillin-clavulanate or an oral cephalosporin such as cefuroxime or cefdinir is appropriate to continue treatment for a possible bacterial uvulitis. Noninfectious causes of uvulitis can be treated with conservative supportive care. Evidence to support the role of corticosteroid therapy in the management of uvulitis is not apparent in the medical literature.

Patient Course

The patient was admitted for 1 day for observation. Testing showed a white blood cell count of 12.0×10^3/mcL (12.0×10^9/L) with 65% neutrophils, 26% lymphocytes, and 7.8% monocytes. His hemoglobin measured 12.8 g/dL (128 g/L), hematocrit was 36.5% (0.365), and platelet count was 295×10^3/mcL (295×10^9/L). Neck radiographs did not show any evidence of epiglottitis (Figure 58.2). He received intravenous ampicillin-sulbactam at 200 mg/kg/d in 4 divided doses and dexamethasone 0.5 mg/kg for 3 doses every 8 hours after an otolaryngology consultation. His blood and throat cultures were negative. He was able to eat and drink without difficulty, and he did not have any oxygen desaturations or fever throughout his inpatient stay. He was discharged on the second inpatient day receiving oral amoxicillin-clavulanic acid 500 mg twice a day for 10 days for presumed bacterial uvulitis.

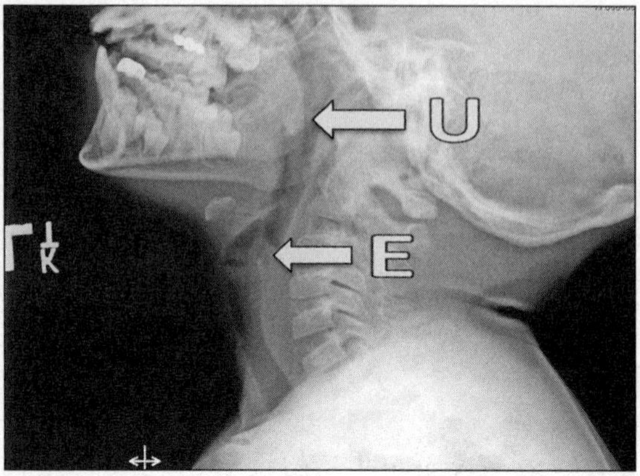

Figure 58.2. Neck radiograph documenting a lack of epiglottitis. E = esophagus, U = uvula.

References

1. Woods CR. Uvulitis: clinical features and treatment. UpToDate Web site. http://www.uptodate.com/contents/uvulitis-clinical-features-and-treatment. Updated Jan 10, 2014. Accessed October 29, 2015
2. McNamara RM. Clinical characteristics of acute uvulitis. *Am J Emerg Med.* 1994;12(1):51–52
3. Wynder SG, Lampe RM, Shoemaker ME. Uvulitis and *Haemophilus influenzae* b bacteremia. *Pediatr Emerg Care.* 1986;2(1):23–25
4. Brook I. Uvulitis caused by anaerobic bacteria. *Pediatr Emerg Care.* 1997;13(3):221
5. Holden JP, Vaughan WC, Brock-Utne JG. Airway complication following functional endoscopic sinus surgery. *J Clin Anesth.* 2002;14(2):154–157
6. Boyce SH, Quigley MA. Uvulitis and partial upper airway obstruction following cannabis inhalation. *Emerg Med.* 2002;14(1):106–108

Summary

- Uvulitis is an infrequently recognized pediatric condition.
- The diagnosis should be considered for the patient who presents with a sore throat, dysphagia, and an erythematous, edematous uvula in the absence of other, more serious disorders such as retropharyngeal or peritonsillar abscess.

Nirav Shastri, MD, FAAP, Assistant Professor of Pediatrics, and Gretchen Black, DO, Assistant Professor of Pediatrics, University of Missouri, Kansas City, MO; Children's Mercy South Urgent Care Center, Overland Park, KS

Milton A. Fowler Jr, MD, FACEP, University of Missouri, Kansas City, MO; Section Chief, Children's Mercy South Urgent Care Center, Overland Park, KS

CHAPTER 59

Sore and Stiff Neck, Jaw Pain, Drooling, Difficulty Swallowing, and Stiffness of Right Leg in a 9-Year-Old Boy

Presentation

A 9-year-old Amish boy presents with a 3-day history of a sore and stiff neck, jaw pain, drooling, difficulty swallowing, and stiffness of his right leg. Three days ago, he began to complain of jaw stiffness and a sore neck. Yesterday, his neck was canted to the right and his right leg felt sore. Today, he is unable to walk and is brought to the emergency department. He has received no immunizations.

On physical examination, the boy has severe right torticollis and trismus and is drooling. There is no evidence of respiratory compromise. He has painful muscle spasms triggered by movement as well as generalized increased muscle tone and brisk-to-hyperactive deep tendon reflexes. His abdomen is tense and firm to palpation. His cognitive abilities are intact. He has a 6.0 × 1.0–cm gaping wound in the left parietal region of his scalp that extends to the galea aponeurotica. The wound bed is moist and red, and there is serous drainage.

Laboratory results reveal a total white blood cell count of 11.0×10^3/mcL (11.0×10^9/L) with 82% neutrophils and 7% lymphocytes, hemoglobin of 14.3 g/dL (143.0 g/L), and platelet count of 327.0×10^3/mcL (327.0×10^9/L). His creatine kinase concentration is 228 U/L. His electrolyte and liver enzyme values are within reference range. A clinical diagnosis is made that is confirmed later by a laboratory result.

- **What is your differential diagnosis at this point?**
- **Are there any elements of history or physical examination that would help you?**
- **What additional diagnostic studies would you like performed?**

Discussion

On further questioning, the boy's parents recounted that 11 days ago he was hit on his head by a metal part of a wagon. The wound was cleaned at home with hydrogen peroxide, and a cultural home remedy, a poultice of red pepper, was applied. A clinical diagnosis of generalized tetanus was made. The boy received 3,000 U of tetanus immunoglobulin (TIG), one dose of penicillin G, and tetanus toxoid. The head wound was debrided and, thereafter, cleaned twice daily.

His muscle spasms continued to worsen and were treated with intravenous diazepam, with doses titrated upward to 15 mg every 3 hours. He was placed on strict "minimal stimuli" precautions, and the diazepam was changed to "as needed" dosing. He later was placed on baclofen, 15 mg orally every 8 hours. His spasms reduced on the baclofen treatment, and the need for frequent diazepam decreased. Intravenous metronidazole was administered at a dosage of 500 mg every 8 hours.

Wound cultures were negative for growth of anaerobic organisms, and there was light to moderate growth of *Staphylococcus aureus,* coagulase-negative staphylococci, and *Enterobacter cloacae.*

Three days after admission, the boy began to show improvement in his muscle stiffness. On day 6 of admission, he underwent a bedside swallowing evaluation by the speech therapist, and a modified pureed diet was started. One week after admission, his muscle stiffness was greatly improved, and physical therapy was begun. He was discharged 9 days after admission on oral baclofen, diazepam, and metronidazole.

Polymerase chain reaction analysis performed after discharge revealed *Clostridium tetani* in the red pepper poultice used to treat the scalp laceration.

The Condition

Tetanus in the United States is an infrequent but critical disease that occurs mostly among unvaccinated or inadequately vaccinated individuals. Tetanus is a toxin-mediated infection, caused primarily by tetanospasmin, an exotoxin produced by the anaerobic bacterium *C tetani.* Tetanospasmin affects the muscle neurons and the central nervous system to cause skeletal muscle spasms. *C tetani* is found in animal and human intestines, and its spores are ubiquitous in the soil. The organism multiplies in contaminated wounds. The incubation period of tetanus can range from days to months; most cases occur within 14 days of infection.

Toxin secretion by *C tetani* is facilitated by necrotic tissue that has a favorable oxidation gradient. Thus, wounds due to trauma (eg, crush injury), surgical wounds, suppurative wounds, and wounds containing a foreign body have been known to develop tetanus infection. Wound contamination with soil or manure makes infection more likely. Wounds inflicted by objects capable of causing deep penetration together with tissue damage (especially wounds tainted with rust, dirt, or foreign debris, including material from socks and shoes) are particularly susceptible to infection by *C tetani*. Wounds that do not involve tissue injury, such as simple needle sticks, are less prone to develop tetanus. Up to 25% of those who have tetanus do not report recent evidence of a wound.

The clinical picture varies with the different forms of the disease. In localized tetanus, localized muscle spasms occur, usually in areas contiguous to the wound. In generalized tetanus, the spasms often start with trismus, which can progress to risus sardonicus (a characteristic grinning facial expression). The muscle spasms then progress to involve the entire body and are triggered by minimal external stimuli. Cephalic tetanus can also occur, is associated with head and neck wounds, is characterized by cranial nerve dysfunction, and may progress to generalized tetanus.

Neonatal tetanus, seen primarily in developing countries, is associated with umbilical stump contamination and manifests with poor suck and opisthotonos. Risk factors for neonatal tetanus in that setting include inadequate immunization of mothers, birth in an unhygienic environment, unclean birthing instruments, and the use of culturally encouraged cow dung poultices or of rags or animal skin dressings (contaminated with mud, manure, animal or human feces) to cover the umbilical stump.

The differential diagnosis of tetanus includes orofacial infection, dystonic drug reaction, hypocalcemia, hysteria, strychnine poisoning, seizures, rabies, and meningitis. The diagnosis of tetanus remains primarily clinical. Laboratory studies are of little help in diagnosis, with a low yield of positive findings from wound cultures.

Management and Prognosis

Standard management of tetanus includes neutralization of unbound toxin, treatment of infection, supportive care, and active immunization. A single dose of TIG in a dosage of 3,000 to 6,000 U intramuscularly is administered to neutralize unbound tetanospasmin, although some recommend a smaller dose of 500 U. Tetanus antitoxin and intravenous immune globulin can be used if TIG is unavailable. Oral or intravenous metronidazole is the antibiotic of choice; parental penicillin G is an acceptable alternative. Antibiotic treatment for 10 to 14 days is recommended.

Wounds should be debrided, and excision of necrotic tissue may be required. Drugs such as benzodiazepines, phenothiazines, anticonvulsants, magnesium sulfate, and baclofen have been used for supportive care, specifically muscle relaxation and sedation. In certain cases, therapeutic paralysis and mechanical ventilation are necessary.

The overall case fatality rate for tetanus ranges from 10% to 70%. Shorter incubation periods are associated with a poor prognosis. Recovery in most cases of tetanus is expected to be complete, with return to normal function in most cases. However, there are reported cases of residual physical or psychological effects. Neonatal tetanus may result in developmental disability.

Prevention

Prevention is primarily through active immunization with tetanus toxoid–containing vaccines throughout life (DTaP, Tdap, DT, or Td). Childhood tetanus immunization should consist of 5 doses of DTaP at 2, 4, 6, and 15 to 18 months and 4 to 6 years. For children 11 or 12 years of age, a single dose of Tdap is recommended. This preparation can also be given in place of one Td booster in adolescents and adults ages 19 through 64 years. Tetanus toxoid efficacy ranges from 80% to 100%, and effective immunity is achieved in most children after 3 doses have been given. Booster doses are required to provide long-lasting immunity.

Measures to prevent neonatal tetanus include educating pregnant women on the dangers of using cultural poultices and educating midwives on aseptic obstetric practices and immunization of pregnant women. Following a tetanus-prone injury, secondary prevention is attempted with prompt treatment of deep wounds and use of tetanus toxoid or TIG, depending on the nature of the wound and the immunization history (Table 59.1). Tetanus infection does not produce reliable natural immunity, and an immunization series should be completed after clinical infection.

Table 59.1. Guide to Tetanus Prophylaxis in Routine Wound Management

History of Tetanus Toxoid Doses	Clean, Minor Wounds		All Other Wounds	
	Td or Tdap[a]	TIG	Td or Tdap[a]	TIG
<3 or unknown	Yes	No	Yes	Yes
≥3	No[b]	No	No[c]	No

Abbreviation: TIG, tetanus immunoglobulin.

[a] Tdap is preferred to Td for adolescents who have never received Tdap. Td is preferred if person received Tdap previously or if Tdap is unavailable.

[b] Yes if ≥10 years since last tetanus-containing vaccine.

[c] Yes if ≥5 years since last tetanus-containing vaccine.

Adapted from American Academy of Pediatrics. Tetanus (lockjaw). In: Kimberlin DW, Brady MT, Jackson MA, Long SS, eds. *Red Book: 2015 Report of the Committee on Infectious Diseases.* 30th ed. Elk Grove Village, IL. American Academy of Pediatrics; 2015:775.

Tetanus toxoid is very safe, even in immunodeficient patients. Minor reactions may include local pain, erythema, fever, and malaise. Severe adverse effects following tetanus toxoid administration are uncommon.

Lessons for the Physician

When dealing with unvaccinated children, a high degree of suspicion must be maintained. Tetanus is a clinical diagnosis, and once the diagnosis is made, immediate treatment is necessary without waiting for laboratory results. Primary prevention by active immunization remains the best method of preventing this disease.

Stella U. Kalu, MD, University of Texas Medical Branch, Galveston, TX

Bradley J. Sullivan, MD, PhD, Marshfield Clinic, Marshfield, WI

CHAPTER 60

Right Ankle Pain in an 11-Year-Old Girl

Presentation

An 11-year-old girl presents to the emergency department with a 4-day history of right ankle pain. Her pain is worse with movement of the ankle as well as with weight bearing. Earlier in the week, she had similar symptoms in her left wrist and elbow. She has no history of trauma, fever, or rash. She has had occasional shortness of breath and chest pain over the past week.

Physical examination reveals a well-appearing girl whose axillary temperature is 101.4°F (38.6°C), heart rate is 122 beats/min, respiratory rate is 16 breaths/min, and blood pressure is 97/60 mm Hg. There is swelling around her right ankle as well as tenderness to light touch and pain on flexion and extension of that joint.

Her ankle radiograph is read as normal. Results of laboratory studies include white blood cell count, 18.4 × 10^3/mcL (18.4 × 10^9/L) with 79% neutrophils, 14% lymphocytes, and 7% monocytes; hemoglobin, 9.7 g/dL (97 g/L); platelet count, 370 × 10^3/mcL (370 × 10^9/L); erythrocyte sedimentation rate, 105 mm/h; and C-reactive protein, 222 mg/dL (2,114.3 nmol/L). Magnetic resonance imaging suggests tenosynovitis but cannot exclude osteomyelitis. The joint is aspirated, fluid is sent for culture, and intravenous antibiotics are started. A development during hospitalization leads to further studies and the diagnosis.

- **What is your differential diagnosis at this point?**
- **Are there any elements of history or physical examination that would help you?**
- **What additional diagnostic studies would you like performed?**

Discussion

On the fifth day of hospitalization, a new grade 2/6 holosystolic murmur is heard at the cardiac apex. Electrocardiography demonstrates first-degree heart block. Echocardiography shows mild mitral and trace aortic regurgitation as well as mild pericardial effusion with normal valve architecture and normal ventricular function. Her antistreptolysin O and anti–deoxyribonuclease B titers are elevated.

She is diagnosed with acute rheumatic fever accompanied by arthritis and carditis and is treated with intramuscular penicillin and high-dose aspirin. Her arthritis improves markedly and almost immediately. She is discharged from the hospital with oral penicillin and high-dose aspirin.

The Condition

Although acute rheumatic fever is seen less often than in the past in developed countries, it remains one of the most common causes of acquired heart disease in much of the world. The prevalence of acute rheumatic fever has declined dramatically in the United States from 5 to 10 cases per 1,000 in the early 1900s to 0.05 cases per 1,000 currently. Typically, affected children and adolescents are between 5 and 15 years of age; fewer than 5% are younger than age 5 years.

Acute rheumatic fever is a delayed nonsuppurative complication of group A streptococcal (GAS) pharyngitis, which is a mandatory precedent to the diagnosis. The initial GAS infection is followed by a latent period of 2 to 4 weeks before symptoms of the disease appear. The clinical manifestations vary but typically include polyarthritis, carditis, subcutaneous nodules, erythema marginatum, or chorea. Prompt diagnosis and treatment of acute rheumatic fever are important to prevent the serious sequelae of rheumatic heart disease. Mitral regurgitation is the most common valvular lesion in children; mitral stenosis is most common in adults, resulting from previous bouts of rheumatic fever and ongoing valvulitis.

Differential Diagnosis

The differential diagnosis for a child presenting with arthritis is extensive and includes infectious, inflammatory, rheumatologic, and oncological causes. The history and physical examination are essential to direct additional evaluation with laboratory or imaging studies.

Children who have fever and joint pain should be evaluated for infectious causes. Osteomyelitis and septic arthritis need to be identified and treated emergently with intravenous antibiotics to prevent joint and bone destruction. Lyme arthritis may present months to years after the initial infection. A history of residence in or travel to an endemic area may be elicited, and diagnosis is confirmed with laboratory evidence of infection with *Borrelia burgdorferi.*

Pain in the lower extremities may be a presenting symptom in children who have tumors, such as leukemia, neuroblastoma, or bone malignancies. Juvenile idiopathic arthritis should be considered in patients who have chronic insidious joint pain. Toxic or transient synovitis, a diagnosis of exclusion, is suggested by a preceding viral upper respiratory tract infection. The sterile joint inflammation is typically self-limiting over 7 to 10 days.

Diagnosis

Acute rheumatic fever remains a clinical diagnosis that is based on the modified Jones criteria, which consist of major criteria, minor criteria, and evidence of a preceding GAS infection. A patient has a high likelihood of acute rheumatic fever if he or she fulfills the modified Jones criteria (Box 60.1).[1]

Box 60.1. Modified Jones Criteria

Major Manifestations

1. Polyarthritis
2. Carditis
3. Subcutaneous nodules
4. Erythema marginatum
5. Sydenham chorea

Minor Manifestations

1. Fever
2. Arthralgia
3. Elevated erythrocyte sedimentation rate or C-reactive protein level
4. Prolonged PR interval

Evidence of Preceding Group A Streptococcal Infection

- Positive throat culture
- Positive rapid antigen test for group A *Streptococcus*
- Elevated streptococcal antibody (antistreptolysin-O, anti–deoxyribonuclease B, anti-hyaluronidase) titer

Acute Rheumatic Fever

Two major *or* 1 major and 2 minor manifestations *plus* evidence of a preceding group A streptococcal infection

Adapted from *Rheumatic Fever and Rheumatic Heart Disease: Report of a WHO Expert Consultation.* Technical Report Series No. 923. Geneva, Switzerland: World Health Organization; 2004. https://extranet.who.int/iris/restricted/handle/10665/42898. Published 2004. Accessed October 29, 2015.

The polyarthritis of acute rheumatic fever is typically migratory, with sequential cycles of inflammation and resolution in involved joints. Large joints, such as the knees and ankles, are affected more commonly. The patient usually experiences intense pain that makes it difficult to tolerate the slightest touch or passive movement. It is important to note that premature therapy of monoarthritis with anti-inflammatory agents may mask subsequent development of polyarthritis.

The cutaneous manifestations of acute rheumatic fever include subcutaneous nodules and erythema marginatum. Subcutaneous nodules are round, firm, mobile, painless lesions found most commonly over bony prominences, such as the knees, ankles, and elbows, or extensor tendons. Such nodules can also be seen in patients who have granuloma annulare, rheumatoid arthritis, and systemic lupus erythematosus. Erythema marginatum is a painless, nonpruritic erythematous macule or papule that spreads in a circular pattern on the trunk and proximal extremities. The rash may be difficult to appreciate, especially on dark-skinned individuals, and can be elicited by the application of heat to the skin. The presence of subcutaneous nodules or erythema marginatum in rheumatic fever is usually associated with carditis.

Sydenham chorea may have a longer latent period, occurring many months after the initial GAS infection. Chorea is a neurologic disorder characterized by rapid irregular involuntary and uncoordinated movements. Some patients may also have muscle weakness and emotional lability. The duration of symptoms lasts from weeks to months, and most children recover completely. Due to the long latent period, evidence of a preceding GAS infection or other clinical manifestations of rheumatic fever may no longer be present.

In addition to the major clinical manifestations, certain laboratory data support the diagnosis. It is mandatory to establish the presence of a preceding GAS infection by using one of several laboratory studies. A rapid streptococcal antigen test has high specificity (>95%) but variable sensitivity of 80% to 90%. Throat culture may be obtained for GAS if the rapid streptococcal antigen test is negative, but culture results are negative in approximately 75% of patients by the time acute rheumatic fever manifests. Antistreptococcal antibody titers (most commonly, antistreptolysin O, anti–deoxyribonuclease B, and antihyaluronidase) peak around the time of onset of acute rheumatic fever and, therefore, are more useful. Elevated erythrocyte sedimentation rate and C-reactive protein levels indicate ongoing inflammation.

Acute rheumatic fever can cause inflammation of the pericardium, myocardium, and endocardium. Accordingly, patients should undergo a thorough cardiac evaluation and echocardiography in a qualified center. Valvulitis can be appreciated on physical examination by auscultating the apical systolic murmur of mitral regurgitation or the early diastolic murmur of aortic regurgitation. Cardiomegaly may be seen on chest radiography. An electrocardiogram may reveal varying degrees of heart block. Echocardiography should be obtained in all patients who have acute rheumatic fever to look for signs of carditis, mitral or aortic regurgitation, myocardial dysfunction, or pericardial effusion. Approximately 5% to 10% of patients who have rheumatic fever have severe myocarditis that results in heart failure and should be treated aggressively.

Group A streptococcal pharyngitis with associated arthralgia is not rheumatic fever.

Treatment

Treatment of the GAS pharyngitis must be initiated within 9 days of onset to prevent acute rheumatic fever. Penicillin is the drug of choice, administered as either a single intramuscular dose or oral dosing for 10 days. For patients allergic to penicillin, a 5-day course of oral azithromycin, 12 mg/kg/d, may be used to eradicate GAS. All household contacts should be evaluated for GAS pharyngitis and treated if infected. Long-term antibiotic prophylaxis is important to prevent additional infection with GAS pharyngitis, recurrence of rheumatic fever, and increased risk of developing rheumatic heart disease. This is different from and not to be confused with subacute bacterial endocarditis prophylaxis.

The unique clinical manifestations of each patient should be treated accordingly. Short-term anti-inflammatory therapy with high-dose aspirin (100 mg/kg/d) is provided to patients who have arthritis. Patients and their parents should be taught to recognize signs and symptoms of aspirin toxicity. Moderate to severe carditis may be treated with corticosteroids. Patients who have heart failure are usually treated with digoxin, diuretics, or afterload reduction therapy. Management of chorea involves the use of sedatives such as haloperidol and phenobarbital.

Reference

1. *Rheumatic Fever and Rheumatic Heart Disease: Report of a WHO Expert Consultation.* Technical Report Series No. 923. Geneva, Switzerland: World Health Organization; 2004. https://extranet.who.int/iris/restricted/handle/10665/42898. Published 2004. Accessed October 29, 2015

Lessons for the Physician

Physicians should be vigilant in diagnosing and treating group A streptococcal pharyngitis to prevent the sequelae of rheumatic fever and rheumatic heart disease. The clinical manifestations of acute rheumatic fever vary widely and may mimic other, more common disease processes. In this particular case, repeated physical examinations were important in diagnosing the true underlying condition.

Heather Liu, MD, Morgan Stanley Children's Hospital of New York-Presbyterian, New York, NY

CHAPTER 61

16-Year-Old Boy With Severe Pain in Right Knee

Presentation

A 16-year-old boy limps into the clinic complaining of severe pain in his right knee, which has been swollen and painful for 5 days. He cannot bear much weight or straighten the leg. One week ago, he fell onto his right wrist and right knee. Two days later, his wrist was improving, but he had pain in his left ankle. Radiographs of the ankle revealed no fracture. Yesterday his right shoulder started to hurt. All joints are better now except his right knee.

He has had fevers since yesterday, chills today, nausea and a decreased appetite for 1 week, but no vomiting or diarrhea. He had a mild sore throat 2 weeks ago. A red rash started yesterday on his right knee and appeared briefly on his neck. The boy lives with his mother; they have hamsters, guinea pigs, a cat, a dog, and a pet rat, purchased just 2 days ago.

The patient had unprotected heterosexual sex 2 months ago. He denies dysuria, frequency, penile discharge, or a history of sexually transmitted infection. His sister has "small joint" rheumatoid arthritis, his mother has Marfan syndrome, and a grandmother has had rheumatic fever.

On physical examination, the boy appears uncomfortable. His temperature is 102.0°F (38.9°C) orally, pulse is 90 beats/min, respirations are 20 breaths/min, and blood pressure is 115/58 mm Hg. Remarkable findings include mild pain on full abduction of his right shoulder; a slightly swollen but nontender left ankle; and a markedly swollen right knee that has limited flexion, is exquisitely tender, and has an area of salmon-colored macular erythema over the patella that fades within the hour.

Laboratory results include white blood cell count, 10,500/mm^3 (10.5 × 10^9/L), with 8% band forms, 74% segmented neutrophils, 9% lymphocytes, and 9% monocytes; hemoglobin, 14.4 g/dL (144 g/L); platelet count, 283 × 10^3/mm^3 (283 × 10^9/L);

and erythrocyte sedimentation rate, 41 mm/h. Results of urinalysis are normal, and a rapid antigen test for group A *Streptococcus* from a throat swab is negative. Preparations are made to aspirate the patient's right knee effusion.

- **What is your differential diagnosis at this point?**
- **Are there any elements of history or physical examination that would help you?**
- **What additional diagnostic studies would you like performed?**

Discussion

Differential Diagnosis

This adolescent has a migratory polyarthritis affecting his larger joints and associated with fever and rash. The causes of polyarthritis are many and include infectious, postinfectious, reactive, rheumatoid, and a variety of systemic etiologies. The diagnosis that needs to be entertained most emergently is a septic joint. Although *Staphylococcus aureus* is the most common cause of septic arthritis overall, it is unusual for this organism to cause a migratory polyarthritis. Specific infectious etiologies of polyarticular infection include the *Neisseria* species (*Neisseria gonorrhoeae* and *Neisseria meningitidis*), *Streptococcus pneumoniae, Haemophilus influenzae,* group G *Streptococcus, Streptobacillus moniliformis,* and *Mycoplasma pneumoniae.* Lyme disease can cause an infectious arthritis, but this patient had not been near an endemic area recently. The migratory nature of his arthritis suggests gonococcemia or meningococcemia as well as acute rheumatic fever, systemic lupus erythematosus (SLE), and viral arthritis.

Because this patient had had unprotected sexual intercourse, both gonococcemia and Reiter syndrome are possible. Although disseminated gonococcal infections occur more frequently in women than in men, neisserial arthritis is usually polyarticular, migratory, and associated with fever and chills. Often a rash is noted on extensor surfaces, consisting of scattered crops of vesicopustules on an erythematous base. Reiter syndrome typically presents as a reactive polyarthritis affecting large joints of the lower extremities and following a variety of enteric infections, but it can also occur after infection with *Chlamydia trachomatis.* However, fever is usually not prominent during the arthritis of Reiter syndrome, and this patient had not complained of the other 2 classic (although variably present) symptoms of this syndrome: eye pain and dysuria. This boy had polymerase chain reaction analysis of his urine for both gonorrhea and *C trachomatis.*

In addition to gonococcemia, another neisserial infection, meningococcemia, can present with migratory polyarthritis and fever in its subacute or chronic forms, and in rare patients, it can present without meningococcal sepsis or meningitis.

Two other sexually transmitted diseases that can cause polyarthritis and fever are syphilis, which can do so in its secondary stage, and human immunodeficiency virus infection. However, this patient does not have the maculopapular rash on the palms and soles that is characteristic of secondary syphilis. Human immunodeficiency virus is associated with several patterns of arthropathy, but the best-described acquired immunodeficiency syndrome–associated arthritis is characteristically a persistent, symmetric, nonmigratory polyarthritis.

A number of other viral infections can cause arthritis. Hepatitis B virus can present with arthritis and fever prior to the onset of hyperbilirubinemia; the diagnosis is suggested by elevated aminotransferase levels and confirmed by detection of viral surface antigen. Both rubella and parvovirus B19 can present with fever and arthritis, but more typically in young women, and the arthritis is more often symmetric and in the hands.

In addition to Reiter syndrome, other postinfectious and reactive arthritides are associated with fever. Arthritis occurring 1 to 2 weeks after infection with *Mycobacterium tuberculosis, Mycoplasma,* and varicella has been described (although none of these disorders is usually associated with a migratory polyarthritis) in addition to poststreptococcal reactive arthritis. Whether the latter is distinct from acute rheumatic fever (ARF) is controversial. Certainly this patient comes from a rheumatogenic family, and he does give a history of a sore throat preceding this illness by 2 weeks. In addition, his knee appears to have the exquisite pain that is described by patients who have this disease. The diagnosis of ARF requires the presence of 2 major Jones criteria (carditis, polyarthritis, Sydenham chorea, erythema marginatum, subcutaneous nodules) or 1 major and 2 minor criteria (fever, polyarthralgias, previous ARF, elevated erythrocyte sedimentation rate or C-reactive protein level or leukocytosis, prolonged PR interval) in conjunction with evidence of a preceding streptococcal infection (positive throat culture or rapid antigen test or elevated antistreptolysin O or anti–deoxyribonuclease B titers). Before this patient was admitted to the pediatric ward, serum was obtained for titers, and an electrocardiogram revealed a normal sinus rhythm with a normal PR interval.

Rheumatologic causes of arthritis should be considered in this patient. Rheumatoid arthritis is a possibility, but the polyarthritis of this disease is usually not migratory and is not associated with fever. The patient's sister has pauciarticular juvenile rheumatoid arthritis, but the boy's high fever and evanescent rash are more suggestive of systemic-onset juvenile rheumatoid arthritis or Still disease. Juvenile rheumatoid arthritis can occur in 4 patterns: (1) systemic-onset, characterized by an evanescent, salmon-pink, macular rash; arthritis; hepatosplenomegaly; leukocytosis; and polyserositis; (2) polyarticular (adult pattern), with chronic pain and swelling of many joints in a symmetric pattern but typically without fever; (3) pauciarticular, with chronic asymmetric arthritis of a few large joints and sometimes associated iridocyclitis of the eye; and (4) HLA-B27–positive pauciarticular disease, which can progress to spondyloarthropathy. Fever is also prominent in polyarticular gout, although this patient is young for that disease. The diagnosis of gout is confirmed by the presence of sodium urate crystals in the synovial fluid.

Finally, a number of systemic illnesses are associated with arthritis and fever. Rash and arthritis of the lower extremities is seen in Henoch-Schönlein purpura, but this patient has no petechiae or purpura, is not complaining of colicky abdominal pain, and has no evidence of nephritis on urinalysis. Patients who have Henoch-Schönlein purpura do not usually have fever. Wegener granulomatosis rarely begins with fever and polyarthritis before progressing to the more common pulmonary symptoms. Although much more common in girls, SLE can present with polyarthritis and fever; the antinuclear antibody (ANA) test is a sensitive but not particularly specific diagnostic tool for this disorder. A patient should meet 4 of 11 diagnostic criteria for SLE: malar rash, discoid rash, photosensitivity, oral ulcers, nonerosive arthritis, pleuritis or pericarditis, proteinuria or casts in the urine, seizures or psychosis, hematologic disorder (decrease in at least 1 blood cell line), a positive ANA, and other positive antibodies. A large joint arthritis can occur in association with inflammatory bowel disease and not necessarily when the patient is symptomatic with gastrointestinal symptoms. The large joint effusions that are seen in patients who have inflammatory bowel disease tend not to be very painful. Two other systemic processes that can cause a migratory arthritis are acute leukemia (for which there is no evidence on this boy's peripheral blood smear) and Whipple disease, which is extraordinarily rare in a young person.

Making the Diagnosis

The patient's knee was aspirated and 60 mL of yellow, straw-colored fluid removed. The synovial effusion contained a white blood cell count of 34,100/mcL with 82% polymorphonuclear white blood cells, 10% lymphocytes, and 8% monocytes. No crystals were seen under the microscope, and a Gram stain of the fluid revealed white blood cells but no organisms.

Results of other tests reported at this time were negative for ANA, antistreptolysin O factor, rheumatoid factor, and polymerase chain reaction test for *N gonorrhoeae* and *C trachomatis.* The lack of evidence for current or recent streptococcal infection and normal findings on heart examination and electrocardiography made rheumatic fever unlikely, and negative ANA results made SLE very unlikely. Because of the moderate number of white blood cells in his knee effusion, his problem could have been either a multifocal septic arthritis or a rheumatologic or reactive process, although the negative Gram stain made it unlikely that the causative agent was a staphylococcal or streptococcal agent. Disseminated *Gonococcus* typically causes joint effusions that yield negative results on Gram stains, and affected patients often also have negative urethral cultures. Because gonococcemia remained high on the differential diagnosis list, the patient was treated with intravenous cefotaxime pending the results of a blood culture.

The following morning, he was much improved. He had been afebrile overnight and denied any knee pain. Furthermore, he could now walk without a limp. The blood culture was negative at this point, but the knee aspirate was growing an organism that on Gram stain appeared as a pleomorphic gram-negative rod. The microbe was oxidase- and catalase-negative, features highly suggestive of *Streptobacillus moniliformis,* the causative agent of rat-bite fever. The culture was sent to the Centers for Disease Control and Prevention for confirmation. Because of this new information, the patient was asked if he could have been bitten by a rat any time in the past few months. He reported that he worked in a pet store until 2 weeks ago, and on his last day of work, one of the rats in the store bit him on his left index finger. There had been some bleeding, but the wound had healed quickly and had not bothered him since.

Clinical Presentation

Rat-bite fever is a zoonotic infection caused by either *S moniliformis* (almost all cases in the United States) or *Spirillum minus* (a spirochete found primarily in Asia). The former is transmitted by the bite or scratch of rats, squirrels, mice, and, rarely, cats or weasels, as well as by carnivores that prey on those small rodents. When infection follows ingestion of contaminated milk or water, the infection is called Haverhill fever. Typically, the initial bite heals without sequelae. After an incubation period of up to 3 weeks, the patient experiences the abrupt onset of fever or chills, muscle aches, headache, and a rash that can be petechial or maculopapular and predominantly affects the extremities (often the palms and soles). Infection by *S minus* can cause a distinctive rash of red or purple plaques. Approximately 50% of patients experience a nonsuppurative migratory polyarthritis. If untreated, complications include destructive joint disease, multiple abscesses, pneumonia, endocarditis, parotitis, pancreatitis, and pericarditis. Without antibiotics, the mortality rate is 10%, due primarily to the complications of endocarditis.

Diagnosis

As demonstrated in this case, *S moniliformis* can be isolated from synovial fluid, blood, and other body fluids. Special culturing techniques using enriched media are required, and laboratory personnel should be notified that rat-bite fever is suspected. Darkfield microscopy is another technique for identifying the organism. Given the many causes of migratory arthritis and the rarity of this infection, initial evaluation of patients who have a clinical presentation typical of rat-bite fever is likely to include testing for a number of disorders.

Therapy

The treatment of choice for rat-bite fever remains penicillin. Because of the invasive nature of the disease, intravenous penicillin G is recommended for 7 to 10 days, followed by oral penicillin V for an additional 7 days. If the patient has had the typical prompt response and is much better in 5 to 7 days without evidence of endocarditis, the transition to oral penicillin can be made at that time. For patients who are allergic to penicillin, a tetracycline may be used—the safest may be doxycycline—assuming that the patient is younger than 8 years (or when the benefits outweigh the low risk of dental staining from only one treatment course).

This patient was asymptomatic when he was discharged after 1 week in the hospital to complete his week of oral therapy. He missed his scheduled follow-up appointment but was seen in the hospital emergency department 3 weeks later for minor trauma, at which time he had no fever or joint complaints.

When patients are bitten by rodents that may carry the threat of rat-bite fever, the physician should clean the wound well, determine the patient's need for tetanus immunization, and consider a few days of penicillin prophylaxis.

Lessons for the Physician

- This case illustrates 3 important clinical points. First, when presented with a patient who has fever and a swollen joint, it is essential both to obtain fluid from the joint to make the diagnosis and to treat the patient for a presumed septic joint until the diagnosis proves otherwise. Second, as is so often the case, the clue to the diagnosis is usually in the history. In this case, a good pet history was obtained but not the key fact that a rat had bitten the patient 2 weeks prior to admission. Finally, this microorganism is extremely fastidious; it does not grow on blood or MacConkey agar and requires 10% to 20% rabbit or horse serum, defibrinated blood, or ascites fluid to sustain growth. This difficulty in laboratory confirmation requires the physician to have a strong suspicion of rat-bite fever based on the history and, in many cases, to treat empirically despite negative cultures.
- It is estimated that 50% to 100% of rats in the United States, both laboratory and wild animals, harbor *Streptobacillus moniliformis* as normal nasopharyngeal flora. Up to 10% of rat bites of humans result in transmission of the organism, and 50% of all cases in this country involve children or adolescents. Although the disease is unusual, it is not disappearing and probably underdiagnosed. When presented with a patient who has unexplained fevers and rash associated with arthritis, especially if there are rats in the history, include rat-bite fever in the differential diagnosis!

Simon J. Hambidge, MD, PhD, and John W. Ogle, MD, Denver Health Medical Center, University of Colorado School of Medicine, Denver, CO

CHAPTER 62

16-Year-Old Girl With Generalized Seizures

Presentation

A 16-year-old girl from Ghana is admitted to the hospital after an episode of generalized seizures. She complains of headache and tiredness at the time of admission. She has had seizures since September 2004, when she immigrated to the United States from a refugee camp in Somalia. She is treated with carbamazepine because she developed Stevens-Johnson syndrome while taking phenytoin. She has a past medical history of malaria, anemia, and peripheral blood eosinophilia (38%), for which she received empiric mebendazole therapy. Her mother has latent tuberculosis.

At admission, the girl's vital signs are stable, and there are no abnormalities on physical examination. Complete blood cell count reveals a hemoglobin of 8.7 g/dL (87 g/L) with 28% eosinophils and an absolute eosinophil count of 1,590 cells/mm^3. Electroencephalogram and computed tomography scan of her head yield normal results. Urinalysis shows a large number of red blood cells but is negative for white blood cells and protein. Tuberculin testing is negative. Additional laboratory evaluation identifies the cause of her hematuria.

- **What is your differential diagnosis at this point?**
- **Are there any elements of history or physical examination that would help you?**
- **What additional diagnostic studies would you like performed?**

Discussion

Abdominal ultrasonography showed normal kidneys with sessile masses in the bladder wall (Figure 62.1). Cystoscopy showed significant bladder edema, several sessile masses, and multiple sandy patches throughout the bladder (Figure 62.2). Multiple biopsies of the bladder were taken during cystoscopy. Stool and urine

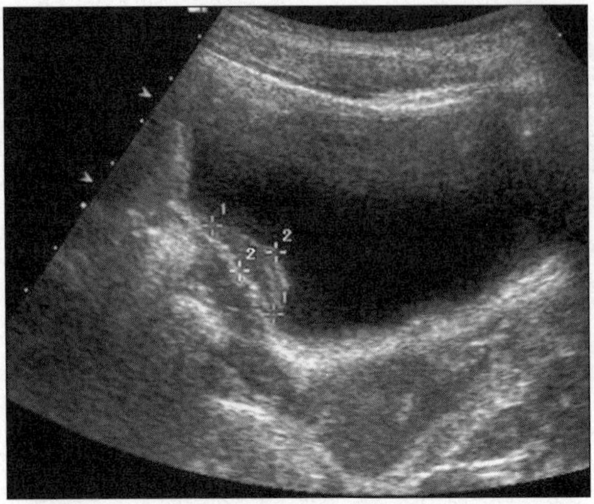

Figure 62.1. Ultrasonography of bladder showing the sessile lesions.

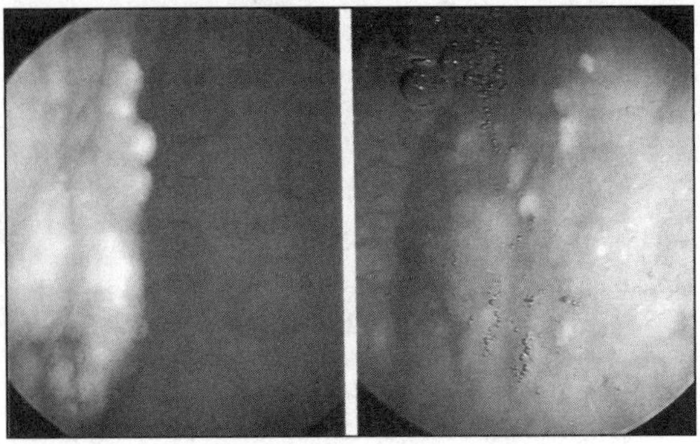

Figure 62.2. Cystoscopy showing the intraluminal lesions of schistosomiasis.

were examined for *Schistosoma* eggs because of the history of emigration from an endemic area, hematuria, and bladder lesions; results of these examinations were negative. However, the serum *Schistosoma* antibody (IgG) was positive at 1.75 optical density. Compression preparations were made of freshly obtained unfixed bladder biopsies, and oval eggs that have terminal spines were seen under the microscope. The eggs contained viable developing or mature miracidia, indicated by actively moving cilia of the flame cells located in the center of the miracidia. A miracidial hatching test was performed by adding fresh water to this slide, and after 1 minute, a number of the eggs hatched, releasing the miracidia, thereby providing additional proof that the eggs were viable.

Bladder biopsies showed hyperplastic transitional epithelium with polyp formation. The subepithelium contained clusters of oval eggs with terminal spines surrounded by a granulomatous response consisting of epithelioid histiocytes, eosinophils, lymphocytes, plasma cells, and occasional giant cells (Figure 62.3). Most of the eggs had clear, delicate outer shells, and some eggs were calcified. The histologic findings were consistent with a chronic active *Schistosoma hematobium* infection.

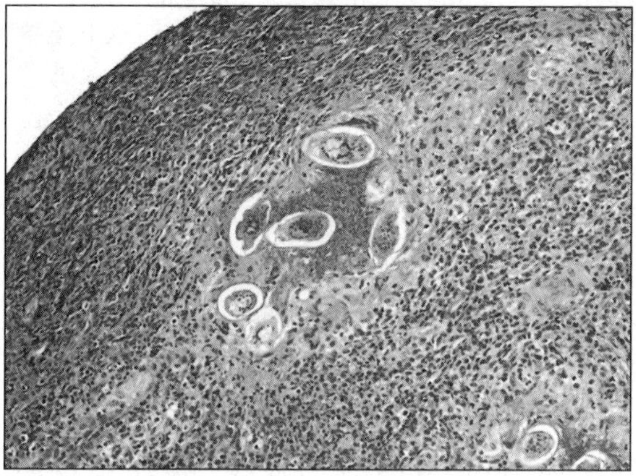

Figure 62.3. Histopathology of bladder biopsy showing *Schistosoma* eggs and surrounding inflammatory cells.

The girl was treated with praziquantel. Her seizurelike episodes were diagnosed as pseudoseizures. At 3-month follow-up, her hematuria and abdominal pain had resolved with treatment. The patient was lost to long-term follow-up.

The Condition

Schistosomiasis is a parasitic infestation in which infecting larvae (cercariae), which have developed in certain species of snails, penetrate the skin of individuals who enter infested waters. The cercariae develop into mature worms in the bloodstream and lay eggs. Inflammation and fibrosis caused by the eggs account for a wide variety of symptoms that affect the gastrointestinal tract, bladder, lungs, and central nervous system. The eggs are passed in urine and feces and hatch into miracidia, a motile form of the parasite that infects the snails.

A World Health Organization report estimates that 500 to 600 million people in 74 countries are at risk for schistosomiasis and that more than 200 million people in these countries are infected. It is estimated that 20 million individuals have severe consequences of this chronic and debilitating disease, which is responsible for at least 500,000 deaths per year.[1] Infestation exceeds 90% in some endemic regions of the world (Nigeria and Ghana). Because of the absence of the necessary species of snails, the United States is free of endemic schistosomiasis. However, an estimated 400,000 cases exist in the United States, chiefly among emigrants from endemic foreign countries. Schistosomiasis is expected to be seen with increasing frequency in the United States with the influx of emigrants and increasing numbers of travelers from endemic areas.

Hematuria is the first sign of established bladder disease, appearing 10 to 12 weeks after infection. Other signs include urinary frequency and dysuria. Chronic infection can evolve to fibrosis or calcification of the bladder and lower ureters, resulting in hydroureter, hydronephrosis, parenchymal damage, and renal failure. Obstructive uropathy is the most common complication of *S hematobium* infection of the interstitial and juxtavesicular portions of the ureter. Nephrotic syndrome, immune complex–mediated glomerulonephritis, and chronic renal failure may be the result of chronic infection. Squamous cell carcinoma of the urinary bladder due to chronic inflammation is a late complication that may occur 10 to 20 years after infection.[2]

Diagnosis

The initial evaluation of a child presenting with hematuria involves a history and examination, including urinalysis, culture, and complete blood cell count. A high degree of suspicion for schistosomiasis is required in a patient who has emigrated from an endemic area and has hematuria and eosinophilia. Employing microscopy to detect *S hematobium* eggs in urine is a sensitive and cost-effective test considered to be the criterion standard for diagnosing this form of schistosomiasis.[3] Because the excretion of schistosome eggs into the urine is not uniform over time, random collection and a single void may not show eggs. Therefore, multiple urine specimens are required for detecting ova and parasites. Urine specimens collected between 10:00 am and 2:00 pm are more likely to be positive because the eggs are shed when the patient is mobile for a few hours. Microscopic examination of urine reveals eggs that have the characteristic species-specific morphology.

Serologic tests detect IgG, IgM, or IgE antibodies against soluble worm or crude egg antigens. Seroconversion occurs within 4 to 8 weeks of infection and remains positive for at least 2 years after cure. Antibody-based assays are sensitive but are not useful in distinguishing prior exposure from active infection or reinfection. The antibodies also cross-react with other helminths and thus may give false-positive results.

In the early phase, cystoscopy reveals mucosal hemorrhages, whereas in chronic infection, punctate white calcifications (sandy patches) are seen in the bladder wall. Biopsy of affected tissues provides specimens for ova identification in cases in which eggs are not shed in urine.

Management

Praziquantel, a pyrazinoisoquinoline derivative, is the mainstay of treatment and community-based schistosomiasis control. The drug disturbs the ionic exchange through the worm's membrane, resulting in tetanic paralysis and reduced glucose absorption. Successful therapy requires 2 to 3 doses of 20 mg/kg of body weight given 6 to 8 hours apart. Community-based control programs usually treat patients with a single dose of 40 mg/kg. Reexamination of feces or urine 1 month after treatment is recommended to assess the success of therapy. Praziquantel cures 60% to 90% of patients; those who are not cured have a 90% to 95% reduction in egg burden. Treatment should be repeated in patients who continue to shed viable eggs; such retreatment is usually successful.

Vaccines directed against the newly identified surface protein Sm29 from the helminth may provide long-term immune response. The tetraspanin family of integument protein from *Schistosoma* is also considered a candidate for vaccine targeting. It is hoped that genomics and proteomics will help identify more candidate antigens for successful vaccine development.

References

1. Chitsulo L, Engels D, Montresor A, et al. The global status of schistosomiasis and its control. *Acta Trop.* 2000;77(1):41–51
2. Koraitim MM, Metwalli NE, Atta MA, et al. Changing age incidence and pathological types of schistosoma-associated bladder carcinoma. *J Urol.* 1995;154(5):1714–1716
3. Feldmeier H, Poggensee G. Diagnostic techniques in schistosomiasis control. A review. *Acta Trop.* 1993;52(4):205–220

Lessons for the Physician

- Schistosomiasis is not encountered commonly in the United States.
- Schistosomiasis should be considered in a child or adolescent who has hematuria and has emigrated from or traveled to areas where schistosomiasis is endemic.
- Early diagnosis and treatment of schistosomiasis is critical in preventing complications of renal failure and bladder cancer.

Poonam Sharma, MBBS, and Meera Varman, MD, Creighton University School of Medicine, Omaha, NE
Joseph T. Snow, MD; Nancy E. Cornish, MD; and John Donovan, MD, Children's Hospital, Omaha, NE

CHAPTER 63

Rash and Headache in a Wrestler

Presentation

A 17-year-old boy presents with severe headache and progressive rash. He complains of chills, sore throat, anorexia, eye pain, and blurry vision. Before the onset of these symptoms, he was healthy and competing in wrestling matches. Today, he reports disabling fatigue and intense pain.

Physical examination reveals a tired-appearing, muscular adolescent boy who has a temperature of 102.0°F (38.9°C), heart rate of 86 beats/min, respiratory rate of 24 breaths/min, and blood pressure of 143/64 mm Hg. His pupils are equal and reactive with intact extraocular movements, but he exhibits photophobia, excessive tearing, and conjunctival injection limited to the right eye. Prominent lymphadenopathy is evident throughout his head and neck. He experiences discomfort with neck movement. His head, neck, right arm, and right trunk are densely covered with clusters of monomorphous vesicles on erythematous bases and 2- to 4-mm crusted erosions (Figure 63.1). A few pustules are visible on his face. No skin lesions are apparent on the remainder of his body, including his genitals.

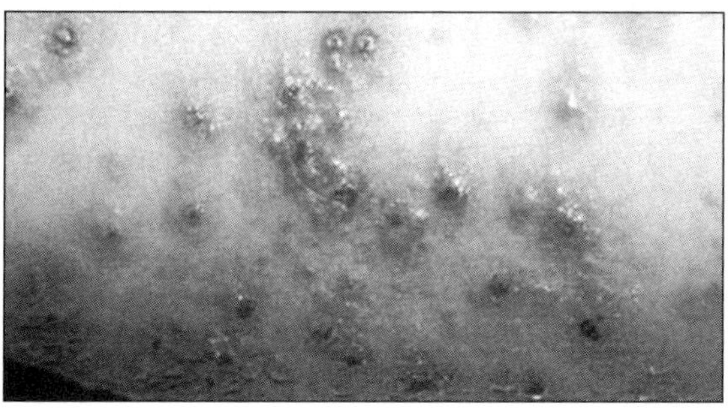

Figure 63.1. Clusters of monomorphous vesicles on erythematous bases.

Results of laboratory studies include white blood cell count of 6.5×10^3/mcL (6.5×10^9/L), with 71% neutrophils, 15% lymphocytes, and 13% monocytes; hemoglobin of 15.8 g/dL (158 g/L); platelet count of 132×10^3/mcL (132×10^9/L); alanine aminotransferase of 24 U/L (0.40 mckat/L); aspartate aminotransferase of 18 U/L

(0.30 mckat/L); and C-reactive protein of 124 mg/dL. Cerebrospinal fluid analysis reveals 1 white blood cell, 3 red blood cells, glucose concentration of 52 mg/dL (2.9 mmol/L), protein concentration of 32 mg/dL, and no organisms on Gram stain. After unroofing a vesicle, fluid is obtained for cultures. Additional history and laboratory testing confirm the diagnosis.

- **What is your differential diagnosis at this point?**
- **Are there any elements of history or physical examination that would help you?**
- **What additional diagnostic studies would you like performed?**

Discussion

The patient remembered that another wrestler in a competition had a "blister" above his lip, and his mother was notified that 4 other boys who participated in recent wrestling meets were hospitalized with similar symptoms. He denied a history of herpes labialis or genital herpes, and he was not immunocompromised. He had primary varicella infection as a child.

Clinical Course and Management

The appearance and distribution of vesicular skin lesions led to a diagnosis of herpes gladiatorum. Because the boy complained of severe headache, photophobia, and neck stiffness, he was admitted for intravenous acyclovir therapy. The ophthalmologist found no evidence of herpetic corneal involvement, uveitis, or retinal pathology. *Human herpesvirus 1* (HSV-1) was cultured from the skin lesions. Cerebrospinal cultures and cerebrospinal HSV polymerase chain reaction tests had negative results. He was transitioned to oral valacyclovir after 2 days of intravenous acyclovir. At that time, all existing lesions were dry and crusted and he was discharged.

The Condition

Herpes gladiatorum, also known as "scrumpox" (named for the scrum team formation in rugby), is a cutaneous HSV-1 infection transmitted by close skin-to-skin contact in sports such as wrestling, rugby, and judo. The National Collegiate Athletic Association estimates that the incidence of herpes gladiatorum among Division I wrestlers is between 20% and 40%. Infection rates as high as 70% have been reported from intense high school wrestling training camps. The attack rate is approximately twice as high for athletes who have had no prior exposure to herpes.

The HSV-1 virus is introduced into the skin via abrasions through direct skin-to-skin contact with an infected player or by self-inoculation. Conditions that impair the barrier function of the skin, such as eczema, may further increase an individual's susceptibility to cutaneous herpes infection. Skin lesions appear 4 to 11 days after exposure. With primary HSV infections, fever, malaise, anorexia, sore throat, and lymphadenopathy are common and typically precede the development of skin lesions by 2 days. Significant associated weight loss has been reported. Skin lesions evolve from vesicles to crusted erosions and eventually heal over the course of 10 to 14 days. In general, the lesions heal without scarring. After the infection resolves, HSV-1 virus remains dormant in nerve tissue and can reactivate in the future. Recurrences of skin lesions are generally less severe than the primary infection.

In wrestlers, herpes gladiatorum skin lesions classically develop on the ventral aspect of the head, neck, arm, and trunk on the side of the body that reflects their handedness. This pattern of distribution has been attributed to the commonly employed “lock-up” position, which places the face, neck, and arms of opponents in close contact.

Herpetic eye involvement can result in serious ocular complications such as blepharitis, scleritis, follicular conjunctivitis, keratoconjunctivitis with dendritic ulcer formation, and uveitis. Reactivation of the dormant herpesvirus along the ophthalmic branch of the trigeminal nerve can result in keratitis with subsequent corneal scarring and vision loss. In one outbreak at a high school wrestling camp, 5 of 60 attendees who had herpes gladiatorum developed ocular complications.[1]

Diagnosis

Other skin infections that should be considered in the differential diagnosis for this patient include folliculitis and impetigo. Variations in the number of herpetic lesions, the presence of secondary bacterial infections, and the evolution of the herpes skin eruption may make herpes gladiatorum difficult to distinguish from these conditions. Viral and bacterial skin cultures, the Tzanck test, and HSV direct fluorescent antibody assay are helpful diagnostic techniques. Direct fluorescent antibody assay is performed frequently as an initial diagnostic test because it offers rapid immunologic identification of HSV in samples collected by swabbing a skin lesion with a Dacron viral culture swab. If the direct fluorescent antibody assay result is negative, the specimen is submitted for viral culture.

Treatment and Prevention

Treatment of active skin infection with oral valacyclovir twice daily for 7 days reduces the duration of both symptoms and viral shedding. Valacyclovir is the preferred oral agent because of better bioavailability than acyclovir. Strict “return to play” rules require that an affected athlete take at least 5 full days of antiviral therapy before resuming competition or practice. In addition, the athlete must have no new lesions in the past 72 hours, and all existing lesions must be dry with adherent crust. Coaches and athletic trainers perform skin checks of athletes before competition in an effort to prevent transmission of the virus. In addition, athletes are encouraged to shower with soap and water immediately after practice and to wash clothes and equipment daily.

Data suggest that prophylactic treatment with antiviral agents may help reduce the number of competition days lost for individual athletes who have had prior cutaneous HSV-1 infection and may help decrease transmission. Prophylactic dosing of valacyclovir has been shown to decrease the number of outbreaks per wrestling season in patients who have recurrent herpes gladiatorum.[2] In one study, introduction of nearly universal antiviral prophylaxis into a large wrestling camp program significantly reduced the total number of herpes gladiatorum cases compared to the number of cases that occurred in previous years.[3]

References

1. Belongia EA, Goodman JL, Holland EJ, et al. An outbreak of herpes gladiatorum at a high school wrestling camp. *N Engl J Med.* 1991;325(13):906–910
2. Anderson BJ. The effectiveness of valacyclovir in preventing reactivation of herpes gladiatorum in wrestlers. *Clin J Sport Med.* 1999;2(2):86–90
3. Anderson BJ. Prophylactic valacyclovir to prevent outbreaks of primary herpes gladiatorum at a 28-day wrestling camp. *Jpn J Infect Dis.* 2006;59(1):6–9

Lessons for the Physician

- Herpes gladiatorum can be a serious health concern for wrestlers.
- It is critical for coaches and athletes to be educated about prevention of human herpesvirus transmission.
- At present, human herpesvirus keratoconjunctivitis is the major cause of blindness from an infectious agent in the United States. When herpes gladiatorum is suspected, any signs or symptoms of ocular involvement warrant immediate referral to an ophthalmologist.

Raegan Hunt, MD, PhD, and Pranita Tamma, MD, The Johns Hopkins Hospital, Baltimore, MD

CHAPTER 64

Congenitally Deaf 17-Year-Old Boy With a 1-Year History of a Rash

Presentation

A congenitally deaf 17-year-old Filipino boy comes to your clinic with a 1-year history of a rash. Because he communicates in sign language, his mother gives the history. He was born in a rural area of the Philippines. At age 16 years, 2 years after immigration to North America, he noted a pale patch surrounded by an erythematous margin on his chest. Similar lesions slowly began to appear, first on his trunk, then on his upper and lower extremities. He sought medical care from numerous physicians, who suggested a variety of conditions, including ringworm and eczema. Several topical therapies did not help.

The current lesions are large, hypopigmented patches, some as large as 8 × 12 cm, on his chest, back, arms, and legs, in a roughly symmetric distribution. Most of the lesions are well-defined, although some have indistinct borders. The lesions on his thighs have erythematous, thickened borders. Other findings of the physical examination support the provisional diagnosis, which is confirmed by a specific laboratory test.

- **What is your differential diagnosis at this point?**
- **Are there any elements of history or physical examination that would help you?**
- **What additional diagnostic studies would you like performed?**

Discussion

Physical examination revealed thickened ulnar and posterior tibial nerves bilaterally as well as decreased strength in the ulnar distribution of the boy's left hand. Many of his skin lesions were hypoesthetic to touch and pinprick sensation. A skin biopsy, as well as slit skin smears, confirmed the diagnosis of borderline lepromatous leprosy (Hansen disease).

Leprosy is a chronic disease caused by *Mycobacterium leprae.* It is endemic in most parts of the developing world, particularly Asia. Although the mode of transmission has not been defined fully, the disease is probably transmitted by droplet spread from the nasal mucosa of infected patients. The usual incubation period is 4 to 6 years. Most people who are infected recover naturally and develop no signs or symptoms of disease.

Clinical Spectrum

In those who develop the disease, the clinical pattern depends on the host's cell-mediated response to the organism. The clinical spectrum ranges from tuberculoid to lepromatous leprosy. In tuberculoid disease, patients mount a good immune response, which is manifested clinically as a few well-defined, hypopigmented, anesthetic, hairless macules and enlarged peripheral nerves. Patients who develop lepromatous leprosy have poor immunity and present with multiple symmetric, poorly demarcated lesions that have normal sensation. These patients develop involvement of multiple organs, including the eyes, upper respiratory tract mucosa, testes, and kidneys. Neural involvement occurs late in the disease. With disease progression or treatment, patients can move up or down this clinical spectrum. As in this boy's case, definitive diagnosis is made by skin biopsy.

The major morbidity in leprosy is due to neuritis, which occurs as a consequence of diminished cell-mediated immunity, leading to anergy for *M leprae* and allowing uncontrolled multiplication of the mycobacteria. Sensory, autonomic, and motor components are affected. Marked anesthesia of the extremities causes delayed detection of injury, with consequent burns, wounds, and infections. Muscle imbalance from damage to motor nerves results in joint deformities and contractures. A claw hand is the most common example.

Treatment

An expert should supervise treatment of leprosy because patients may have a sudden, overexuberant immunologic response ("upgrading of immunity"), leading to erythema nodosum or irreversible nerve damage on a hypersensitivity basis. Drugs used in treatment include dapsone, rifampin, clofazimine, and ethionamide. Prevention of nerve damage is the most important therapeutic goal. If nerve damage has already occurred at the time of diagnosis, patients need extensive physical rehabilitation, counseling about avoiding injury, appropriate footwear, and prosthetic devices. It is important to remember the great social stigma of this disease, particularly in areas of the world where it is endemic. In many communities, affected people are rejected by society and live in social and physical isolation. Fear and misconceptions about leprosy can jeopardize their care seriously.

This patient was started on a triple-drug regimen and is doing well. He will require at least 2 years of therapy. His mother had difficulty coming to terms with the diagnosis because she felt her son was already stigmatized by his deafness. This boy did not develop permanent nerve damage, which is particularly important because his hands are his only means of communication.

Lessons for the Physician

Leprosy should be suspected in adolescents coming from endemic areas who present with chronic hypoesthetic skin lesions or numbness or weakness of the extremities. Early diagnosis is essential to prevent nerve damage and disability. Most patients in North America have sought many medical opinions, sometimes over several years, before the diagnosis finally is considered. This disease offers another example of how the immune response of the host governs the clinical manifestations of infection. A poor immunologic response will allow the infection to become more extensive, but an inappropriately exuberant reaction will damage tissue and harm the individual.

Marina Salvadori, MD, The Hospital for Sick Children, Toronto, Ontario, Canada

COMMENTARY BY DR DEEPAK KAMAT, GLOBAL HEALTH SPECIALIST, CHILDREN'S HOSPITAL OF MICHIGAN

In certain parts of the world leprosy remains an important communicable disease, in spite of aggressive programs to control and eradicate leprosy. Children make up approximately 10% of all leprosy cases in endemic regions. To contract the disease, individuals have to be in close contact with the contagious case for prolonged periods of time because the incubation period of leprosy is long. Adolescents and young adults with leprosy are likely to have contracted the illness as a child. Children exhibit the entire spectrum of leprosy. Even in 2015, skin histopathology is still considered the "gold standard" for the diagnosis of leprosy. However, newer diagnostic modalities such as serologic test for detection of antibodies to the *Mycobacterium leprae*-specific phosphoglycolipid-1, polymerase chain reaction for detecting specific nucleic acid sequences of *M leprae*, immunocytochemistry and in situ hybridization on biopsied skin tissue are also available to assist in making the diagnosis of leprosy. As with the patient described in this report, patients with leprosy are treated with a combination of 3 or 4 drugs. However, in spite of using multiple drugs, resistant strains of *M leprae* are emerging. Leprosy is a global problem. While it's endemic in only a few countries, a large number of immigrants are moving from endemic countries to non-endemic countries. The diagnosis of leprosy is delayed in non-endemic countries because of low awareness of the disease due to lack of training in global health during medical education.

Part 11

Nephrology

CHAPTER 65

Urinary Frequency in a 6-Year-Old Boy

Presentation

A 6-year-old boy is brought to the pediatric clinic with a 1-week history of urinary frequency. He urinates every 15 to 20 minutes. In spite of voiding just before leaving home, he had to stop at a restroom on the way to the clinic. The frequency has occurred both at home and at school, with his teacher reporting that he disrupts class by leaving the room frequently to use the restroom. He urinates once or twice nightly but less frequently than during the day.

The child produces only a small amount of urine with each void. His stream, urine color, and urine odor are normal. There has been no daytime incontinence, nocturnal enuresis, or polydipsia. The patient denies dysuria and flank or abdominal pain. His appetite and activity level have been normal, and his bowel movements are regular. There is no history of urinary tract infection.

Findings on physical examination and urinalysis are normal. Urine culture results are negative. Further history reveals that his best friend's father recently drowned in a boating event.

- **What is your differential diagnosis at this point?**
- **Are there any elements of history or physical examination that would help you?**
- **What additional diagnostic studies would you like performed?**

Discussion

The patient began to exhibit urinary frequency shortly after learning of the death of his friend's father. His mother recalled that the condition also worsened 2 days later, when she left him with a babysitter while she and her husband attended the memorial service. He has not talked about the event frequently at home, and his parents have been hesitant to discuss it with him at length. His teacher, however, has stated that he has seemed a bit more withdrawn at school and has been preoccupied with the topic of the drowning. The history of primarily daytime frequency, associated temporally with an emotional trigger in an otherwise asymptomatic child, is consistent with the diagnosis of extraordinary urinary frequency.

The Condition

Extraordinary urinary frequency is a benign, self-limiting condition that presents as the sudden onset of urinary frequency in a previously toilet-trained child who has no polyuria or evidence of infection. The terms *pollakiuria* and *extraordinary daytime urinary frequency* are also used.

Most patients have only daytime frequency, although approximately 25% also have nocturia. The nocturia is typically much less frequent than the daytime symptoms. A smaller percentage of patients develops secondary nocturnal enuresis. Urgency and frequency occur as often as every 5 minutes, and urine volumes are small. Incontinence and dysuria are usually absent. Findings on the physical examination and urinalysis are characteristically normal.

The condition is reported more commonly in boys, and the peak age is 5 to 6 years, with a range from 3 to 14 years. Symptoms may resolve spontaneously within a few days or persist for months. Cases have been reported that lasted for more than 3 years, with a relapsing, remitting course.

Cause

There is likely more than one cause for benign urinary frequency in childhood, and the lack of physical or laboratory findings makes the determination difficult. Nonbacterial cystitis and hypercalciuria have been discovered in a few patients, and chemical urethritis and heightened bladder sensitivity during cold-weather months have been proposed as possible causes.

Several series of patients having extraordinary urinary frequency have been reported. Most studies identified significant social or emotional stressors in at least some patients, with a range of 19% to 100%. Moreover, subsequent stressors may exacerbate frequency in prolonged cases or cause relapses in patients who have had a previous episode that resolved. Frequency may occur only in the stressful environment, and improvement in symptoms following counseling or resolution of the stressful situation has been reported. In some children, the frequency seems to disappear when the child is intensely focused, as when participating in a sporting event. This patient's frequency occurred somewhat less at school than at home and seemed more urgent when he was riding in the car.

The most frequently described psychogenic triggers are school problems, such as academic difficulties or bullying, and a perceived threat to self or a loved one. Parental divorce and moving have also been cited as precipitating events.

Diagnosis

Taking a careful history and performing a physical examination, urinalysis, and urine culture are all that are necessary to arrive at the diagnosis of extraordinary urinary frequency.

The history of small-volume voids, absence of polydipsia, normal urine specific gravity, and absence of urine glucose are reassurance against metabolic disorders such as diabetes mellitus or diabetes insipidus. Similarly, an absence of dysuria, normal findings on urinalysis, and a negative urine culture are important in ruling out urinary tract infection. The differential diagnosis includes neurogenic bladder and constipation, which can be ruled out by history and physical examination.

Ultrasonography and voiding cystourethrography have not revealed anatomic abnormalities in patients who have the solitary symptom of urinary frequency and, therefore, are not routinely recommended. Urodynamic measurements and other more invasive procedures should be reserved for patients who have progressive symptoms or who develop incontinence.

Treatment

The only treatment necessary is to reassure the parents and the child that there is no underlying medical cause and that extraordinary urinary frequency usually resolves over days or weeks. Anticholinergic medications such as oxybutynin and propantheline are useful for treating incontinence but are not as effective against isolated frequency. Electromyographic biofeedback may help shorten the course of refractory cases.

Identification of an emotional trigger for the frequency may offer the parent or physician the opportunity to allay the child's anxiety and reassure the parents that the condition can be explained.

School-aged children who encounter death may fear that something similar will happen to their parents and may worry about the possibility of separation but may not vocalize these concerns. Parents sometimes avoid discussing death with a child for fear that it may make him or her uncomfortable, but taking the opportunity to dispel some of the child's misconceptions may alleviate some of the child's worries.

In this case, the boy's mother was advised to give him an opportunity to talk about his feelings about the drowning and any concerns that he may have. She was also encouraged to explain the rarity of such deaths to her son and to reassure him that his parents are safe and that he will always be loved and cared for. On follow-up 1 week later, the patient's frequency had resolved fully.

Bradley S. Hood, MD, Madigan Army Medical Center, Tacoma, WA

PEDIATRICS IN REVIEW EDITOR'S NOTE

For years, my partners and I have encountered patients who have the sudden onset of urinary frequency. Evaluation reveals no infection, diabetes, or other discernible disease. More than 50% of the patients are boys, and the peak incidence is in the middle of winter. They all get better in a matter of weeks or a few months. Our local urologists refer to this condition as dysfunctional urinary frequency syndrome (affectionately labeled "dufus") and speculate that it might have a viral cause, given the time of year, sudden onset, and spontaneous resolution. Obvious stress factors have not been common in our patients, but perhaps we have not looked hard enough. What we see is very much like the condition described in this case. The authors state the likelihood that benign urinary frequency has more than one cause. Suffice it to say that self-limited urinary frequency is a real phenomenon; the cause is not clear, but stress plays a role in at least some cases, and the cornerstone of therapy is reassurance.—LFN

COMMENTARY BY AMRISH JAIN, MD, PEDIATRIC NEPHROLOGIST, CHILDREN'S HOSPITAL OF MICHIGAN

The 6 year-old-boy presented has a condition called pollakiuria (Greek word *pollakis*, meaning "often"), or extraordinary daytime urinary frequency (EDUF). The International Children's Continence Society defined EDUF as (1) a child voiding at least once hourly and with small volumes during the daytime only; (2) incontinence is not a usual or necessary ingredient; (3) nocturnal bladder behavior is normal for the age of the child; (4) the condition occurs from the age of daytime bladder control or 3 years. The common differential diagnosis of this condition includes urinary tract infection, diabetes mellitus, diabetes insipidus, constipation, and bladder detrusor instability. Pollakiuria is often associated with emotional events like death in the family, although this trigger may not be present in all the cases.

Bergmann et al reported a systematic analysis of 19 peer-reviewed case series in children (n = 1–19) with EDUF. The average age of presentation of EDUF was 6 years and the condition persisted for an average of 6 months. Most reports suggest that reassurance and counseling of parents and child regarding the stressor event is most important in management of this condition. Dietary approaches that have been described include liberal intake of water, reducing intake of acidic juices (apple, orange, grape, or tomato), oxalate-rich beverages (tea), and caffeine. The nonsteroidal anti-inflammatory drugs (indomethacin) and anticholinergic agents (oxybutynin) have been proposed or studied in treatment of EDUF, but may be indicated only in severe and long-standing cases. In some reports, biofeedback has been found to be helpful and deserves further consideration in management of EDUF. Timed voiding is useful in children with dysfunctional voiding. However, in older children with EDUF, instructions to voluntarily delay voiding (timed non-voiding) may be beneficial.

CHAPTER 66

Severe, Sudden, Bilateral, Throbbing Headaches in an 11-Year-Old

Presentation

An 11-year-old previously healthy boy develops severe, sudden, bilateral, throbbing headaches, occurring several times a day for the past 2 weeks. He had never complained of headaches before this time. The headaches seem to be precipitated by urination. They resolve when he lies down for 15 minutes. He denies visual disturbances, nausea, or sweating. There is no family history of migraines or thyroid disorders. He is taking no medications and has experienced no recent stressors.

On physical examination, the boy's temperature is 98.4°F (36.9°C), heart rate is 80 beats/min, and blood pressure is 125/65 mm Hg. He is alert and oriented and currently has no headache. No goiter, heart murmur, or abdominal masses are present. Findings on the rest of his examination, including neurologic and funduscopic evaluations, are normal.

On a recent visit to an emergency department for headache, computed tomography of his head was performed. His mother was told that everything was normal and that he probably had a migraine. An imaging study reveals the diagnosis.

- **What is your differential diagnosis at this point?**
- **Are there any elements of history or physical examination that would help you?**
- **What additional diagnostic studies would you like performed?**

Discussion

Results of magnetic resonance imaging of the boy's pelvis revealed a small mass within the left lateral wall of the bladder. Metaiodobenzylguanidine radio nucleotide scan confirmed the diagnosis of a pheochromocytoma and demonstrated the lack of metastatic disease. Both plasma dopamine and urinary homovanillic acid levels were elevated. The patient was placed on phenoxybenzamine prior to undergoing a partial cystectomy. Subsequent measurements of urinary catecholamines have revealed normal values, and his signs and symptoms have resolved.

Evaluating Headache

Although migraines account for 75% of headaches in children who seek medical attention, a family history of migraine can be obtained in approximately 90% of cases. The pain may be one-sided or bilateral, but it builds in intensity and is usually accompanied by severe nausea and photophobia. In addition, the pain typically persists for 2 to 6 hours. These discrepancies make the diagnosis of migraine unlikely in this case.

The history of multiple discrete attacks per day raises the possibility of cluster headaches. These uncommon headaches occur as bursts of pain lasting 30 to 90 minutes, repeat 2 to 6 times per day for several weeks, and then vanish for a period of months to years. However, the definitive feature of a cluster headache is its unilateral nature, beginning behind one eye and spreading to the rest of the hemicranium, making it an unlikely diagnosis in this patient.

The sudden nature of this patient's headaches suggests the possibility of paroxysmal headaches triggered by sudden rises in systemic blood pressure. Compared with chronic hypertension, there are only a few causes for sudden hypertension. After ruling out unusual causes such as cocaine abuse, the 2 primary causes are thyroid storm and pheochromocytoma. In this patient, the precipitation of headache by urination points to a disease process that originates in the pelvis, which induced his physicians to obtain images of that area.

Clinical Presentation

Pheochromocytomas are rare tumors in childhood and adolescence. They occur primarily between the ages of 6 and 14 years, with a slight predominance in boys. Most occur spontaneously, although perhaps 10% are part of a heritable disorder, such as multiple endocrine neoplasia 2A or 2B.

Pheochromocytomas occur wherever chromaffin tissue is found, with 85% located in the adrenal medulla. Another 10% are found in the organs of Zuckerkandl, aggregates of norepinephrine-secreting cells forming 2 masses along the sides of the abdominal aorta. Finally, a small percentage may occur within the wall of the urinary bladder. Although up to one-third of affected children may have multiple discrete tumors at diagnosis, fewer than 10% of pheochromocytomas are truly malignant, as defined by the tendency to spread into lymphatics, bone, liver, lung, or cranium.

Pheochromocytomas produce catecholamines, which explains their cardinal symptom of hypertension. However, only 70% to 80% of patients have sustained high blood pressures with or without paroxysms. The remainder have only paroxysms of high blood pressure. The classic symptom triad of a paroxysm is hypertension, sweating, and palpitations. Anxiety, tremors, nausea, abdominal or chest pain, and visual disturbances may all occur. Between paroxysms, orthostatic hypotension is fairly common, resulting from inadequate neurovascular functioning.

Clinical examination may reveal hypertension and its consequences, such as cardiomegaly and retinopathy. The tumor is usually too small to palpate. Initial laboratory evaluation may reveal hyperglycemia and hypercalcemia.

Diagnosis

Once a clinical suspicion is raised, the confirmatory tests include output measurement of 24-hour urine catecholamines and their metabolites (metanephrine and vanillylmandelic acid). Plasma catecholamine levels should also be obtained. Elevated levels of plasma dopamine or urine homovanillic acid (its metabolite) suggest the diagnosis of either a pheochromocytoma or a neuroblastoma. For patients who have brief and infrequent paroxysms, carefully controlled stimulation with glucagon may be required to collect a diagnostic sample of blood and urine.

The tumor should be localized with a nuclear medicine scan using I 131–labeled metaiodobenzylguanidine. This scan will detect most cases of pheochromocytoma as well as any metastases. Finally, precise localization can be obtained with magnetic resonance imaging.

Treatment

Once the diagnosis is confirmed, alpha-adrenergic blockade should be initiated, typically with phenoxybenzamine. Occasionally, the addition of small amounts of propranolol may be required to control reflex tachyarrhythmias. After several days of this preoperative preparation, the vascular bed expands, and the tumor can be removed safely. Postoperative management includes careful monitoring of blood pressure, fluid status, and blood glucose levels. Children who have had pheochromocytomas deserve careful long-term follow-up. The signs and symptoms may reappear later in life, most likely because of the tendency of these tumors to be multifocal in a significant number of patients.

Lessons for the Physician

This case highlights the importance of obtaining a detailed history when evaluating headaches. Frequently, the story alone will point to the correct diagnosis, allowing the physician to avoid costly and inappropriate tests. This case also reminds physicians that headaches of sudden onset are unusual in children and warrant further evaluation for underlying disease. As in this case, the astute physician should notice when a patient's baseline systolic blood pressure is at the 95th percentile for age, necessitating, at the very least, repeat measurements and evaluations that might eventually lead to the detection of underlying disease.

Christopher Dvorak, MD, Lucile Packard Children's Hospital at Stanford, Palo Alto, CA

CHAPTER 67

Fatigue, Weakness, Body Aches, and Metabolic Alkalosis in a 15-Year-Old Boy

Presentation

A 15-year-old boy presents with a 4-day history of fatigue, intermittent mild headache, and a 1-day history of generalized weakness, body aches, sleepiness, dizziness, and 3 episodes of nonbilious, nonbloody vomiting. He denies cough, shortness of breath, palpitations, or chest pain, as well as abdominal pain, joint pain, rash, vision changes, weight loss, polyuria, polydipsia, or change in urine color. He currently takes methylphenidate for attention-deficit/hyperactivity disorder and sertraline for depression. He denies any over-the-counter or illicit drug use.

Physical examination reveals a well-developed, tired-appearing adolescent. His temperature is 100.6°F (38.1°C) with otherwise normal vital signs, including blood pressure. Physical examination of the heart, lungs, and abdomen are within reference range. His proximal muscle strength is 4 of 5; the rest of his neurologic examination is within reference range.

Initial laboratory examination includes the following levels: sodium, 133 mEq/L; potassium, 2.4 mEq/L; chloride, 90 mEq/L; bicarbonate, 30 mEq/L; urea nitrogen, 9 mg/dL; creatinine, 0.5 mg/dL; glucose, 103 mg/dL; calcium, 9.4 mg/dL; magnesium, 2.0 mg/dL; and phosphorus, 4.3 mg/dL. Complete blood cell count, liver function test results, and hepatic enzyme levels are normal. Electrocardiography shows a prolonged QT interval at 550 milliseconds.

On admission, the patient receives a potassium bolus, followed by maintenance intravenous fluids containing potassium chloride. He has no vomiting or diarrhea on his first hospital day. A follow-up laboratory examination of his chemistry studies shows persistence of his initial abnormalities.

- **What is your differential diagnosis at this point?**
- **Are there any elements of history or physical examination that would help you?**
- **What additional diagnostic studies would you like performed?**

Discussion

This adolescent had an initial laboratory evaluation hallmarked by a hyponatremic, hypokalemic, hypochloremic metabolic alkalosis that persisted despite normal saline infusion and potassium correction. Furthermore, he denied gastrointestinal losses or diuretic use. In addition, he was not hypertensive, as would be expected in primary hyperaldosteronism. Because of the unexplained hypokalemic metabolic alkalosis, ongoing renal loss was suspected, and spot urine electrolyte testing revealed the following values: sodium, 193 mEq/L; potassium, 61 mEq/L; chloride, 272 mEq/L; and calcium, 0.5 mg/dL. These urine electrolytes demonstrate high levels of potassium and chloride despite low serum levels. In children and adolescents who have metabolic alkalosis with chloride loss secondary to vomiting or diarrhea, the urine chloride concentration should be low because of chloride retention.

The clinical picture of elevated urine chloride in conjunction with a hypochloremic metabolic alkalosis suggests either ongoing diuretic therapy or a renal tubular disorder mimicking diuretic therapy, which would include diseases such as Bartter syndrome and Gitelman syndrome. Both of these conditions have hyperreninemia- and hyperaldosteronism-associated hypokalemia. However, this patient's overall clinical presentation, including age of presentation, normal growth and development, and hypocalciuria, makes Gitelman syndrome the more likely diagnosis.

The Condition

Gitelman syndrome is 1 of 2 rare inherited forms of hypokalemic-hypochloremic metabolic alkalosis caused by disorders of the renal tubular electrolyte transport. The other is Bartter syndrome, which has a similar presentation and overlapping physiology.

The inheritance pattern in children and adolescents born with Gitelman syndrome is autosomal recessive but may be sporadic. The prevalence is difficult to assess but is estimated to be 1 in 40,000. There is no ethnic or sex predilection.

Gitelman syndrome presents typically in adolescence and early adulthood. The most common presenting symptoms in patients who have Gitelman syndrome are salt craving, musculoskeletal complaints such as muscle weakness and cramps, and constitutional complaints such as fatigue and dizziness. Notably absent are the features of polydipsia, polyuria, and growth retardation seen in Bartter syndrome. The spectrum of symptoms ranges from being asymptomatic to the extremes of tetany and rhabdomyolysis. These symptoms do not seem to correlate with the degree of hypokalemia. Gitelman syndrome is characterized by hypokalemia and metabolic alkalosis. These patients have hyperreninemia and hyperaldosteronemia but are not hypertensive. Serum calcium levels are normal, with low or normal serum magnesium levels. In Gitelman syndrome, a low urinary calcium level is a hallmark, compared with patients who have Bartter syndrome, in whom hypercalciuria predisposes to nephrocalcinosis.

Pathogenesis

The pathophysiology in Gitelman syndrome is a loss of function of the thiazide–sensitive sodium chloride cotransporter located in the distal convoluted tubule, which leads to defective sodium and chloride reabsorption. Bartter syndrome is caused by a mutation affecting the Na-K-2Cl cotransporter in the loop of Henle. These mutations mimic the physiology seen in patients taking thiazide and loop diuretics.

In Gitelman syndrome, the impaired reabsorption of sodium and chloride at the thiazide–sensitive sodium chloride cotransporter effectively leads to some degree of hypovolemia. Hypovolemia in turn activates the renin-angiotensin-aldosterone system, ultimately increasing levels of aldosterone to maintain intravascular volume. The increase in aldosterone results in hypokalemia and metabolic alkalosis, as potassium and hydrogen ions are excreted in exchange for sodium. Despite the upregulation of the renin-angiotensin-aldosterone system, children and adolescents who have Gitelman syndrome have normal or low blood pressure.

Filtered calcium reabsorption is coupled to the Na-K-Cl channel, which is dysfunctional in Bartter syndrome. In Bartter syndrome, this impaired reabsorption leads to urinary calcium wasting and hypercalciuria, in contrast with Gitelman syndrome, in which marked hypocalciuria occurs. Lastly, hypermagnesuria leading to hypomagnesemia is often seen in Gitelman syndrome, but the pathophysiologic mechanism is unclear.

Treatment

The treatment of Gitelman syndrome is geared toward correcting hypokalemia and hypomagnesemia if needed. Patients benefit from oral magnesium and a potassium-sparing diuretic, such as amiloride or spironolactone, to counteract distal tubular potassium secretion.

Lessons for the Physician

- Analysis of urine electrolytes, including chloride, is essential in distinguishing the etiology of hypochloremic-hypokalemic metabolic alkalosis.
- Gitelman syndrome is a rare, inheritable cause of renal tubular dysfunction at the thiazide–sensitive sodium chloride cotransporter in the distal convoluted tubule, leading to hypokalemic-hypochloremic metabolic alkalosis.
- Gitelman syndrome presents in adolescence or adulthood, with a spectrum ranging from an asymptomatic state to severe fatigue and a potential for tetany and rhabdomyolysis.

Gunjan Kamdar Tiyyagura, MD, Yale Department of Pediatric Emergency Medicine, New Haven, CT

Janienne Kondrich, MD, NYU School of Medicine, Bellevue Hospital Center, Division of Pediatric Emergency Medicine, NY

Part 12

Neurology

CHAPTER 68

5-Week-Old Boy With 2 Days of Coughing That Worsens After Feeding

Presentation

A 5-week-old boy is brought to the emergency department because of 2 days of coughing that worsens after feeding. The neonate was born by cesarean section because of breech presentation after an uncomplicated term pregnancy. His birthweight was 2.89 kg. He is a poor feeder and does not suck as vigorously as his siblings did; he has gained only 0.28 kg since birth.

Physical examination reveals an irritable, ill-looking neonate who has erythematous eyes and slight nasal discharge. The neonate's weight, height, and head circumference plot on the 5th percentile. His muscle tone is decreased, and his deep tendon reflexes are reduced. He is breathing with nasal flaring, minimal retractions, and a respiratory rate of 50 to 60 breaths/min. His lungs are clear on auscultation. Cardiac and abdominal examinations yield normal findings.

Initial diagnostic possibilities include respiratory syncytial virus infection, bronchiolitis, sepsis, and gastroesophageal reflux. A rapid antigen test for respiratory syncytial virus is negative. A radiograph of the chest shows mild hyperinflation of the lungs. Cultures are obtained and antibiotics, started. The neonate is given oxygen and seems to improve.

After 48 hours of antibiotic therapy, results of the neonate's neurologic examination do not improve. He has an episode of choking and coughing, and a repeat radiograph shows a right upper lobe infiltrate consistent with aspiration. The family history reveals Jewish ancestry and suggests a procedure that reveals the diagnosis.

- **What is your differential diagnosis at this point?**
- **Are there any elements of history or physical examination that would help you?**
- **What additional diagnostic studies would you like performed?**

Discussion

Diagnosis

Both sweat testing and thyroid function testing produced normal findings. Because of the constellation of poor suck, poor gag, and aspiration, a histamine response test was performed, which involves subdermal injection of a miniscule amount of histamine and observation of the patient's response. A normal response to this test would be a notable axon flare and pain in addition to a wheal at the area of injection. Failure to respond to the pain and lack of an axon flare, as was the case with this patient, serves as an indication of Riley-Day syndrome (familial dysautonomia [FD]). This diagnosis was supported by the results of radiography with barium swallow, which revealed gastric reflux and aspiration, common findings in this condition.

Familial dysautonomia is an autosomal recessive disorder that occurs most commonly in people of Ashkenazi Jewish descent. The frequency of individuals who are heterozygotes for the disorder is 1 in 30 among that population. Richard Lawrence Riley and Conrad Milton Day recognized the condition initially in 1949. The FD gene has been identified and appears to be located on the distal q31. Sufficient DNA markers have been recognized to allow for prenatal diagnosis and carrier identification of individuals who have the genetic abnormality. Clinically, the disease manifests primarily as a disorder of the peripheral nervous system, although there appear to be central nervous system defects as well.

Clinical Presentation

Most of the signs and symptoms associated with FD are attributed to defects in the sensory nervous system. Because these fibers are disturbed, the patient exhibits a weakened response to pain, inability to taste, and poor temperature regulation. The autonomic nervous system is also affected by a decrease in the number of nerve fibers, mainly in the sympathetic division. This pathologic situation contributes to the inappropriate temperature regulation and causes such signs as decreased tearing, blotching of the skin, and postural hypotension. A decrease in large myelinated afferent nerve fibers from muscle spindles and Golgi tendon organs accounts for diminished deep tendon reflexes and decreased muscle tone, causing the patient to have difficulties with gait and proprioception from a young age.

The earliest signs of illness occur shortly after birth, when the patient presents with a poor sucking reflex and difficulty swallowing, which can lead to poor weight gain and aspiration pneumonia. The loss of pain fibers facilitates injuries to the skin, including lacerations, bedsores, burns, and injuries to the joints. Skeletal deformities occur in approximately 90% of FD patients who survive beyond early childhood, with the most common problem being scoliosis. Unique features of the disease include the absence of lingual fungiform papillae and decreased production of tears. Corneal ulcerations occur in some patients because the corneas generally lack sensation and tears. Corneal disease is one of the reasons for impaired vision in FD, although optic nerve degeneration appears to be associated with the condition later in life. Another interesting finding is that patients who have FD have a decreased occurrence of herpes simplex virus type 1 and varicella virus infections, a characteristic attributed to their deficiency in type C sensory nerve fibers. The virus normally spreads and is reactivated through these fibers; apparently a lack of such fibers confers protection against these infections.

Children who can overcome the frequent episodes of pulmonary infection and other complications in childhood usually present with further neurologic and circulatory problems in adulthood. These difficulties can include deteriorating peripheral sensory function, worsening orthostatic hypotension, the development of supine hypertension, occasional bradyarrhythmias, poor balance, unsteady gait, and difficulty with concentration. They demonstrate a tendency toward depression, anxieties, and phobias.

Etiology

The molecular basis of the disease seems to involve a decreased amount of dopamine β-hydroxylase, which converts dopamine (DA) to norepinephrine (NE). This lack of NE is the reason for the inappropriate autonomic response to a challenge. Because DA is being synthesized but not converted to NE, there tends to be a large ratio of homovanillic acid to vanillylmandelic acid, the respective breakdown products of DA and NE. These breakdown products are important clinically because their levels can help in the diagnosis of the disease. The embryologic basis for the lack of both sensory and sympathetic ganglia seen in FD may involve the absence of a specific nerve growth factor during development.

Prognosis

The prognosis for the disease is dim, with death in childhood being very likely. A number of treatments have improved survival, leading to an increased number of adults who have FD. Nissen gastrotomy performed very early in infancy is recommended to prevent aspiration. Diazepam, chlorpromazine, and bethanechol are used to decrease the severity of dysautonomic vomiting, decrease blood pressure, and prevent enuresis. Methylcellulose eyedrops or topical ocular lubricants can prevent corneal ulcerations by replacing tears. Patients should also be followed by orthopedists for scoliosis and joint disorders and must be protected against injuries.

Lessons for the Physician

The future of the treatment of this disease is encouraging because of new advances in genetic detection that could allow prenatal diagnosis and the earliest possible treatment of neonates and infants born with familial dysautonomia. In addition, improvements in gene therapy may ameliorate the condition of patients who currently have the disease. A good review of the condition and how treatment has evolved is the following article: Axelrod FB. Familial dysautonomia: a 47-year perspective: how technology confirms clinical acumen. *J Pediatr.* 1998;132(3 Pt 2):S2–S5.

John Harrington, MD; Eugenia Gianos, MSIII; and Marc Stiefel, MSIII; New York Medical College, Valhalla, NY

COMMENTARY BY DR LALITHA SIVASWAMY, PEDIATRIC NEUROLOGIST, CHILDREN'S HOSPITAL OF MICHIGAN

The familial dysautonomia gene has been identified as *IKBKAP* and is located on chromosome 9q31. Mutations in the gene affect the production of a protein called IKK complex associated protein, the deficiency of which leads to failure of the brain cells and peripheral nerves to perform certain vital functions.

The cornerstone of treatment has remained unchanged over the years, with symptomatic approaches such as control of labile blood pressure, protecting the child from extremes of temperature, management of gastric dysmotility, prevention of corneal ulcers, and periodic screening for renal function continuing to be of paramount importance. Half of all individuals with familial dysautonomia survive into their 30s thanks to improved anticipatory therapies. Nonetheless, sudden death due to cardiorespiratory arrest is not uncommon. However, clinical trials of compounds that increase IKAP levels are underway and have the potential to slow disease progression.

CHAPTER 69

Poor Weight Gain in a 14-Month-Old Boy

Presentation

A 14-month-old Caucasian boy is seen by the gastroenterology service because of poor weight gain. At age 9 months, his weight started to plateau and was at the 15th percentile. He has gained only 0.45 kg over the last 5 months. His mother and maternal grandmother report that he eats well with them but question whether his father feeds him adequately.

Birth and past medical histories are unremarkable. There is no family history of gastrointestinal disorders, cystic fibrosis, failure to thrive, seizures, or developmental delay. He lived with his mother, who now attends rehabilitation for alcohol abuse, until age 10 months when his father obtained legal custody. Subsequently, he sees his mother only on weekends. His paternal grandfather and "other people" live at the father's house. His father is described as abusive of alcohol and marijuana. An ongoing custody battle continues.

On physical examination, the boy appears emaciated, with decreased subcutaneous fat, but is very active and happy. His weight is 8.67 kg (below the 3rd percentile), length is 82.5 cm (75th–90th percentile), and head circumference is 49 cm (90th–95th percentile). Vital signs are normal. He has a broad forehead, and his face appears triangular, with a small, pointed chin and a thin-lipped, wide mouth. The rest of his physical findings are normal.

All laboratory findings are within reference range. A celiac screen, chloride sweat test, and fecal elastase determination are normal. An upper gastrointestinal series with small bowel follow-through does not reveal any abnormalities.

- **What is your differential diagnosis at this point?**
- **Are there any elements of history or physical examination that would help you?**
- **What additional diagnostic studies would you like performed?**

Discussion

This child was emaciated and had an unusual facial appearance (Figure 69.1). The social situation was believed to be the cause of his failure to thrive (FTT). He did not gain weight over the next month despite the recommended high-caloric intake. Admission was advised for aggressive nutritional supplementation employing overnight tube feedings to ensure meeting 100% of his needs. Despite meeting 100% of his daily caloric and protein requirements for several days, he still lost weight.

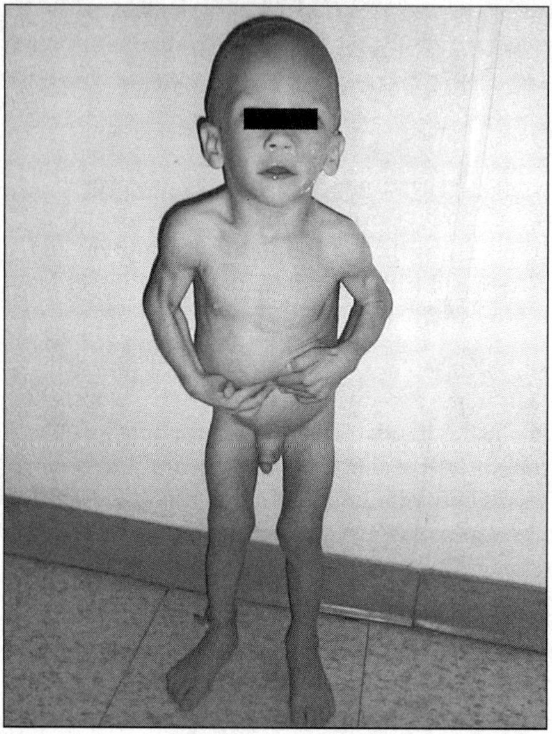

Figure 69.1. Emaciated child who has unusual facial appearance.

A pediatric neurologic assessment revealed no abnormalities. Magnetic resonance imaging of the head revealed a solid, intensely enhancing suprasellar mass lesion located in the region of the hypothalamus and third ventricle, measuring approximately 1.5 × 1.7 × 2.3 cm, with no surrounding edema (Figure 69.2). The mass was believed to represent an astrocytoma or germinoma. Diencephalic syndrome was diagnosed. Because of the tumor location, biopsy and surgical excision were not options. A short time after diagnosis, chemotherapy was begun. The boy began to gain weight consistently, and his weight is now where it belongs on the growth chart. His regaining of weight has been accompanied by a normalization of his facial appearance. He is followed regularly by the pediatric oncology service.

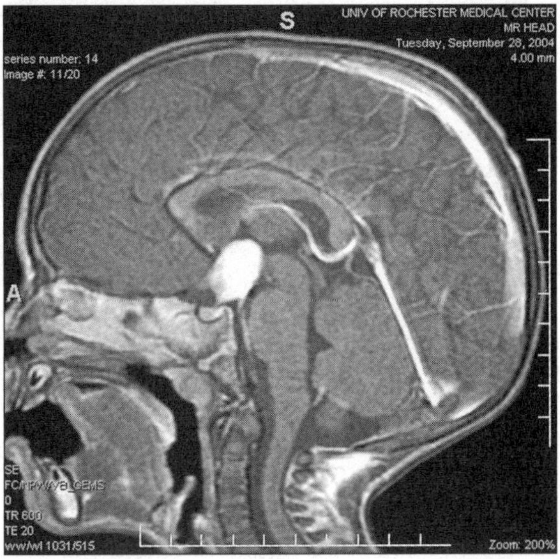

Figure 69.2. Magnetic resonance image showing a solid, intensely enhancing suprasellar mass lesion located in the region of the hypothalamus and third ventricle.

The Disorder

Diencephalic syndrome results from a brain mass, in most cases located in the hypothalamic-optic chiasm region. It is almost exclusively a disease of infants and young children. The mass can be an astrocytoma, germinoma, craniopharyngioma, or lesion of histiocytosis.

The mean onset of signs and symptoms occurs between 6 and 12 months, with about only 15% of cases diagnosed after the age of 2 years. As with this patient, severe wasting, hyperactivity, and euphoria are characteristics of the syndrome. Early experiments demonstrated that lesions confined to the dorsomedial thalamic nuclei can induce euphoria and hyperactivity. In spite of the emaciation, linear growth is maintained or even accelerated.

Other features of the syndrome include nystagmus, pallor without anemia, autonomic dysfunction with profuse sweating, erratic temperature control, hypotension, tremor, and endocrine dysfunction. The head circumference is usually normal, although 33% to 58% of patients have obstructive hydrocephalus at diagnosis. Even in those who do not have hydrocephalus, the marked loss of facial adipose tissue often creates a pseudohydrocephalic appearance.

The space-occupying lesion of the hypothalamic-optic chiasm region is usually a low-grade astrocytoma and generally slow growing. Therefore, the neurologic signs appear slowly, which may explain why this patient's neurologic findings were normal. Visual signs such as nystagmus and optic pallor have been observed in several series, occurring on average in 55% to 65% of cases. In animal studies, lesions in the anterior hypothalamus caused an increased level of growth hormone, which stimulates lipolysis and may explain the loss of subcutaneous fatty tissue.

Most patients experience weight loss despite having a normal or increased appetite. Disruption of appetite control is due to the location of the tumor in the ventromedial hypothalamus where the satiety center is located. Caloric expenditure is increased due to the hyperactivity and euphoria caused by the tumor in this location. A secondary problem is the inability of affected children to tolerate the food intake necessary to maintain energy balance or growth.

Misleading Factors

The presence of psychosocial issues and questionable nutritional intake in this severely emaciated child led his physicians to believe that his FTT was caused by these factors. With unremarkable findings on the neurologic examination, an intracranial lesion ranked low in the differential diagnosis. However, the patient's failure to gain weight while in the hospital under strict intake and output monitoring and despite the use of nasogastric feeding necessitated expansion of the evaluation.

Differential Diagnosis

Growth failure can have organic or nonorganic causes. Stress and psychosocial factors frequently contribute to FTT. Parental anxiety or depression can lead to feeding behavior problems and FTT. Issues such as unusual feeding behaviors (food fads, excessive juice, etc), low income, food shortages, neglect due to parental drug and alcohol abuse, and a disturbed parent-child relationship were considered as causes of inadequate nutrition in this case.

Malabsorption should always be investigated by screening for celiac disease, performing a sweat test for cystic fibrosis, and checking a stool fecal elastase-1 for pancreatic insufficiency. Changing to semielemental or elemental formula is recommended if cow's milk–protein allergy is suspected.

Hypermetabolic states such as hyperthyroidism can cause FTT. Chronic renal disease, chronic infection (human immunodeficiency virus), immunodeficiencies, or even malignancy are other causes.

This patient appeared somewhat dysmorphic, and a genetic syndrome or congenital anomalies were considered after the evaluation failed to supply an explanation. Mechanical feeding difficulties caused by oromotor dysfunction and even severe reflux were other diagnostic possibilities.

Finally, although low on the differential diagnosis list, diencephalic syndrome from a central nervous system lesion should be considered.

Evaluation

Neuroimaging is used to diagnose diencephalic syndrome and will reveal a space-occupying lesion, most often in the hypothalamic-optic chiasm area. Of course, suspicion of this diagnosis is necessary to suggest the imaging.

Therapy

The treatment of diencephalic syndrome is surgical excision of the mass, if possible. Radiation and chemotherapy have been reported to reduce the size of the mass effectively in many patients. The ultimate prognosis is related to how well the tumor can be eliminated. Many affected children have masses deep in the brain in proximity to critical areas, making cure difficult.

Lessons for the Physician

Growth failure results most often from inadequate nutrition that is due to psychosocial factors. Serious disease also can cause failure to thrive and may not only manifest in other ways but also coexist with social problems. Failure to gain weight associated with emaciation, loss of subcutaneous fat, euphoria, and hyperactivity suggests diencephalic syndrome. Even without finding neurologic abnormalities on the physical examination, children suspected of having diencephalic syndrome should receive neuroimaging.

Juan F. Villalona, MD; Rebecca K. Lehman, MD; Marilyn R. Brown, MD; Koorosh Kooros, MD; and Jennifer M. Kwon, MD, Golisano Children's Hospital at Strong, University of Rochester Medical Center, Rochester, NY

CHAPTER 70

Seizurelike Activity Precipitated by Loud Noise in a 2-Year-Old

Presentation

The neurology consultant examines a 2-year-old boy in the outpatient clinic for "passing-out seizures." His mother indicates that in response to loud sounds her otherwise healthy child experiences episodes of generalized, nonrhythmic, tonic muscle contractions characterized by "stiffness and back arching," collapse, and apnea. The episodes last 30 to 45 seconds, and in a typical day, the boy experiences 3 to 4 events. No other family members experience similar bouts. Findings on electrocardiography, echocardiography, and 23-hour cardiac monitoring are unremarkable.

Physical examination reveals an alert child who interacts appropriately with his mother and has no obvious signs of sensory or motor deficit. To evaluate the events, the child is admitted to the epilepsy monitoring unit. Examination of the electroencephalogram (EEG) reveals normal background rhythm. During the admission, 2 "typical" episodes are recorded. Following a loud sound for the first event and following frustration for the second, the child cries and holds his breath in expiration. Subsequently, bradycardia is observed on the electrocardiographic lead of the EEG (Figure 70.1). Bradycardia is followed rapidly by asystole lasting 13 to 16 seconds (Figure 70.2). Eleven seconds after the cardiac arrest, the background EEG becomes slow and then flat (Figure 70.2). A few seconds after the heart starts beating again, the brain's electrical activity slowly returns to baseline (Figure 70.3). During asystole, the patient adopts an opisthotonic posture: back arching, overextension of the upper extremities, and flexion of the legs at the hip (Figure 70.2). The episodes are not associated with EEG signs of seizures.

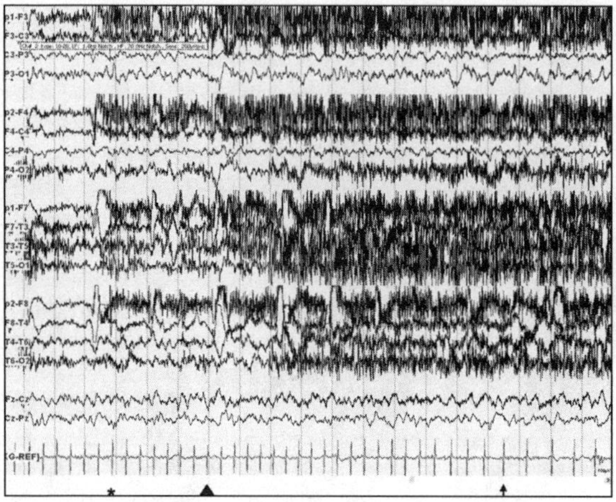

Figure 70.1. The child was stimulated (asterisk) and soon thereafter began crying (arrowhead). The electrocardiographic lead of the electroencephalogram (read tracing) shows subsequent progressive bradycardia (arrow).

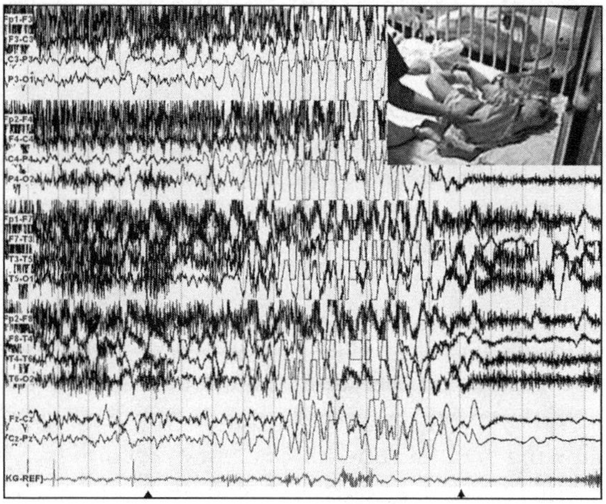

Figure 70.2. Twenty seconds after stimulation (see Figure 70.1), bradycardia evolved to a 16-second period of asystole (arrowhead). This was accompanied by flattening of the electroencephalogram (arrow) and opisthotonic posture (picture insert).

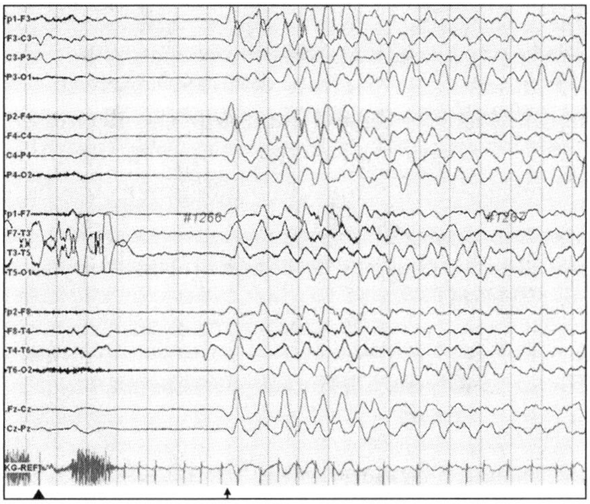

Figure 70.3. Following 17 seconds of asystole, the heart rate returned spontaneously (arrowhead). Electroencephalographic activity followed 6 seconds later (arrow). The tracing revealed generalized slowing, with gradual return to baseline background activity.

- **What is your differential diagnosis at this point?**
- **Are there any elements of history or physical examination that would help you?**
- **What additional diagnostic studies would you like performed?**

Discussion

Interview with the child's mother made the consultant suspect the diagnosis of hyperekplexia or "stiff baby" syndrome. Analysis of the events captured during the video-EEG recording confirmed that the episodes were not consistent with seizures. Instead, the record was characterized by muscle artifact, bradycardia leading to asystole, and near-flattening of electrical brain activity. The clinical history and these findings are consistent with the diagnosis of "major" hyperekplexia.

The Condition

Hyperekplexia, or "stiff baby" syndrome, is a rare congenital condition characterized by excessive response to unexpected stimuli. The term comes from the Greek and means "to startle excessively." Bakker and associates[1] consider hyperekplexia to be the most severe of a group of disorders characterized by an abnormal response to startling events. They limit use of the term hyperekplexia to the congenital form of the condition. Neuropsychiatric startle syndrome and startle-induced epilepsy are other events that fall under the rubric "startle syndromes."

Two primary types of hyperekplexia have been identified: major and minor. Major hyperekplexia, which frequently is identified in the neonatal period, is characterized by a disproportionate response to common and innocuous stimuli (sound, touch) in the form of generalized muscle contractions and startle-associated falls. Breath-holding spells and anoxic seizures also have been described in this condition, making the diagnosis difficult at times. This form of the condition has a well-established genetic cause: mutations in the gene for the α-1 subunit of the glycine receptor (*GLRA1*) on chromosome 5q33.1. The most common *GLRA1* defect leading to major hyperekplexia is an autosomal dominant missense mutation. However, *GLRA1* mutations also can have recessive inheritance. Finally, mutations of genes other than *GLRA1*, ones coding for glycinergic synapse proteins, also have been linked to sporadic cases of major hyperekplexia.

Minor hyperekplexia is also characterized by exaggerated startle responses but without tonic muscle contractions. The genetic basis of minor hyperekplexia is yet to be determined.

Genetic testing of this child failed to reveal *GLRA1* mutations. Such a finding is not surprising because the defect is identified most commonly in patients who have the disease's hereditary form. Sporadic hyperekplexia has been linked to abnormalities of other genes, such as that coding for the glycine-receptor beta-subunit (*GLRB*); the gene coding for gephyrin (*GPHN*), a protein responsible for clustering of glycine receptors at inhibitory synapses; and the gene coding for collybistin (*ARHGEF9*), a protein that interacts with gephyrin. Regardless of genetic flaw, most forms of hyperekplexia have a glycine-gated chloride-channel defect as a common denominator.

Animal models of hyperekplexia include knockout and naturally occurring examples. The former group comprises mice that have mutations in genes coding for either the α- or the β-subunit of the glycine receptor or for gephyrin. The latter group includes cattle born with a *GLRA1* nonsense mutation. Specifically, Poll Hereford cattle exhibit spontaneous and startle-evoked myoclonic jerks leading to death because the calves are unable to stand and feed. In addition, a missense mutation in the *SLC6A5* gene, encoding the presynaptic glycine transporter 2 (GlyT2), causes hyperekplexia in the Belgian blue cattle. These animals die in the perinatal period from apnea due to muscle rigidity. This last example is unique because the defect, unlike those involving the glycine receptor, is presynaptic, which leads to decreased glycine reuptake.

Differential Diagnosis

In children, the differential diagnosis of hyperekplexia includes stimulus-induced seizures, tetanus, Tourette syndrome, and anxiety disorder. Stimulus-induced seizures are, as the name implies, convulsions that are triggered by external stimuli. These events, which have a correlating EEG pattern, are common in children who have severe brain damage. Signs and symptoms of tetanus include, in addition to muscle contractions, fever and a history of an infected wound. In the case of

Tourette syndrome, tics are not triggered by stimuli but by an internal urge. Finally, the exaggerated startle response seen in patients with anxiety disorder has been deemed to be related to a state of hyperarousal.

Treatment

Clonazepam has become the treatment of choice for all forms of hyperekplexia. The medication's use is predicated on 2 counts. First, as a γ-aminobutyric agonist, clonazepam is assumed to compensate for the glycine-gated chloride channel defect. Thus, the medication increases postsynaptic hyperpolarization and synaptic inhibition. Second, clonazepam has anxiolytic properties. The latter effect cannot be underestimated because children who have hyperekplexia have been reported to shy away from bicycle riding, running, and climbing for fear of falls and injury. This patient has been treated with clonazepam, and his response to the medication has been encouraging.

Lessons for the Physician

- Although hyperekplexia can be a clinical diagnosis, this case illustrates the contribution of video-electroencephalogram monitoring in diagnosing paroxysmal events.
- Like breath-holding spells, hyperekplexia is a disturbance of autonomic regulation in response to adverse stimuli.
- Breath-holding spells and hyperekplexia are involuntary responses; they cannot be attributed to a child's temperament.

Reference

1. Bakker MJ, van Dijk JG, van den Maagdenberg AMJM, Tijseen MAJ. Startle syndromes. *Lancet Neurol.* 2006;5(6):513–524

Nathan Lehman, Keck School of Medicine/University of Southern California, Los Angeles, CA

L. Nandini Moorthy, MD, MS, University of Medicine and Dentistry of New Jersey, New Brunswick, NJ

CHAPTER 71

6-Year-Old Boy With Leg Pain During Times of Inactivity

Presentation

A 6-year-old boy complains of leg pain during times of inactivity. The pain is diffuse, affects both legs simultaneously, and feels like "pins and needles." The episodes occur intermittently throughout the day and are more intense at night, preventing sleep. In the last week, the discomfort has occurred during sleep, waking him. Massage and movement usually bring relief, with occasional need for acetaminophen.

The episodes began 1 year ago, happened 1 to 2 times per month, and now occur several times per week and are more intense. He is noted to be "squirming" while sitting still. His past medical history is free of significant illness, including trauma or sleep disturbances. He is an excellent student. Two aunts have chronic leg pain and associated sleep disturbance.

Physical findings are normal. His legs show no muscle abnormalities, redness, swelling, masses, or pain on palpation. Radiographs of the legs are normal. He has a normal white blood cell count count but has anemia (hemoglobin, 10.4 g/dL [104 g/L]) and iron deficiency (serum ferritin, 40 µg/L). Red blood cell indices reveal a mean corpuscular volume of 76 fL and mean corpuscular hemoglobin of 26.4 pg/cell. Antinuclear antibody titer is negative, and erythrocyte sedimentation rate is 1 mm/h.

- **What is your differential diagnosis at this point?**
- **Are there any elements of history or physical examination that would help you?**
- **What additional diagnostic studies would you like performed?**

Discussion

A therapeutic trial of iron (ferrous sulfate, 6 mg/kg/d) resulted in immediate and complete cessation of the boy's symptoms. When the iron therapy was stopped, the leg discomfort recurred and subsequently disappeared when iron was restarted. He was kept on iron until his blood tests showed a complete return to normal concentrations, at which time the medication was discontinued. He has continued to do well, but his mother now feels that she has the same condition and is seeking treatment.

The Condition

Restless legs syndrome (RLS) and *periodic leg movement disorder* (PLMD) are closely related and are believed to be a continuum of the same disorder, with the terms often used interchangeably. Restless legs syndrome occurs during the waking state and is diagnosed clinically. Periodic leg movement disorder is a sleep disorder that is diagnosed on the basis of findings on polysomnography (PSG) as well as clinical symptoms (insomnia or excessive daytime sleepiness).

Restless legs syndrome is characterized by dysesthesias (uncomfortable sensations) and paresthesias (abnormal sensations) in the lower extremities that are exacerbated by rest and relieved with movement of the affected extremity. The sensations are described as "creepy and crawly" feelings, "pins and needles," tingling, burning, throbbing, electric current, "worms crawling under the skin," and heebie-jeebies. Patients report an almost irresistible urge to move the legs. In severe cases, the arms may also be affected. Most episodes of RLS occur during periods of rest or inactivity, such as lying in bed attempting to fall asleep. Describing these sensations may be difficult for children and may be interpreted by parents as bedtime resistance.

The limb movements of PLMD are defined as repetitive, stereotypical dorsiflexions of the great toe, with fanning of the small toes, accompanied by flexion of the ankle and knee, that occur at 5- to 90-second intervals with a duration of 0.5 to 5 seconds. At least 4 movements must be counted per episode to meet PSG criteria for PLMD. Severity of PLMD based on PSG evaluation has been classified arbitrarily according to the number of limb movements per hour of sleep: fewer than 5 hourly movements is considered normal; 5 to 24 hourly movements, mild; 25 to 49, moderate; and 50 or more, severe.

Studies in adults indicate that 70% to 90% of patients who have RLS also have PLMD; only 20% of patients who have PLMD also have RLS. Ten of 11 children attending a pediatric neurology clinic that had an emphasis on attention-deficit/hyperactivity disorder and had been diagnosed as having growing pains met criteria for RLS.[1] Several other studies in referral centers have reported an incidence of PLMD in as many as 25% of children with attention-deficit/hyperactivity disorder.

Pathophysiology

The cause of primary RLS is unknown, but a recent study indicates that the disorder may be due to low brain iron concentration caused by a dysfunction of iron transportation from serum to the central nervous system.[2] Serum ferritin is a sensitive indicator of total body iron stores. Evidence is substantial that dopaminergic dysfunction is involved.[3] Interestingly, iron is required for tyrosine hydroxylation, which is the rate-limiting step in the biosynthesis of dopamine. A genetic link for primary RLS has been postulated, with an autosomal dominant pattern suggested by a high familial incidence of 92% and the prevalence of RLS 6 to 7 times that of the general population in first-degree relatives of patients who have early-onset RLS.

Several disorders are associated with secondary RLS, including iron deficiency, renal failure, neuropathies, myopathies, pregnancy, and drugs (caffeine, selective serotonin reuptake inhibitors, tricyclic antidepressants, dopamine blockers). Iron deficiency and a strong family history have been identified as characteristics of childhood-onset RLS.[4] Davis and colleagues[5] identified 29% of pediatric patients on dialysis as having RLS or PLMD.

Diagnostic Criteria

The criteria for diagnosing RLS include 4 primary features: (1) unpleasant limb sensations, with the desire to move the limbs, usually associated with paresthesias and dysesthesias; (2) motor restlessness, with the patient feeling compelled to move; (3) symptoms precipitated by rest and relieved by activity; and (4) symptoms worse in the evening or at night.[6,7]

For a definitive diagnosis of childhood RLS, the child must meet all 4 essential adult criteria for RLS and provide a description in his or her own words consistent with leg discomfort. Alternatively, the child must meet all 4 adult criteria and have 2 of the following features: (1) sleep disturbance for age, (2) biological parent or sibling who has RLS definitively, or (3) documented PSG with PLMD (≥5/h of sleep).[7] Diagnostic criteria for childhood PLMD include evidence of a clinical sleep disturbance for age as manifested by sleep onset problems, sleep maintenance problems, or excessive sleepiness with leg movements not accounted for by sleep-disordered breathing or medication effect (using the same PSG criteria used in the adult population).[7]

Treatment

Treatment of RLS and PLMD ranges from correcting iron deficiency and treating other underlying secondary causes to providing sleep aids. Iron supplementation should be started in patients who have ferritin levels lower than 50 mc/L. Other therapies commonly used for treatment are dopaminergic agents (carbidopa-levodopa), dopamine agonists (pergolide, pramipexole, ropinirole), benzodiazepines, anticonvulsants, and opioids. Treatment should be individualized and behavioral therapy considered.

References

1. Rajaram SS, Walters AS, England SJ, Metha D, Nizam F. Some children with growing pains may actually have restless legs syndrome. *Sleep.* 2004;27(4):767–773
2. Mizuno S, Mihara T, Miyaoka T, Inagaki T, Horiguchi J. CSF iron, ferritin and transferrin levels in restless legs syndrome. *J Sleep Res.* 2005;14(1):43–47
3. Comella CL. Restless legs syndrome: treatment with dopaminergic agents. *Neurology.* 2002; 58(4 Suppl 1):S87–S92
4. Kotagal S, Silber MH. Childhood-onset restless legs syndrome. *Ann Neurol.* 2004;56(6):803–807
5. Davis ID, Baron J, O'Riordan MA, Rosen CL. Sleep disturbances in pediatric dialysis patients. *Pediatr Nephrol.* 2005;20(1):69–75
6. Allen RP, Picchietti D, Hening WA, et al. Restless legs syndrome: diagnostic criteria, special consideration, and epidemiology. A report from the restless legs syndrome diagnosis and epidemiology workshop at the National Institutes of Health. *Sleep Med.* 2003;4(2):101–119
7. NIH/RLS Foundation Workshop. *RLS: Diagnosis and Diagnostic and Epidemiological Tools.* Bethesda, MD: National Institute on Aging; 2002

Lessons for the Physician

Pediatric sleep medicine is an evolving field, with recognition of more sleep disorders in childhood. Growing pains in children have long puzzled physicians, but research suggests that they are related to restless legs syndrome (RLS) in children. Long-term studies evaluating RLS and periodic leg movement in children and adolescents do not exist. Most likely these are chronic, lifelong disorders in patients who have a genetic predisposition, with periods of relapse when the underlying condition is exacerbated. The most common association of this disorder during childhood is iron deficiency, making it important to measure ferritin level. Physicians caring for children need to be cognizant of RLS and periodic leg movement and the high correlation with attention-deficit/hyperactivity disorder.

Kevin Turner, MSIII, University of California Irvine School of Medicine, Irvine, CA

Michael Ozaki, MD, Huntington Beach, CA

Don Hayes Jr, MD, University of Wisconsin Hospital and Clinics, Madison, WI

CHAPTER 72

Increasing Knee and Back Pain in a 6-Year-Old Boy

Presentation

A 6-year-old boy comes to an urgent care facility because of increasing knee and back pain. Yesterday, while swimming, he sustained a light kick to the middle-back. Hours later, he developed intermittent sharp pain behind his knees that resolved with ibuprofen. This afternoon he began crying abruptly, complaining of sharp, midline, lower back pain and bilateral anterior thigh pain. He refuses to walk. He has experienced 3 febrile seizures in the past and still wets the bed at night.

On examination, the boy appears in marked distress and is unable to lie still. His heart rate is 110 beats/min, respiratory rate is 28 breaths/min, blood pressure is 92/68 mm Hg, and temperature is 98.1°F (36.7°C). Evaluation of his back reveals point tenderness over L4 and L5 and mildly reduced flexibility but no birthmarks, bruising, redness, or swelling. His left patellar reflex is graded at 3+/4; the remainder of his reflexes are 2+/4. The Babinski reflex is absent. The muscle tone in his legs is good, with strength graded at 5/5, but he can take only 3 shuffling steps, and his movements are limited by pain. His white blood cell count is 8.6×10^3/mcL (8.6×10^9/L), erythrocyte sedimentation rate is 20 mm/h, and urinalysis is significant only for ketone levels of 15 mg/dL. A lumbosacral spine radiographic series shows normal findings.

A diagnostic imaging study reveals the diagnosis.

- **What is your differential diagnosis at this point?**
- **Are there any elements of history or physical examination that would help you?**
- **What additional diagnostic studies would you like performed?**

Discussion

The patient was admitted for pain control and further imaging. He responded well to low-dose intravenous morphine and was able to lie still for magnetic resonance imaging with and without gadolinium contrast. This imaging revealed an intramedullary lesion within the distal spinal cord at the T11 to T12 level (Figure 72.1). On the T2-weighted sequence, the signal intensity was most consistent with an acute hematoma or hemorrhage, measuring 2.0 cm vertically and 1.0 to 1.5 cm horizontally. There was also a large-caliber, serpiginous-enhancing structure communicating with the inferior portion of the lesion and descending into the lumbosacral

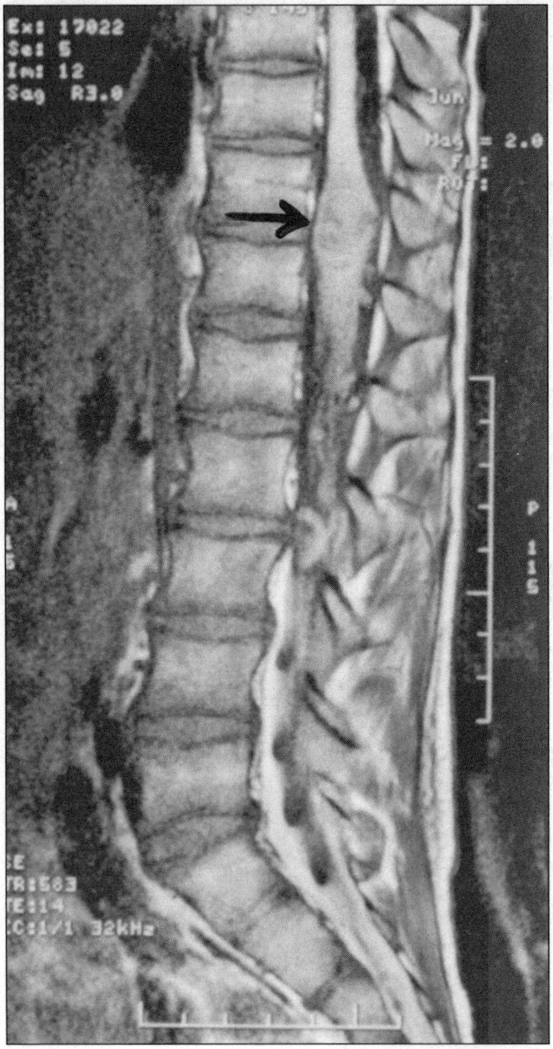

Figure 72.1. Intramedullary lesion (arrow) in the distal spinal canal.

region. More of these structures were visible above the lesion. These findings were consistent with a vascular malformation (arteriovenous malformation or fistula) that had hemorrhaged acutely. After the patient returned from undergoing magnetic resonance imaging, he began limping and favoring his right leg. His right patellar reflex diminished to 1/4, and his right leg strength decreased. These acute changes raised the fear that he was beginning to bleed again. He was sent to a pediatric neurosurgeon for immediate consultation. Fortunately, he remained stable and did not require surgery.

The Symptom

Back pain is an unusual problem in childhood that mandates concern. Unlike adults, in whom back pain is commonly due to mechanical or psychological factors, an organic cause is found in 85% of children who have back pain within 2 months of presentation. A careful history and physical examination are essential and should include not only the characteristics of the pain but also a thorough review of symptoms, highlighting the genitourinary and neurologic systems.

Red flags include young age, progressive or persistent pain, radicular pain, muscle weakness, gait abnormalities, sensory changes, bowel and bladder abnormalities, and systemic signs and symptoms such as fever, malaise, and weight loss. The physical examination should include a careful evaluation of strength, gait, straight-leg raising ability, and reflexes. Sensation testing should evaluate touch, pain, temperature, proprioception, and vibration. The examiner should look for spinal deformities, loss of curvature and motion, spasm, and areas of tenderness. Areas of erythema should be sought, with and without the patient performing the Valsalva maneuver. The examiner should listen for bruits over the spine.

Differential Diagnosis

The differential diagnosis of back pain in childhood is extensive. The initial evaluation evolves from the results of the history and physical examination. Obtaining plain radiographs, including posterior-anterior, lateral, and oblique views of the areas of concern, is usually the first step. Complete blood cell count with differential and erythrocyte sedimentation rate may be followed as the symptoms evolve, and tests for juvenile rheumatoid arthritis and ankylosing spondylitis may be necessary.

Infectious causes of back pain include vertebral osteomyelitis, spinal epidural abscess, and pyelonephritis. Among the inflammatory and rheumatologic diseases are diskitis, pancreatitis, pauciarticular juvenile rheumatoid arthritis, Reiter syndrome, and psoriatic arthritis. More common in adolescents are spondylolysis, spondylolisthesis, Scheuermann syndrome, scoliosis (in which the pain is associated with overcompensation due to the spinal curvature, rather than the curvature itself), overuse syndromes, vertebral stress fractures, and herniated disks.

A primary urologic cause is nephrolithiasis. Neoplastic diseases involving the spine are most often metastatic, including metastases from a primary brain tumor, such as medulloblastoma, acute lymphoblastic leukemia, solid tumors such as neuroblastoma, and lymphoma. Rarely, primary tumors are a source of back pain, examples being osteogenic sarcoma of the vertebrae, lipoma, and osteoid osteoma. Factors that suggest psychiatric disorders may be noted early in the evaluation, and emotional conditions should be discussed with the family as the clinical appraisal proceeds. However, it is incumbent on the physician to consider the broad range of serious physical disorders before deciding that the patient's signs and symptoms have a psychological origin.

The Specific Disorder

Spinal cord hematoma is a rare condition that usually results from rare predisposing conditions, such as spinal cord vascular malformations, coagulopathy (either congenital or pharmacologically induced), spinal cord tumors, inflammatory myelitis, abscess, or syringomyelia. Spinal cord trauma and postsurgical complications are also causes of bleeding.

Regardless of the underlying cause, excruciating back pain related to the location of the underlying lesion is the most common presentation of a spinal cord hematoma. The neurologic deficits may lag behind the onset of pain and increase over the ensuing days. The risk of rebleeding from a vascular malformation is about 3% within the first 24 hours and then 3% per year for life. However, these malformations commonly self-destruct during the initial or subsequent hemorrhages and no longer pose a risk of recurrence.

Arteriovenous malformations of the spinal cord are not common in the pediatric population; they are more likely to occur in the second and third decades of life. Physicians should recognize that changes in micturition and progressive weakness may be early signs caused by these malformations (as well as other spinal cord lesions). There may be a combination of both upper and lower motor neuron findings, and sensory deficits do not match a radicular pattern.

Treatment

If the bleeding and its resolution destroy the malformation only partially, embolization may be beneficial, providing that no critical feeder vessels exist. Progressive neurologic impairment may mandate direct neurosurgical intervention. This patient is currently receiving intensive physical therapy and will have spinal angiography to determine the need for embolization after the acute edema resolves. Because this condition presents only rarely in the pediatric age group, there are no data on the prognosis or outcome in children.

Lessons for the Physician

Back pain in children must be evaluated carefully because it carries a high probability of being caused by a serious condition. Findings gathered by performing a thorough history and physical examination will direct the remainder of the evaluation, which must include imaging if a lesion in the spine is suspected.

Jennifer A. Hunt, MD; Richard Friederich, MD; and Peter S. Palka, MD, Spangdahlem Air Base, Germany

CHAPTER 73

Vomiting, Unsteadiness, Vision Problems, and Unresponsiveness in a 10-Year-Old Boy

Presentation

While watching television, a 10-year-old boy suddenly feels nauseated and vomits once. Then he develops unsteadiness and complains that he cannot see properly. He becomes silent and stares into space. There is no seizure activity or any history of trauma, medication use, or substance abuse. His neonatal period and development were normal. Like his mother, grandfather, and uncle, he was diagnosed 2 years earlier as having migraine with visual aura and without focal neurologic deficit.

On examination 1 hour later, the boy's eyes are open but he is responsive only to pain. Vital signs are in the normal range, and oxygen saturation is 99%. There are no meningeal signs, and neurologic findings are normal except for the sensorial changes and reduced muscle tone. Results of a complete blood cell count, liver function tests, and toxicology studies are normal, as are levels of glucose, calcium, magnesium, urea, creatinine, electrolytes, ammonia, lactate, amino acids, and organic acids.

Thirty minutes after hospital admission, the boy develops flexion posturing, his Glasgow Coma Scale decreases to 4, and his respiratory rate drops to 4 breaths/min without signs of respiratory distress, laryngospasm, or aspiration. Radiographs of the chest, cranial computed tomography, and electroencephalography all yield normal results. Cerebrospinal fluid findings are normal, including cultures and polymerase chain reaction studies.

The patient is ventilated and given intravenous cefotaxime and acyclovir. His respiratory efforts and consciousness improve over 6 hours, and he progresses to complete recovery. A diagnosis is made, he is prescribed medication, and he has remained well.

- **What is your differential diagnosis at this point?**
- **Are there any elements of history or physical examination that would help you?**
- **What additional diagnostic studies would you like performed?**

Discussion

Coma has many etiologies, including cerebrovascular injuries, cerebral edema, and space-occupying lesions, as well as infectious, metabolic, toxic, and convulsive disorders, all of which were excluded in this child. In addition, his past and family history suggested autosomal dominant migraine with aura. Because of his rapid normalization on supportive therapy, familial hemiplegic migraine (FHM) was considered to be responsible for his transient neurologic and respiratory depression. This diagnosis was made by exclusion. The boy was prescribed medication for prophylaxis of migraine and has had no further episodes.

Variations

Although migraine is estimated to occur in 15% to 29% of the general population, coma and respiratory depression are exceedingly rare complications. In acute confusional migraine, patients may be confused, but unlike this patient, they are alert, have rapid fluent speech, are unable to form new memories, and have a variable degree of retrograde amnesia. Coma has not been described. In basilar artery migraine, recurrent episodes of coma may occur during attacks, but unlike the situation in this patient, these episodes are associated with severe occipital headaches, dizziness, vertigo, visual disturbances, ataxia, and dysarthria. The coma may last from 3 to 10 days, with subsequent slow improvement.

Familial hemiplegic migraine is a rare disorder, is genetically heterogenous, and has an autosomal dominant mode of inheritance. The condition is associated with genes mapped on chromosome 1q21–23 and on chromosome 19p, where mutations have been described in the *CACNA1A* gene, which encodes the voltage-gated P/Q-type calcium channels in neurons. Aura, paresthesias, or transient motor deficits are common in this form of migraine, and complications such as fever, meningismus, dysphasia, coma, seizures, respiratory arrest, and cerebral edema may be precipitated by mild head trauma, strenuous exercise, or cerebral angiography. These effects are usually reversible, but permanent sequelae may occur. The pathophysiology of FHM is not well understood, although hemodynamic or metabolic abnormalities and cortical spreading depression have been postulated.

Respiratory arrest in autosomal dominant FHM is very rare and has not been reported in the nonhemiplegic forms. In one case report, the respiratory arrest led to a persistent vegetative state and death 4 months later. Microinfarcts were found in the basal ganglia but not in the brainstem nuclei associated with respiration, leaving unexplained the mechanism of the arrest. Even without respiratory depression, FHM may lead to irreversible brain damage and cerebral atrophy, probably due to cortical hypoperfusion.

Familial hemiplegic migraine with coma may be confused with cerebral autosomal dominant arteriopathy with subcortical infarcts and leukoencephalopathy, but unlike FHM, the latter condition is characterized by abnormalities on neuroimaging studies.

Although the effect of migraine prophylaxis on the reduction of coma or respiratory depression has not been studied, prevention of migraine attacks seems prudent in patients who have had these dramatic effects.

Lessons for the Physician

Although some are rare, many effects can result from migraine episodes, including coma and respiratory depression. After excluding traumatic, cerebrovascular, infectious, neoplastic, convulsive, and metabolic causes as well as mitochondrial brain disorders, the physician should consider migraine as a cause of altered consciousness or respiratory depression, especially in the presence of a past or family history of migraine with aura.

Hassib Narchi, MD, and Linda Edwards, MB, ChB, Sandwell General Hospital, West Bromwich, United Kingdom

COMMENTARY BY DR LALITHA SIVASWAMY, PEDIATRIC NEUROLOGIST, CHILDREN'S HOSPITAL OF MICHIGAN

Familial hemiplegic migraine is a rare disorder, is genetically heterogenous, and has an autosomal dominant mode of inheritance. The condition is associated most commonly with *CACNA1A* gene mapped on chromosome 19p (referred to as *FHM1*), which encodes the voltage-gated P/Q-type calcium channels in neurons. More recently, mutations in the *ATP1A2* gene mapped on chromosome 1q21-23 (*FHM2*) and *SCN1A* gene mapped on chromosome 2 (*FHM3*) have been noted to be associated with forms of familial hemiplegic migraine.

Genetic testing may prove helpful in establishing a diagnosis of hemiplegic migraine and instituting appropriate treatment. Serotonin agonists such as sumatriptan and rizatriptan that are commonly used as abortives in children with migraine should be avoided in the setting of hemiplegic migraine. Flunarizine, a long-acting calcium channel blocker, has been found to be an effective prophylactic agent in over three-fourths of children with hemiplegic migraine. Mood swings and weight gain are common adverse effects. Unfortunately, flunarizine is not commercially available in the United States. The *International Classification of Headache Diseases* is a valuable resource for practitioners who have a special interest in headache medicine.

CHAPTER 74

Weakness and Inability to Walk in an 11-Year-Old Boy

Presentation

An 11-year-old boy is brought to the emergency department because of weakness and inability to walk. He has been well prior to this morning, when he tried to get out of bed and could walk only a few feet before falling. There is no history of fever, cough, diarrhea, shortness of breath, loss of sensation, drug ingestion, or recent travel.

On physical examination, the boy appears alert and friendly. His temperature is 98°F (36.7°C), pulse is 115 beats/min, blood pressure is 117/61 mm Hg, respiratory rate is 18 breaths/min, and oxygen saturation by pulse oximetry is 98%. He has decreased strength in his shoulders and hips (level 3/5) and decreased reflexes in the arms but no change in tone or sensation. No goiter is palpated and no exophthalmos, noted. His white blood cell count is 7.9×10^3/mcL (7.9×10^9/L), hemoglobin level is 13.3 g/dL (133 g/L), and platelet count is 315×10^3/mcL (315×10^9/L). Additional laboratory findings and elements of his past medical history and family history reveal the underlying diagnosis.

- **What is your differential diagnosis at this point?**
- **Are there any elements of history or physical examination that would help you?**
- **What additional diagnostic studies would you like performed?**

Discussion

The patient's serum sodium level was 141 mEq/L (141 mmol/L), potassium was 1.9 mEq/L (1.9 mmol/L), chloride was 105 mEq/L (105 mmol/L), and bicarbonate was 24 mEq/L (24 mmol/L). Levels of urea nitrogen, creatinine, glucose, and liver function chemistries were normal. A detailed family history revealed that this adopted boy's biological father had experienced similar periodic attacks of weakness and paralysis as an adolescent, all of which were associated with hypokalemia. In addition, the patient had a similar "attack" 6 months ago, but he experienced only weakness, and he improved without sequelae after consuming potassium-rich foods.

During this episode, the patient had been given a banana at home without improvement. An intravenous bolus of potassium was administered in the emergency department. The patient had normal electrocardiographic findings throughout; within a few hours of receiving the potassium, he was able to get out of bed and go to the restroom on his own. His physical findings normalized, and his potassium level rose to be 4.5 mEq/L (4.5 mmol/L). The low potassium of 1.9 mEq/L (1.9 mmol/L) along with the family history confirmed the diagnosis of familial periodic paralysis (FPP).

The Condition

Familial periodic paralysis is a relatively rare autosomal dominant inherited disorder that can be characterized as being hypokalemic, normokalemic, or hyperkalemic. The hypokalemic form, as seen in this boy, presents as acute systemic weakness in association with a low serum potassium level. There is a male predominance of 3 to 1. The age of onset generally is in adolescence, and the condition occurs most frequently in Caucasians. Episodes are most common at night, with patients typically awakening unable to walk. The potassium deficiency most seriously affects the neuromuscular system, and the weakness is generally limited to the limbs and limb girdles. The respiratory muscles are rarely involved, but deaths from respiratory failure and cardiac arrhythmias have been reported in the literature.

Hyperkalemic periodic paralysis is also inherited in an autosomal dominant pattern. Affected patients have episodic weakness but also experience myotonia. It is believed that this disorder is caused by a mutation in chromosome 17 that affects a sodium channel, which then influences potassium transport. In normokalemic periodic paralysis, the signs and symptoms are the same, but there is no change in the serum potassium level. Many similarities exist between the normokalemic and hyperkalemic disorders, such as the mutation affecting the sodium channel, the same triggers (cold weather, exertion, oral potassium ingestion), and improvement with the intake of sodium.

The paralysis in this disorder is related to serum levels of potassium, although total body potassium stores remain adequate. Potassium moves into the muscle cells in FPP (the exact method of this translocation of potassium is unknown), thereby causing a decrease in the serum potassium level, which causes the weakness. The hypokalemia is exacerbated by exercise followed by rest, a high-carbohydrate diet, or a glucose and insulin infusion. In this case, there was no obvious trigger. The boy had exercised the day before but not more than usual. There also appears to be a relationship between the development of paralysis and increased endogenous mineralocorticoid.

On physical examination, deep tendon reflexes are typically absent or diminished, but sensation and level of consciousness are generally unaffected. Muscle weakness, especially in the lower extremities and limb girdles, can be appreciated, but tone remains normal. The weakness may last up to 36 hours, and the symptoms usually remit spontaneously.

Differential Diagnosis

The differential diagnosis of acute weakness is extensive, and a few disease processes should be considered. Guillain-Barré syndrome is a possibility, but the paralysis in this condition is usually ascending, which was not present in this case. Also, there was no apparent preceding viral illness. Myasthenia gravis is another cause of muscle weakness, but the most common initial features are ptosis and diplopia, and the deep tendon reflexes are usually preserved. Adult botulism can present with acute weakness, but it also is characterized by a relatively rapid progression of cranial nerve dysfunction, which was not present in this case.

Any disease that results in the loss of potassium is potentially capable of producing hypokalemic paralysis. Potassium can be lost in the urine in nephrotic syndrome, in acute tubular necrosis, and during treatment of diabetic ketoacidosis. Potassium can be lost from the gastrointestinal system in severe diarrhea associated with celiac disease, bacterial or parasitic enteritis, and malabsorption due to short bowel syndrome.

Thyrotoxic periodic paralysis (TPP) occurs when the onset of hyperthyroidism coincides with a hypokalemic paralytic attack. This condition usually occurs in males (20:1), and more than 90% of cases have been reported in Asian people. As with FPP, there is translocation of potassium into muscle cells, but the mechanism appears to differ from that of FPP. Acetazolamide, which is the preventive treatment of choice for FPP, exacerbates the attacks of paralysis in TPP. The attacks in TPP can be blocked with propranolol. Treatment of TPP is the same—the administration of potassium—but attacks are prevented best by treating the hyperthyroidism.

Barium poisoning can also cause an intracellular shift of potassium. This toxicity does not result from the barium sulfate used in radiologic studies but from barium chloride or barium carbonate used for glazing pottery and sometimes found as a contaminant in flour or salt.

Renal tubular acidosis is a syndrome of abnormal urine acidification. There is an associated hypokalemia (due to serum potassium deficit) in type 1 and type 2. The pathogenetic mechanism has not been defined totally but appears to be related in part to the decreased rate of hydrogen secretion and potassium absorption by the distal nephron. Treatment involves correction of the hypokalemia and the chronic acidosis.

In primary hyperaldosteronism (Conn syndrome), an increase in aldosterone excretion leads to increased secretion of potassium and hypokalemia as well as hypertension. The preferred treatment is to remove the aldosterone-secreting tumor. If that is not possible, spironolactone therapy is an alternative to surgery.

Chronic licorice ingestion can result in electrolyte imbalance seen in heperaldosteronism. The licorice contains glycyrrhizic acid, which has mineralocorticoid activity that can produce sodium retention and hypokalemia.

Treatment

Hypokalemic attacks associated with minimal weakness can be managed with the oral administration of 130 mEq of potassium over 24 hours. Intravenous supplementation is required to treat frank paralysis. Prophylaxis against recurrent attacks has been successful by using low-carbohydrate diets, oral potassium supplementation, spironolactone, and acetazolamide. Acetazolamide has been shown to be the most effective prophylactic treatment. The drug works by inducing metabolic acidosis, thereby blunting the intracellular translocation of serum potassium.

Lessons for the Physician

Hypokalemic paralysis is uncommon, but it must be considered in the differential diagnosis of systemic weakness. The family history, age of presentation, race, medications, and underlying disease states may assist the physician in determining the cause of the paralysis. In this case, the father's history of hypokalemic paralysis helped to make the diagnosis and assured prompt and appropriate treatment for this rare, usually benign, but potentially dangerous entity.

Andrea Alexander, MD; Jacob J. Rosenberg, MD; and Sania Wilkins, DO, North Shore University Hospital, Manhasset, NY

COMMENTARY BY DR LALITHA SIVASWAMY, PEDIATRIC NEUROLOGIST, CHILDREN'S HOSPITAL OF MICHIGAN

Hypokalemic periodic paralysis is usually the consequence of mutation in the *CACNA1S* gene mapped to chromosome 1q32. The condition is characteristically precipitated by a carbohydrate-rich meal, emotional stress/excitement, exposure to cold temperatures, or rest after exercise. A specific subtype of hypokalemic paralysis (Andersen syndrome) is associated with prolonged QT interval on electrocardiogram and predisposition to ventricular dysrthymias. Therefore, cardiac screening is an important facet of evaluation of children with periodic paralysis. The differential diagnosis of generalized acute weakness is extensive and a few important disease processes should be considered, including myelopathy of various etiologies such as infections, lesions compressing the spinal cord and demyelinating disorders, acute viral myositis, and tick paralysis.

CHAPTER 75

Excessive Nighttime Eating in a 14-Year-Old Boy

Presentation

A 14-year-old boy is evaluated for excessive nighttime eating. Since early childhood, he awakens every night around midnight and consumes large quantities of food, even those he dislikes. Alarms, locks, and punishment have not stopped this habit. He remembers his eating in the morning but has no remorse or regret. In addition, he eats a small breakfast and a lunch and dinner normal for his age. He has gained 22.5 kg in the last year.

He has been evaluated by a pediatrician, psychologist, psychiatrist, neurologist, and educational specialist; has been diagnosed as having mild autism, obsessive-compulsive disorder (OCD), and learning problems; and has been treated with methylphenidate, divalproex, and clonidine. He was adopted at 6 days of age, and no family medical history is available.

Physical examination reveals an interactive, conversational boy who answers questions appropriately. His vital signs are normal, weight is 7.7 kg (above the 95th percentile), height is 175.3 cm (90th percentile), and body mass index is 25.2 (95th percentile). He has mild hypotonia and mild weakness of the legs. Other than obesity, all other physical findings are normal.

- **What is your differential diagnosis at this point?**
- **Are there any elements of history or physical examination that would help you?**
- **What additional diagnostic studies would you like performed?**

Discussion

This boy had an eating disorder characterized by overeating at night in conjunction with associated psychological problems, including OCD and learning disability. His nighttime eating was causing numerous problems, including a loss of sleep that might be affecting his school performance. The long-term effects on his health from the gain of 22.5 kg in 1 year are significant and could include metabolic syndrome, diabetes, hypercholesterolemia, and coronary artery disease. His eating pattern is troubling socially and has been disruptive to the family.

Differential Diagnosis

Nighttime eating can have many causes, including sleep-related eating disorder (SRED), binge-eating disorder with binges at night, night eating syndrome (NES), and behavioral disorders that have nonconventional eating patterns. Another consideration in this patient who has an associated learning disability is Prader-Willi syndrome, which was ruled out via genetic testing. It should be noted that some nighttime snacking is normal, especially in adolescents, but eating greater than 50% of total calories at night and awakening from sleep to eat are not normal eating behaviors. Discerning the cause of nighttime eating requires clinical judgment aided by a thorough history, including dietary "logs" and eating questionnaires.

Sleep-related eating disorder and NES are similar conditions, but the history can elicit differences. Sleep-related eating disorder is associated with other sleep-related disorders, such as sleep apnea and restless legs syndrome, that are not seen in NES. Polysomnography can aid in differentiating the conditions because the only abnormality usually reported in NES is low sleep efficiency. Patients who have SRED often consume unusual foods and nonfood items, in contrast to the consistent food choices in NES. Another variance between the 2 disorders is that patients who have NES are aware of their eating (and show no remorse), whereas patients who have SRED are often not aware of their eating and do not remember the event.

Bulimia nervosa can also present with nighttime eating binges, often with purging, but purging is not reported typically in NES. The abnormal feature seen in NES is more the timing of food intake than the actual amounts. Intake of massive quantities of food is more characteristic of bulimia, although patients who have NES can eat enough to gain excessive weight.

The Condition

As part of his evaluation, the patient completed a diet log that revealed an average consumption of 1,417 kcal from 10:00 pm to 6:00 am and consumption of 1,388 kcal during the other 16 hours of the day (more than 50% of calories after the evening meal). Nighttime eating was reported during 7 of 7 nights, and he was fully aware of his eating. Anorexia was present each morning. The boy also met criteria for depression (by use of a standard depression scale). This patient, therefore, seemed to fit closely a diagnosis of NES. The diagnosis of NES is difficult in pediatrics because criteria are established only for adults.

Although first described in 1955, NES was not studied extensively until the recent societal increase in obesity, and the disorder is still in the early stages of investigation. Most research has been performed in adults, and pediatric and adolescent diagnostic criteria still are being developed. The major characteristics are evening or night hyperphagia, insomnia with waking to eat at night, and morning anorexia. Birkvedt and associates[1] include additional criteria: consuming greater than 50% of total daily calories at night, awakening at least once per night, consuming a snack during awakenings, having symptoms for at least 3 months, and not meeting the criteria for bulimia nervosa or binge-eating disorder.

Although the criteria for inclusion have changed over the years, the central feature is a delay in the circadian pattern of eating. Circadian oscillators may signal food intake at a different phase than is signaled normally, and the circadian timing of food intake is delayed. Other problems associated with NES include psychological disorders such as depression, anxiety, and low self-esteem. This boy's learning problems and OCD are consistent with such observations about NES. In one study, 5.6% of patients who had NES had OCD as well.

The prevalence of NES is estimated to be 0.5% to 1.6% of the general population and 6% to 14% of patients who attend obesity clinics. Outpatient psychiatric clinics report an incidence of NES as high as 16%. Patients who have NES can be of normal weight as well as obese. The mean body mass index in a study of 106 patients was 30.8.[2]

Treatment

Optimal treatment of NES still is subject to research. The nighttime food preferences primarily seeming to be carbohydrates may signify an attempt to promote sleep or improve mood. Tryptophan uptake is promoted by insulin release after carbohydrate ingestion, and tryptophan is a precursor to serotonin synthesis. Circadian rhythms of eating and sleep are controlled by a part of the hypothalamus that is affected by serotonin. The use of selective serotonin reuptake inhibitors, therefore, has been studied in treating NES. A study by O'Reardon and colleagues[3] showed a decreased number of awakenings, episodes of nocturnal ingestion, and percent of calories eaten after supper after 12 weeks of treatment with sertraline. Approximately 25% of the patients in this study experienced remission and had an average weight loss of 4.8 kg.

References

1. Birkvedt GS, Florholmen J, Sundsfjord J, et al. Behavioral and neuroendocrine characteristics of the night-eating syndrome. *JAMA.* 1999;282(7):657–663
2. de Zwaan M, Roerig DB, Crosby RD, Kraz S, Mitchell JE. Nighttime eating: a descriptive study. *Int J Eating Dis.* 2006;39(3):224–232
3. O'Reardon JP, Sunnkard AJ, Allison KC. Clinical trial of sertraline in the treatment of night eating syndrome. *Int J Eating Dis.* 2004;35(1):16–26

Lessons for the Physician

Night eating syndrome is an unusual form of eating disorder whose pathophysiology, treatment, and prognosis are still being explored and require more study, especially in children and adolescents. As additional research is completed in children, a more concrete set of criteria may be developed for diagnosis in pediatric and adolescent patients. Treatment with selective serotonin reuptake inhibitors offers some promise based on a recent study. This diagnosis should be considered in patients who demonstrate excessive nighttime eating or in those who are obese without clear cause, especially if they have sleep disturbances or other psychological disorders. A history that involves detailed documentation of eating and sleeping habits is the most important diagnostic tool.

Seth Septer, DO; Cristina Fernandez, MD; and Fernando Zapata, MD, University of Nebraska/Creighton University School of Medicine, Omaha, NE

CHAPTER 76

Intermittent Swelling and Arm Pain for 2 Years in an Adolescent Girl

Presentation

A 17-year-old girl presents with intermittent right upper extremity swelling and pain over the past 2 years. Her symptoms began after an episode of Bell palsy. She describes swelling and an "electrical shooting" pain in the right shoulder that radiates toward her hand, followed by a cool feeling of the hand and decreased range of motion of the arm. The episodes occur during both summer and winter and can last anywhere from 2 to 30 days. Initially, between these episodes, she regained normal function, but recently has noted residual weakness. She denies any history of trauma, fever, rash, or muscle weakness.

On examination, there is swelling of the entire right arm. The nails are normal. The right arm is colder in comparison with the left and has decreased hair growth. Peripheral pulses and capillary refill were normal. Pinprick and temperature sensations are intact, without hyperesthesia. Range of motion of the right arm, forearm, and hand is compromised because of pain. Except for her right arm, she is warm, well perfused, and free of joint swelling. The muscle tone is normal, and strength in the other muscle groups is 5/5.

Laboratory studies reveal an erythrocyte sedimentation rate of 15 mm/h, C-reactive protein level less than 0.5 mg/dL, white blood cell count of 6.3×10^3/mcL, and creatine phosphokinase level of 100 U/L. The results of additional laboratory studies, including antinuclear antibody titer, rheumatoid factor, antibody test for *Borrelia burgdorferi*, rapid plasma regain test for syphilis, urine-amplified DNA assay for *Chlamydia* and gonorrhea, hemoglobin electrophoresis, serum lactic acid dehydrogenase level, and uric acid level, are normal or negative.

Radiographs of cervical spine, chest, right elbow, forearm, and hand as well as magnetic resonance imaging of the brain, cervical spine, and entire arm yield normal findings. Right upper extremity vascular duplex ultrasonography shows normal flow without evidence of a deep venous thrombosis.

- **What is your differential diagnosis at this point?**
- **Are there any elements of history or physical examination that would help you?**
- **What additional diagnostic studies would you like performed?**

Discussion

This patient was evaluated thoroughly by consultants from anesthesiology, neurology, and rheumatology. Her pain was poorly controlled with morphine. During her hospitalization, the skin temperature along her right arm became normal, but she developed hyperesthesia and allodynia (perception of pain from a nonpainful stimulus) of her right arm. She also developed tenderness of the right trapezius muscle. She was unable to move her fingers because of weakness. Temperature sensation was decreased over the entire surface of the arm.

After ruling out other possible causes, such as malignancy, postinfectious reaction, and rheumatologic diseases, it was felt that she met criteria for complex regional pain syndrome (CRPS). A trial of gabapentin and amitriptyline was begun and her symptoms improved. Subsequently, she had a nerve block placed, following which she regained use of her arm. She has had some residual weakness, for which she is receiving physical and occupational therapy.

The Condition

Complex regional pain syndrome type 1, formerly known as reflex sympathetic dystrophy syndrome, is a chronic progressive disease characterized by severe pain, swelling, and changes in the skin. Current understanding of this condition is that it is caused by a disruption of the autonomic nervous system. The International Association for the Study of Pain (IASP) has divided CRPS into 2 types based on the detection of a nerve lesion. Type 1 is not associated with an identifiable nerve lesion, whereas type 2, previously known as causalgia, presents evidence of obvious nerve damage. It is unclear what causes the abnormal pain sensations that typify CRPS, but injury of the affected body part and stress seem to play a role.

Most cases of CRPS occur in the fourth decade after birth. However, the incidence of CRPS among children is increasing.

Diagnosis

The most widely accepted criteria for the diagnosis have been published by IASP[1] and are as follows:

1. The presence of an initiating noxious event or a cause for immobilization
2. Continuing pain, allodynia, or hyperalgesia disproportionate to the inciting event
3. Evidence at some time of edema, changes in skin blood flow, or abnormal motor activity in the area of pain
4. Exclusion of the diagnosis by the existence of any condition that would otherwise account for the degree of pain and dysfunction

Criteria 2 through 4 must be present for the diagnosis.

According to the IASP, the diagnostic criteria for CRPS type 2 (also known as causalgia) are as follows:

1. The presence of continuing pain, allodynia, or hyperalgesia after a nerve injury, not necessarily limited to the distribution of the injured nerve
2. Evidence at some time of edema, changes in skin blood flow, or abnormal motor activity in the region of pain
3. Exclusion of the diagnosis by the existence of any condition that would otherwise account for the degree of pain and dysfunction

All 3 criteria must be present to make the diagnosis.

No specific laboratory or imaging studies are available to establish the diagnosis of CRPS, and most experts agree that diagnostic studies are not necessary to make the diagnosis. However, the following tests have been found useful in confirming the diagnosis:

Three-phase bone scan and gadolinium magnetic resonance imaging have been used to diagnose and stage the disease. Although radiographs can yield normal findings in as many as 30% of patients, osteoporosis may be demonstrated as early as 3 to 5 weeks after the onset of the symptoms. Laser Doppler flow studies have been used to monitor background vasomotor control. A cold pressor test performed in conjunction with thermographic imaging may demonstrate a vasoconstrictor response.

Treatment

A number of different treatment modalities are available, including nerve blockades; medications such as topical analgesics, gabapentin, tricyclic antidepressants, and corticosteroids; and psychotherapy. Physical therapy is an essential and nonnegotiable part of treatment. It is extremely important to restore normal function of the affected body part through vigorous and intense physical therapy. Additionally, tactile stimulation can reduce the associated pain and swelling significantly.

Prognosis

The prognosis is good if the condition is treated early, ideally within the first 3 months of onset. Patients may develop permanent muscle, nerve, and skin damage if CRPS is not diagnosed and treated in a timely fashion.

Reference

1. Merskey H, Bogduk N, eds. *Classification of Chronic Pain: Descriptions of Chronic Pain Syndromes and Definitions of Pain Terms.* Seattle, WA: International Association for the Study of Pain Press; 1994

Lessons for the Physician

Complex regional pain syndrome is a diagnosis that is sometimes overlooked but should be considered if there is intense and intractable pain, especially in an isolated area.

For most patients, the diagnosis and treatment are delayed by months and even years.

Early diagnosis and treatment can prevent long-term damage, such as muscle atrophy, joint contractures, and possible permanent loss of function of the affected extremity.

Alfredo Torralbas, MD, Doctors Medical Center & Miami Children Hospital, Miami, FL

Part 13

Pulmonology

CHAPTER 77

2-Month-Old Girl With Protrusion in Neck When Crying

Presentation

A 2-month-old girl is admitted to the hospital following 8 days of vomiting, diarrhea, and dehydration and is rehydrated intravenously. On day 2, a nurse notes a protrusion in the infant's neck when she cries.

Physical examination reveals an alert, vigorous infant in no distress. Her temperature is 98.6°F (37.0°C), pulse is 164 beats/min, respirations are 40 breaths/min, and blood pressure is 72/30 mm Hg. The infant has several abnormal features, including dolichocephaly (premature fusion of the sagittal suture), a large anterior fontanelle, a depressed nasal bridge, low-set ears, downslanting palpebral fissures, a high-arched palate, camptodactyly (permanent flexion of the fingers), and prominent calcanei.

A dynamic bulge protrudes just left of the midline above the clavicle when the infant cries. The mass does not appear on quiet breathing. The infant does not have increased work of breathing or tachypnea, and the remainder of the pulmonary and cardiac findings are normal. She has a reducible umbilical hernia. Her genitalia, muscle tone, and reflexes are normal.

Chest radiograph and computed tomography scan of the chest yield normal findings. Further radiologic studies reveal the diagnosis.

- **What is your differential diagnosis at this point?**
- **Are there any elements of history or physical examination that would help you?**
- **What additional diagnostic studies would you like performed?**

Discussion

Dynamic airway fluoroscopy demonstrated during a Valsalva maneuver that the mass was lung, establishing the diagnosis of a unilateral, apical cervical lung hernia. A search of the literature for a link between the patient's dysmorphisms and the cervical lung hernia failed to reveal an association. The family was reassured that the hernia should resolve eventually without intervention.

The Clinical Challenge

Head and neck lesions are encountered commonly in neonates and infants. The differential diagnosis can be extensive and includes both congenital and acquired conditions. History and physical examination can narrow the differential diagnosis and guide diagnostic testing. Pertinent historical and examination findings include the time when the mass was initially detected, location of the mass, presence of inflammation or drainage, color and character of the mass, transillumination, and the effect of a Valsalva maneuver on the mass. These findings guide further diagnostic efforts (Table 77.1).

Differential Diagnosis

Branchial cleft cysts can present during the first year after birth. Improper branchial arch closure in early gestation results in a cleft cyst or sinus. Branchial cleft cyst can present as a nontender, fluctuant mass in the lateral anterior triangle. The cyst may become inflamed during an upper respiratory tract infection.

Thyroglossal duct cyst presents as a painless mass that moves with tongue protrusion. Such cysts are found in the midline between the base of the tongue and the sternum, most often below the hyoid bone, and may become inflamed during an upper respiratory tract infection. Treatment of both thyroglossal duct cysts and branchial cleft cysts is excision following resolution of infection.

Enlargement of the thyroid can be due to congenital goiter or a mass in the thyroid gland. Defects in fetal thyroxine synthesis or maternal antithyroid medications or iodides during pregnancy can cause congenital goiter. Congenital goiter is always present in congenital hyperthyroidism. Congenital goiter presents as thyroid enlargement (midline mass) at birth that may cause hyperextension of the head. Goiter nodules need nuclear medicine assessment for "hot" or "cold" status. Cold nodules must be evaluated further for malignancy. Treatment of goiters due to hypothyroidism requires immediate replacement of thyroid hormone.

Lymphatic malformations, such as cystic hygroma, are congenital malformations of lymph tissue resulting from failure of the lymphatic primordial buds to establish venous drainage. A lymphatic malformation presents as a soft, smooth, nontender, compressible mass that transilluminates. Typically, lymphatic malformations

Table 77.1. Characteristics and Recommended Imaging Studies for Neck Masses

Condition	Location	Description	Change With Valsalva Maneuver	Transillumination	Imaging
Branchial cleft cyst	Lateral anterior triangle	Nontender, fluctuant May have associated drainage or inflammation	–	–	CT, US
Thyroglossal duct cyst	Midline anterior triangle—tongue to sternum Most commonly at base of hyoid	Painless mass, moves with tongue protrusion, may increase in size with URTI or inflammation	–	–	US, CT, MRI
Lymphatic malformation	Most often in posterior triangle	Soft, smooth, nontender, compressible	–	+	CT, MRI
Hemangioma	Variable	Red or bluish soft mass	+	–	US (Doppler), CT, MRI
Laryngocele	Just lateral to midline	May have associated cough, stridor, hoarseness	+	–	CT, MRI
Cervical lung hernia	Supraclavicular, just lateral to midline	Dynamic mass most noticeable with crying, straining, coughing	+	–	CT, AF
Congenital torticollis	Sternocleidomastoid muscle	Firm, discrete, fusiform mass	–	–	None
Dermoid cyst	Usually suprahyoid	Nontender, smooth, rubbery	–	±	US, CT
Goiter	Midline	Associated with hypothyroidism or hyperthyroidism	–	–	US, TS

Abbreviations: AF, airway fluoroscopy; CT, computed tomography; MRI, magnetic resonance imaging; TS, thyroid scintigraphy; URTI, upper respiratory tract infection; US, ultrasonography.

fluctuate in size with infection or hemorrhage. These masses can cause respiratory compromise and difficulty feeding. Treatment of a lymphangioma is excision or observation, depending on the severity of the lesion.

Hemangiomas are proliferative hamartomas of vascular endothelium that present at birth, grow rapidly during the first postnatal year, and begin to involute slowly by 18 to 24 months of age. Hemangiomas often present as red or bluish soft masses that enlarge with crying or Valsalva maneuvers and do not transilluminate. Surgery or laser therapy may be required if the hemangioma impinges on vital structures of the neck and chest.

A laryngocele is an abnormal dilation or herniation of the saccule of the larynx. Laryngoceles may present in the neonate or infant with hoarseness, stridor, cough, dyspnea, or dysphagia. They are found just lateral to midline and may enlarge with Valsalva maneuvers. Surgical excision is the management of choice.

Congenital torticollis presents as a firm, painless, discrete, fusiform mass within the sternocleidomastoid muscle that slowly increases in size for 2 to 3 months and then regresses slowly for 4 to 8 months. Torticollis usually improves with conservative management, including stretching and exercises of passive and active range of motion.

Lymphoma must be kept in mind when evaluating a neck mass.

The Condition

Cervical lung herniation is defined as the presence of lung tissue outside the confines of the bony thorax. Lung herniation was described first by Roland in 1499. Morel-Lavallée further classified lung hernias based on location and cause (intercostal, cervical, and diaphragmatic).

Twenty percent of all lung hernias are congenital; the remainder follow trauma. Congenital cervical lung hernia manifests during the first year after birth but may not be apparent at birth. The most common location is cervical because of the absence or laxity of the endothoracic fascia (Sibson fascia) in this area.

The presenting sign of a cervical hernia is usually a neck mass noticed while the patient is straining, crying, or coughing. Examination may demonstrate a supraclavicular mass that increases in size with Valsalva maneuvers, representing extrathoracic lung protrusion (Figure 77.1). Cervical lung hernias are spongy and sometimes appear to move with respiration. They are rarely painful but may cause hoarseness, chronic cough, stridor, or superior vena cava syndrome by external compression of the structures within the neck. Patients are at risk for pneumothorax when a central venous catheter is placed.

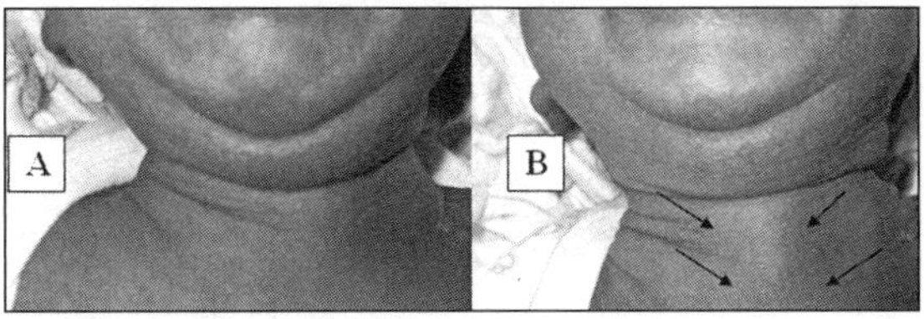

Figure 77.1. Photos taken of the patient during a crying episode. Photo B was taken during a more forceful Valsalva maneuver. Arrows mark the periphery of the visible protuberance caused by the cervical lung hernia, which on examination was located to the left of the midline.

Cervical lung hernias usually resolve spontaneously. Treatment should be pursued if there is incarceration or complications from compression of nearby structures.

Evaluation

Although physicians experienced in managing cervical lung hernias point out that their appearance is usually so characteristic that the diagnosis is apparent, physicians should be aware of the wide spectrum of neck masses and the modalities available for differentiating among them. Imaging studies are often used to delineate the nature of a neck mass. Choice of the best study is guided by history and physical findings (see Table 77.1). The most common modalities for evaluating neck masses include ultrasonography, computed tomography, and magnetic resonance imaging. Important factors guiding the choice of imaging include the size and suspected extent of the lesion, suspicion of vascular or airway involvement, need for a bedside examination, and the perceived risk of sedation.

Lessons for the Physician

History and physical examination often allow the physician to identify the nature of a congenital neck mass. Because the mass in this patient was dynamic, a dynamic study (airway fluoroscopy) was employed to verify the diagnosis. Although many types of neck masses occur in neonates and infants, masses that are intermittent are rare. The dramatic increase with Valsalva maneuver, absence of red or bluish color change, and supraclavicular location helped focus the diagnosis. A cervical lung hernia should be considered when a neck mass behaves as this one did.

Elizabeth Walenz, MD; Michael Weisgerber, MD; and Stephen Conley, MD, Children's Hospital of Wisconsin, Milwaukee, WI

CHAPTER 78

18-Month-Old Girl With Intermittent Fevers, 2.27-kg Weight Loss, and Mild Respiratory Distress

Presentation

An 18-month-old girl presents with a 6-month history of intermittent fevers, 2.27-kg weight loss, and mild respiratory distress. A chest radiograph demonstrates bibasilar infiltrates. Despite treatment with parenteral antibiotics, the symptoms persist and the radiographic changes worsen. She has had no cough, vomiting, food aversion, change in appetite, contact with tuberculosis, or foreign travel. Born at term, she was previously healthy and developing normally.

The girl's weight is 9.07 kg (<3rd percentile), and her height is 200 cm (10th–25th percentile). Her respiratory rate is 30 breaths/min, and oxygen saturation is 91% on room air; she is afebrile. Mild intercostal retractions are noted, and crackles are heard bilaterally. There is no clubbing, organomegaly, or rash. Her neurologic findings are normal. Her white blood cell count is 15.6×10^3/mcL (15.6×10^9/L), with normal differential, pH is 7.42; bicarbonate concentration is 20 mEq/L (20 mmol/L); carbon dioxide partial pressure is 32 mm Hg; and base excess is −3 mEq/L. Blood cultures are sterile, and a tuberculin test is nonreactive. A sweat test yields normal results. Twenty-four–hour esophageal pH monitoring does not show gastroesophageal reflux disease (GERD). An additional bedside clinical assessment followed by radiologic confirmation reveals the diagnosis.

- **What is your differential diagnosis at this point?**
- **Are there any elements of history or physical examination that would help you?**
- **What additional diagnostic studies would you like performed?**

Discussion

A bedside feeding assessment by an occupational therapist revealed increased congestion and upper airway sounds without cough during feeding. Subsequently, asymptomatic ("silent") aspiration was confirmed during a videofluoroscopic swallow study. Endoscopic evaluation of the upper airway and magnetic resonance imaging of the head yielded normal findings. Treatment was initiated with thickening of feedings, which resulted in weight gain and resolution of the fever, pulmonary signs, and radiographic abnormalities.

The Condition

Silent aspiration describes aspiration without cough or obvious acute distress.[1] Infants and young children with this disorder are at increased risk of developing aspiration-induced chronic lung disease, malnutrition, and neurodevelopmental problems. Pulmonary failure due to chronic aspiration is a leading cause of death in children who have severe neurologic impairment. Silent aspiration is commonly associated with aspiration from below (due to GERD). Investigations such as 24-hour pH monitoring can be helpful in excluding this condition.

Silent aspiration can be due to aspiration from above (related to dysphagia) and is often associated with underlying conditions such as prematurity, global neurologic dysfunction, or anatomic anomalies of the upper aerodigestive tract. These conditions put the child at risk for aspiration by interfering with the complex neuromuscular and airway coordination involved in swallowing. However, several studies have suggested that aspiration can occur from oropharyngeal dysfunction in children who have none of these risk factors. Most affected children develop symptoms in the first postnatal year, and many outgrow the condition by the preschool years.[2] Radiographic aspiration in children who aspirate while in a supine position (infants, neurologically impaired children) frequently affects the upper lobes or perihilar regions, but bilateral basilar findings can occur in children who aspirate while in an upright position.

Diagnosis

Silent aspiration should be considered in infants and children who experience unexplained recurrent chest infections or who have a history of wheezing or congestion after feedings. Aspiration should also be considered in children who have respiratory symptoms and a history suggestive of GERD. Less commonly, silent aspiration can present with recurrent undiagnosed fevers, perioral cyanosis or vocal changes with feedings, failure to thrive despite adequate nutritional intake, feeding aversion, or poor control of secretions.

A comprehensive clinical assessment that involves a history, risk factors, and a bedside feeding evaluation by an experienced occupational therapist or speech-language pathologist has been shown to have 92% sensitivity and an 89% negative predictive value for diagnosing aspiration of fluids in children.[3] This assessment can prevent the need for the radiation exposure and cost of additional radiologic assessment in many children. It should be noted, however, that the accuracy of the evaluation depends on the experience of the specialist; speech pathologists or occupational therapists who are highly trained in this area are not immediately available in all locations.

Videofluoroscopic swallow studies are dynamic radiographic examinations of food passing from mouth to pharynx and are considered the standard study for diagnosing aspiration from above in patients who have a positive screening assessment. Findings from the videofluoroscopic swallow study can also help physicians identify safe feeding strategies if the child only aspirates foods of certain consistencies.

Management

Recommended management depends on the underlying cause of the aspiration. For infants and children who have GERD, optimal medical management is successful in many patients and often includes the use of acid suppression with histamine$_2$ receptor antagonists or proton pump inhibitors. Occasionally, prokinetic agents can be helpful, although the evidence for the effectiveness of many of these drugs is weak. Surgical options such as fundoplication and enterostomy tube insertion are viable alternatives for patients who cannot be treated medically.

If the primary problem is dysphagia, a variety of dietary modifications can be employed. Thickening of liquids is often helpful. Other therapies include changing the feeding position (upright versus reclined), slowing the pace of feedings, and altering the feeding schedule (small and more frequent meals). For patients who do not respond to these therapies, a referral to a multidisciplinary feeding and swallowing program is suggested.

References

1. Ramsey D, Smithard D, Kalra L. Silent aspiration: what do we know? *Dysphagia.* 2005;20(3):218–225
2. Lefton-Greif M, Carroll J, Loughlin G. Long-term follow-up of oropharyngeal dysphagia in children without apparent risk factors. *Pediatr Pulmonol.* 2006;41(11):1040–1048
3. DeMatteo C, Matovich D, Hjartarson A. Comparison of clinical and videofluoroscopic evaluation of children with feeding and swallowing difficulties. *Dev Med Child Neurol.* 2005;47(3):149–157

Lessons for the Physician

Silent aspiration should be considered in infants and children who have pulmonary symptoms of unclear cause, particularly those who have risk factors such as gastroesophageal reflux disease, prematurity, or global neurologic dysfunction. Prompt identification can lead to simple therapies that can reduce the degree of aspiration.

Eyal Cohen, MD, and Oscar M. Navarro, MD, The Hospital for Sick Children, Toronto, Ontario, Canada

CHAPTER 79

2½-Year-Old Girl Who Has Cough and Right Pulmonary Abnormalities

Presentation

A 2½-year-old girl presents to an outside emergency department with a 1-week history of nasal congestion and increasing cough. She is sent home on co-trimoxazole but returns the next day with increasing cough, low-grade fever of 100.9°F (38.3°C), and reduced fluid intake. A chest radiograph is reported to reveal a right lower lobe pneumonia with mucus plugging. The antibiotic is changed to azithromycin, and the girl is discharged. Three days later, her symptoms are much improved. Follow-up chest radiographs, performed over the next 2 weeks, show no improvement.

The girl is referred to a tertiary care center where she appears well, with the only reported symptom being cough with exertion. She is afebrile and has a weight of 11.3 kg (5th percentile) and height of 88 cm (10th percentile). Her vital signs are within reference range, with an oxygen saturation of 96% on room air. Her physical examination is completely unremarkable.

Her white blood cell count is 11.5×10^3/mcL, and her aspartate aminotransferase is slightly elevated at 45 U/L (0.75 mckat/L). Serum electrolytes, erythrocyte sedimentation rate, C-reactive protein, and *Mycoplasma* serology are unremarkable. Her most recent chest radiograph reveals a heterogeneous opacity blunting the right side of the heart border, a blunting of the right costophrenic angle, a midline shift to the right, and an elevated right hemidiaphragm (Figure 79.1). Ultrasonography of her chest does not reveal any pleural effusion. One additional investigation identifies the condition.

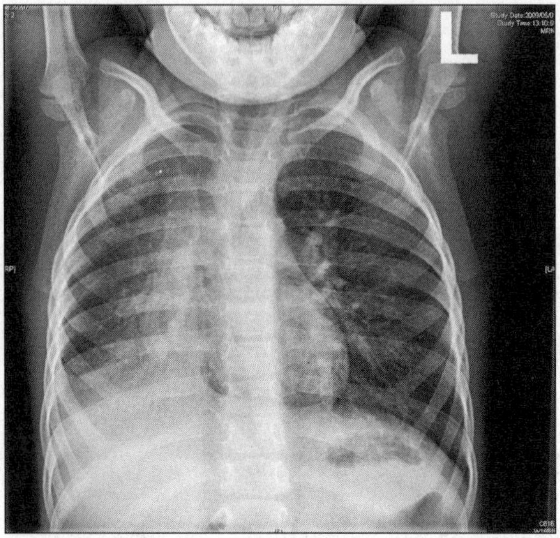

Figure 79.1. Chest radiograph revealing a heterogeneous opacity blunting the right side of the heart border, blunting of the right costophrenic angle, a midline shift to the right, and an elevated right hemidiaphragm.

- **What is your differential diagnosis at this point?**
- **Are there any elements of history or physical examination that would help you?**
- **What additional diagnostic studies would you like performed?**

Discussion

A computed tomography (CT) scan of the chest demonstrated a bilobed right lung, which was hypoplastic and connected with the left lung posterior to the heart, thus forming a horseshoe lung (Figure 79.2). The left lung was unremarkable otherwise.

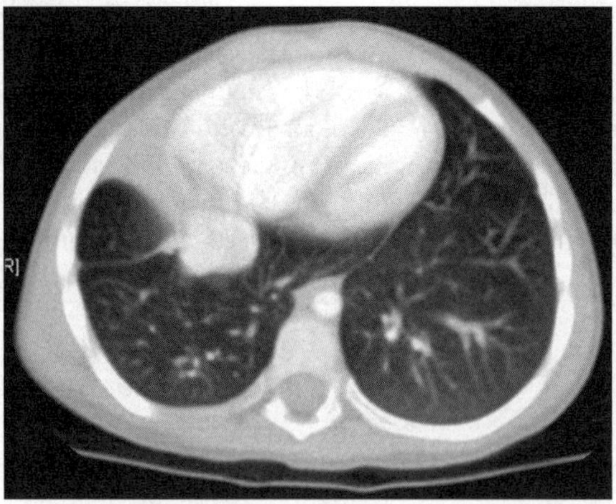

Figure 79.2. Computed tomography scan of the chest revealing a hypoplastic right lung, which is connected with the left lung posterior to the heart, thus forming a horseshoe lung.

The pulmonary arterial supply was normal, with no systemic arterial contribution. Normal pulmonary veins were found on the left, but there was anomalous systemic pulmonary venous return on the right into the suprahepatic inferior vena cava (IVC) (Figure 79.3). This constellation of findings was consistent with Scimitar syndrome.

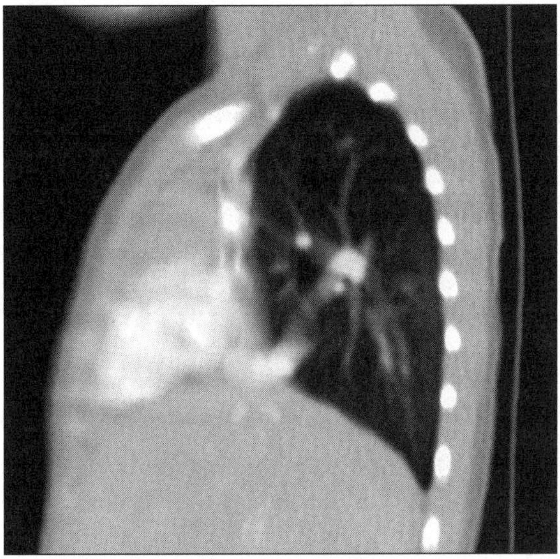

Figure 79.3. Computed tomography scan of the chest reveals an anomalous systemic pulmonary venous return on the right into the suprahepatic inferior vena cava.

The findings on chest radiograph (opacity blunting the right side of the heart border and right costophrenic angle, midline shift to the right, elevated right hemidiaphragm) are likely secondary to the right lung hypoplasia. The vertical radiopacity on the right hemithorax may represent the anomalous veins as they course and coalesce toward the right hemidiaphragm (see Figure 79.1).

Cardiac defects are frequently associated with Scimitar syndrome. Echocardiography demonstrated a moderate ostium secundum-type atrial septal defect, a mildly dilated right ventricle, and the anomalous pulmonary venous return on the right as previously documented on CT. Because of the age of this patient, and because she was symptom-free and had no signs of heart failure, an observational approach to management with regular follow-up was chosen. She will eventually require cardiac catheterization to assess her pulmonary to systemic flow ratio (Qp:Qs) and the corrective surgery.

The Condition

Scimitar syndrome, a variant of partial anomalous pulmonary venous drainage, is a rare congenital disorder, with girls being more frequently affected than boys (1.4–2:1). The hallmark of this condition is a partial anomalous systemic pulmonary venous drainage of a part of or the entire right lung into the IVC-atrial junction, the

IVC, or the right atrium. The anomalous drainage occurs through a single, curved vein, referred to as a "Scimitar vein" because of its crescent shape on frontal chest radiograph, resembling a Turkish scimitar sword, as demonstrated in the chest radiograph of this patient.

Most cases of Scimitar syndrome are associated with a partial or total hypoplastic right lung, which frequently demonstrates lobar anomalies such as a mono- or bilobed- or, more rarely, a horseshoe lung configuration, as in this patient. Other commonly associated conditions include an anomalous systemic arterial supply to the right lung, a hypoplastic right pulmonary artery, dextroposition of the right side of the heart (often obscuring the Scimitar vein on chest radiograph), pulmonary sequestration, and cardiac defects, especially an ostium secundum–type atrial septal defect, but also ventricular septal defect, pulmonary vein stenosis, coarctation of the aorta, and patent ductus arteriosus. Left-sided Scimitar syndrome has also been described, in which some or all of the left pulmonary veins connect to the right side of the IVC.

The clinical presentation of Scimitar syndrome varies with the age at presentation. Infants and young children often have more severe signs related to heart failure and other cardiac or pulmonary conditions. Signs include tachypnea, poor feeding, failure to thrive, cyanosis, and lethargy. One-half of older patients who are diagnosed after 1 year of age remain asymptomatic and are diagnosed when characteristic findings are discovered incidentally on chest radiograph.

Pulmonary hypertension may be present at presentation because of a significant left to right shunt caused by the systemic pulmonary venous drainage and associated cardiac defects. Other factors contributing to the development of pulmonary hypertension may include the presence of a systemic arterial supply to the right lung and a stenosis of the Scimitar vein, which is seen in up to 20% of patients with Scimitar syndrome.

Cardiac catheterization is still regarded by many as the criterion standard for diagnosis. Catheterization allows assessment of the Qp:Qs ratio and simultaneous embolization of an anomalous systemic artery in symptomatic infants. Chest CT or magnetic resonance angiography, however, should also be considered initially because these modalities provide excellent images of the cardiovascular and pulmonary anatomy, are noninvasive, and are usually readily available. Echocardiography is useful to assess cardiac function, associated cardiac defects, and pulmonary hypertension, as well as to confirm the presence of partial anomalous pulmonary venous return.

Management

In general, patients with congestive heart failure, pulmonary hypertension, a Qp:Qs greater than 1.5, and insufficient response to medical treatment warrant a surgical approach to management. However, medical treatment of heart failure should be attempted initially in infants and children without pulmonary hypertension to reduce the higher risks associated with early surgery and to allow time for growth. The surgical repair aims to reroute the blood flow of the anomalous pulmonary vein to the left atrium, to repair associated cardiac defects, and to ligate any anomalous systemic arterial supply to the right lung. Alternatively, especially in the case of associated pulmonary sequestration and recurrent pneumonias, a lobectomy or pneumectomy may be considered. Asymptomatic patients with a minor left to right shunt (Qp:Qs ≤1.5) do not require surgical repair and can be followed conservatively.

Lessons for the Physician

- Scimitar syndrome is a rare form of partial anomalous pulmonary venous return associated in most cases with right lung hypoplasia of varying degrees, lobation anomalies, and cardiac defects, particularly ostium secundum–type atrial septal defect.
- Scimitar syndrome should be considered in patients presenting with signs of heart failure or pulmonary hypertension, as well as in patients who experience recurrent right-sided pneumonias.
- Asymptomatic patients with a small left to right shunt can be followed conservatively. Symptomatic patients and those with a major left to right shunt require surgical intervention.

Dirk E. Bock, MD; April Price, BSc, MD; and Dhenuka K. Radhakrishnan, BSc, MD, Department of Pediatrics, Children's Hospital, London Health Sciences Centre, University of Western Ontario, London Ontario, Canada

Dimas Mateos-Corral, MD, Department of Pediatrics, IWK Health Centre, Dalhousie University, Halifax, Nova Scotia, Canada

CHAPTER 80

Shortness of Breath and Wheezing in a 9-Year-Old Chinese Girl

Presentation

A 9-year-old Chinese girl who has mild intermittent asthma, allergic rhinitis, and sinusitis is evaluated for 2 days of shortness of breath and wheezing following a viral upper respiratory tract infection. Three months ago, she was hospitalized for 3 weeks in China for status asthmaticus; 1 month ago, she was hospitalized again for status asthmaticus.

Physical examination reveals an afebrile, well-nourished child in severe respiratory distress. Auscultation reveals diffuse wheezing and poor air entry. Multiple palpable, painful, purpuric lesions are noted on her shins and feet. Her condition worsens, and she requires intubation and mechanical ventilation. She is placed on albuterol, budesonide, montelukast, azithromycin, and cefotaxime.

Laboratory studies reveal white blood cell count, 25×10^3/mcL (25×10^9/L), with 42% neutrophils, 1% bands, 8% lymphocytes, 45% eosinophils, and 5% monocytes; hemoglobin, 13.5 g/dL (135 g/L); platelet count, 281×10^3/mcL (281×10^9/L); and normal concentrations of immunoglobulins. Antinuclear antibody, circulating antineutrophil cytoplasmic antibody (ANCA), and perinuclear ANCA values are normal. Results of testing for *Coccidioides immitis, Cryptosporidium parvum, Mycoplasma pneumoniae,* and *Legionella pneumophila* are negative. A tuberculin test is nonreactive.

Chest radiography shows bilateral pulmonary interstitial infiltrates and bilateral hilar adenopathy. Chest computed tomography (CT) scan reveals patchy confluent air space disease and nodular densities in the periphery of the lungs. Sinus (CT) scan shows mild bilateral ethmoid and sphenoid sinus disease. Bronchoalveolar lavage reveals eosinophils in the pulmonary parenchyma. This finding, together with the nodular densities noted on CT scan and the peripheral eosinophilia, leads to the diagnosis.

- **What is your differential diagnosis at this point?**
- **Are there any elements of history or physical examination that would help you?**
- **What additional diagnostic studies would you like performed?**

Discussion

Poorly controlled asthma with severe status asthmaticus would have been the most likely diagnosis at presentation for this patient. However, the chronic and severe nature of this child's illness, along with eosinophilia, palpable purpura, and focal imaging findings, necessitated a search for alternate diagnoses.

Differential Diagnosis

Although asthma is typically associated with eosinophilia, the eosinophil count is usually no greater than 10% of the total white blood cell count. Helminthic infections can cause pulmonary eosinophilia. The patient's recent travel history raised suspicion for *Ascaris lumbricoides,* hookworms, and *Strongyloides stercoralis,* organisms endemic to China. Symptomatic patients have coughing, dyspnea, wheezing, weight loss, and fever. Laboratory evidence did not support such infestations.

Some medications and industrial toxins can induce pulmonary eosinophilia and hypersensitivity pneumonitis. The most common medications are nonsteroidal anti-inflammatory drugs, antimicrobials such as minocycline and nitrofurantoin, β-blockers, angiotensin-converting enzyme inhibitors, methotrexate, bleomycin, and phenytoin. Inhalation of toxins such as aluminum metals, sulfite, heroin, and cocaine are also associated with pulmonary eosinophilia. No toxin or drug exposure was elicited in this patient.

Allergic bronchopulmonary aspergillosis is an allergic response to *Aspergillus* that causes respiratory distress, wheezing, and pulmonary eosinophilic infiltrates. The normal concentrations of the patient's total IgE and specific IgE against *Aspergillus* argued against allergic bronchopulmonary aspergillosis. Other causes of pulmonary eosinophilia include tumors rare in the pediatric population, such as adenocarcinoma of the stomach and squamous carcinoma of the vagina, penis, or skin, as well as acute and chronic eosinophilic pneumonia (CEP). Acute chronic eosinophilic pneumonia and CEP present as febrile illnesses with nonproductive coughing and dyspnea. Histopathologic findings in CEP, which was more likely in this patient, given the chronicity of her presentation, include interstitial and alveolar eosinophils and histiocytes and multinucleated giant cells. The bronchoalveolar lavage result was not diagnostic of CEP.

Palpable purpura is a classic example of a vasculitic skin lesion. Churg-Strauss syndrome (CSS) is the only vasculitis that is associated with both peripheral and pulmonary eosinophilia. Churg-Strauss syndrome is a constellation of sinusitis, asthma, and peripheral and pulmonary eosinophilia. Given the clinical history, physical findings, and laboratory results, a clinical diagnosis of CSS was made, and the patient was started on high-dose methylprednisolone. She improved promptly and was extubated. Her pulmonary function stabilized during the next several months with high-dose prednisone therapy, but she currently has many steroid-induced complications.

The Causative Condition

Churg-Strauss syndrome is a small-vessel vasculitis involving multiple organs, especially the lungs, heart, peripheral nervous system, skin, and gastrointestinal tract. The syndrome is characterized by a history of asthma, eosinophilia of more than 10%, neuropathy, pulmonary infiltrates, paranasal sinus syndrome, and extravascular eosinophilic infiltration findings on biopsy.

Churg-Strauss syndrome affects 2 to 7 per 1 million people and is diagnosed most commonly in those between 14 and 75 years of age, although it has been identified in children as young as 4 years of age. Although CSS is rare, its symptoms mimic common pediatric complaints such as asthma and sinusitis.

It has been postulated that CSS occurs in association with the use of leukotriene receptor antagonists (LTA) such as montelukast. The United States Food and Drug Administration reported development of CSS after the use of LTAs in a subset of patients.[1] Churg-Strauss syndrome developed 2 days to 10 months after treatment was initiated. Although the temporal relationship suggests an association, the symptoms of CSS occurred shortly after corticosteroids were tapered in all of the patients. Also, the incidence of CSS in patients receiving LTAs is similar to that of CSS in patients who have asthma and are not receiving LTAs. More likely, CSS was a preexisting condition that appeared after the withdrawal of steroids rather than a disorder caused by a direct effect of LTAs.

Asthma usually arises early in the course of the disease and worsens over time. Asthma and sinus disease precede the onset of pulmonary eosinophilia and vasculitis by years. As the disease progresses, pulmonary infiltrates are seen in most cases. Histologic changes are described as eosinophilic pneumonia, necrotizing vasculitis, and granulomatous inflammation, sometimes occurring in this order.

Most patients with CSS have mononeuritis multiplex or polyneuropathy. Central nervous system involvement is less common and can include cranial nerve palsy, ischemic optic neuritis, cerebral infarction or hemorrhage, seizures, and psychosis. Vasculitis and eosinophilia may also affect the gastrointestinal tract, causing abdominal pain, diarrhea, and hemorrhage. Eosinophils may infiltrate various cardiac layers directly, causing cardiac dysfunction, the leading cause of mortality. Skin lesions are vasculitic and are described as palpable purpura, erythematous macules, and nodules on the trunk and upper and lower extremities. Churg-Strauss syndrome affects the kidneys less commonly.

Making the Diagnosis

Diagnosing CSS is challenging. The association of asthma, rhinitis, or sinusitis along with eosinophilia and vasculitic symptoms suggests CSS. A tissue biopsy revealing vasculitis and eosinophilia confirms the diagnosis. Churg-Strauss syndrome initially may have the histologic appearance of CEP. Laboratory tests are generally not helpful. Peripheral eosinophilia is commonly greater than 10% of all white blood cells but may decline rapidly as the disease course improves or if the patient is treated with steroids for other reasons. Antineutrophil cytoplasmic antibody, especially perinuclear ANCA, is positive in 60% to 70% of patients who have CSS. Chest radiography usually reveals bilateral patchy alveolar infiltrates. A chest CT scan demonstrates interstitial and bronchial wall thickening, diffuse patchy opacities in the parenchyma, or pulmonary nodules. The imaging studies are helpful but nondiagnostic.

Treatment and Prognosis

Most patients who have CSS show a reduction in vasculitic symptoms with corticosteroid therapy alone. In some, additional treatment with cyclophosphamide is needed to achieve remission. Several successful case reports of plasma exchanges, interferon-α, or intravenous immunoglobulin suggest options for patients who are refractory to corticosteroid or cyclophosphamide treatment. The prognosis is fairly good, with 80% to 90% of patients achieving remission, although 26% to 28% of those relapse. The mortality from organ failure is only 3%.

Reference

1. Tuggey JM, Hosker HSR. Churg-Strauss syndrome associated with montelukast therapy. *Thorax.* 2000;25(9):805–806

Lessons for the Physician

The differential diagnosis of pulmonary eosinophilia is extensive, including drug- and toxin-induced eosinophilic lung disease, helminthic infection, allergic bronchopulmonary aspergillosis, sarcoidosis, hypereosinophilic syndrome, acute or chronic eosinophilic pneumonia, hypersensitivity pneumonitis, and Churg-Strauss syndrome (CSS). Churg-Strauss syndrome is often diagnosed clinically because there are no definitive laboratory tests or imaging findings. Physicians must have a high degree of suspicion, especially when the presentations are lengthy and mimic other common diseases. In CSS, asthma and sinusitis occur years prior to the onset of vasculitic symptoms. Most patients who have CSS are responsive to corticosteroid therapy or cyclophosphamide.

Belinda Chan, MD, and Ara Festekjian, MD, Children's Hospital of Los Angeles, Los Angeles, CA

CHAPTER 81

Wet, Mucous Cough for Years in a 12-Year-Old Girl

Presentation

A 12-year-old girl is referred to you because of a "wet, mucous cough for years." She never wheezes and has used salbutamol intermittently without relief. She was treated as a neonate for pneumonia and has had recurrent sinusitis and middle ear effusions; ventilating tubes have been inserted twice. She has never had allergic symptoms, and there are no smokers or pets at home. Her brother has a history of recurrent upper respiratory tract infections, otitis media, sinusitis, and mild asthma.

Physical examination reveals a thin, prepubertal girl who is not acutely ill. Her growth has consistently followed the 25th percentile for height and 10th percentile for weight. She is afebrile and has a respiratory rate of 20 breaths/min. Bilateral middle ear effusions are noted. No wheezes are audible, but crackles are heard in the right middle lobe (RML). Her cardiovascular findings are normal, with the apical beat on the left side. Her liver and spleen are not enlarged. There is no digital clubbing.

Chest radiography reveals normal lung volumes, no calcifications, and alveolar opacification in the RML consistent with pneumonia. Pulmonary function test results, sweat chloride level, findings on immunologic evaluation, IgE levels, and eosinophil count all are normal. A tuberculin test is negative.

Two courses of antibiotics fail to bring improvement. Computed tomography of the chest reveals bronchiectasis in the RML with volume loss as well as mild central bronchiectasis of the lower lobes. A nasal biopsy reveals the diagnosis.

- **What is your differential diagnosis at this point?**
- **Are there any elements of history or physical examination that would help you?**
- **What additional diagnostic studies would you like performed?**

Discussion

Differential Diagnosis

Chronic or recurrent cough in children has multiple causes, including viral infections, pertussis syndrome, chronic sinusitis, and tuberculosis. Often children who have recurrent or persistent cough have asthma. Cystic fibrosis should be considered and ruled out. In younger children, foreign body aspiration or congenital anatomic abnormalities (eg, vascular rings, tracheoesophageal fistulas) must be considered. Recurrent bacterial pneumonias suggest an immunologic disorder. Sometimes school-aged or adolescent patients develop a habitual cough (psychological basis).

Ultrastructural examination of the nasal biopsy of this patient showed abnormalities of the cilia with absence of the inner dynein arms (Figure 81.1). Thus, the disorder in this girl was not asthma but primary ciliary dyskinesia (PCD), formerly called immotile cilia syndrome.

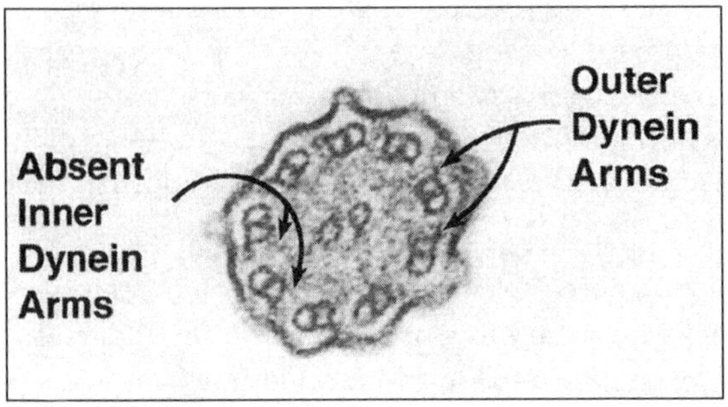

Figure 81.1. Ultrastructural examination of the nasal biopsy shows abnormalities of the cilia with absence of the inner dynein arms.

The Condition

Siewert first described PCD in 1904, but it was closely associated with the Austrian family physician Kartagener, who noted that an unusually large number of his patients had bronchiectasis, recurrent sinusitis, and situs inversus. We now know that only 50% of individuals who have PCD have situs inversus.

Primary ciliary dyskinesia is a relatively uncommon but underdiagnosed cause of chronic cough. The incidence is 1:20,000, with equal distribution in males and females. The incidence of situs inversus in the general population is 1:10,000. In one report from the United Kingdom, there were 130 to 150 cases known to support groups, whereas the population incidence would suggest the existence of about 3,000 cases. At the Montreal Children's Hospital, approximately 30 patients who have PCD are followed, but the population incidence suggests that a much larger number of people actually have the disorder.

Pathophysiology

Figure 81.2 demonstrates schematically the normal ultrastructure of cilia in cross-section. There are 9 microtubule couplets on the periphery and 2 central microtubule couplets. The peripheral couplets have both inner and outer dynein arms, which are essential for normal movement of the cilia. In addition, the peripheral couplets are connected to the center by radial spokes as well as to each other by another protein link, nexin. Functionally, the outer dynein arms affect beat frequency, and the inner ones affect the waveform.

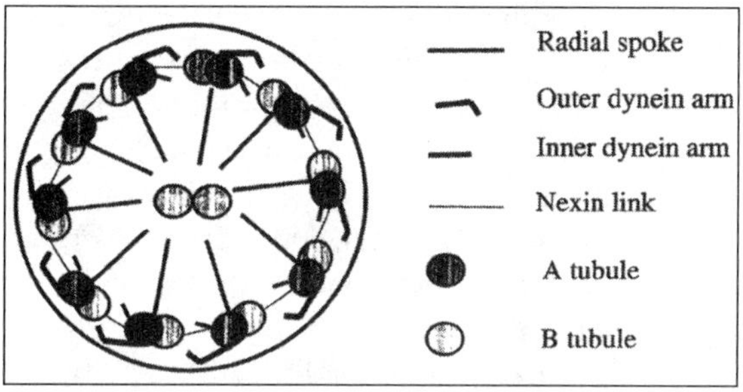

Figure 81.2. Diagram of the ultrastructural components of a cilium, as seen in cross-section.

Cilia line the respiratory tract (including sinuses and middle ear), ependyma of the brain, efferent ductules of the testis, and oviducts. Normal cilia beat metachromatically at 12 Hz, moving the mucus layer toward the oropharynx. Mucus is a complex mixture that forms a viscoelastic layer and traps small particles and bacteria, preventing bacterial colonization. Failure of this defense mechanism results in recurrent otitis media, sinopulmonary infections, and bronchiectasis. Because of abnormal cilia in the efferent ductules and abnormal flagelli in spermatozoa, males who have PCD have impaired fertility.

What is the relationship between abnormal cilia and situs inversus? One hypothesis suggests that the beating of primitive cilia in the embryo plays an important role in the left-right orientation of structures. Abnormal cilia beat randomly and would account for a random left-right orientation, explaining the observation that only about 50% of individuals who have PCD have situs inversus. In one mouse model, an abnormal dynein heavy-chain protein was associated with defects of laterality.

Abnormalities of ciliary ultrastructure can be primary or secondary. Smoking and pollutants can lead to secondary abnormalities. Cilia in patients who have PCD beat at a frequency of 7 to 9 Hz (reference range, 12 Hz) and have abnormal waveforms, resulting in abnormal movement of the mucus defense layer. One study evaluated normal and abnormal cilia quantitatively in normal healthy subjects, atopic nonsmokers, nonatopic nonsmokers, asymptomatic smokers, patients who had cystic fibrosis, people having allergic rhinitis, and patients who had PCD. In all control groups, 4% of cilia were abnormal either ultrastructurally or functionally. In the PCD group, the range was 78% to 95%, with most defects occurring in the dynein arms.

Making the Diagnosis

Diagnosing PCD requires an alert physician. The condition should be suspected if there is unexplained neonatal tachypnea, pneumonia, or recurrent atelectasis without cause in a term neonate who has no risk for congenital infections or in a neonate who has dextrocardia or a family history of PCD. In an infant or older child, recurrent sinusitis, chronic secretory otitis media, persistent ear discharge through ventilating tubes, recurrent pneumonia, or bronchiectasis should raise the possibility of this diagnosis. In adults, a significant number of cases are found in infertility clinics.

If PCD is suspected, the first set of investigations should include a chest radiograph, Computed tomography scans of chest and sinus, a diagnostic test for cystic fibrosis (sweat chloride or cystic fibrosis genotyping), and measurement of immunoglobulins. An alpha$_1$-antitrypsin level might be indicated. When other causes of chronic cough are eliminated, more specific investigations include mucociliary clearance tests, biopsy (nasal mucosal brushings or bronchial brushings), and ultrastructural studies as well as functional assessment of ciliary wave and frequency (some centers can assess ciliary beating from strips of epithelium obtained from mucosal brushings). Theoretically, the measurement of nitrous oxide in exhaled breath might be useful diagnostically. It is markedly lower in PCD but elevated in cystic fibrosis, asthma, and bronchiectasis. The anatomically abnormal cilia characteristic of PCD may have abnormal nitric oxide synthetase as well, accounting for this finding.

Management

The management of PCD is similar to that of cystic fibrosis, requiring a multidisciplinary team of pediatrician, respiratory physician, nurse, and physiotherapist. Increased cough with fever is an indication for antibiotic therapy, which should be maintained for prolonged periods when lung function deteriorates. Bronchodilators are helpful if reversibility is demonstrated with pulmonary function tests. Exercise aids in clearing mucus. Ventilating tubes in tympanic membranes are not indicated and may lead to chronic ear drainage with no improvement in hearing outcome; hearing aids should be used if hearing is a problem during critical phases of language acquisition. Chronic serous otitis tends to improve somewhat with age.

Fertility assistance may be required during the reproductive years in males who have PCD. Respiratory functioning, hearing, and fertility require monitoring. Patients should be followed with regular pulmonary function tests, pulse oximetry, and chest imaging. Sputum cultures for *Staphylococcus aureus, Serratia,* and *Pseudomonas* colonization should be performed periodically. Hearing assessments should be obtained. In young children, inhalation of a saline solution induces sputum production. Sinus drainage may be necessary in some cases.

Lessons for the Physician

Cough is a common presenting symptom in children. Primary ciliary dyskinesia is an uncommon cause of chronic cough in children but should be considered, especially if associated characteristics are present. Not all children referred for persistent cough with a diagnosis of asthma have asthma.

L. Richard Haber, MD, McGill University, Montreal, Quebec, Canada

COMMENTARY BY LOKESH GUGLANI, MD, PEDIATRIC PULMONOLOGIST, DEPARTMENT OF PEDIATRICS AT EMORY UNIVERSITY SCHOOL OF MEDICINE

Several advances have been made in the diagnosis of primary ciliary dyskinesia (PCD). Nasal nitric oxide measurement has now become an accepted screening method and its levels are extremely low (in single digits) in patients with PCD. In patients with cystic fibrosis, the levels are lower than normal controls, but not as low as they are in PCD. Other screening tests that can be utilized for screening patients include qualitative tests of ciliary motion (such as saccharin test), high-speed video microscopy analysis, and immunofluorescence labeling of ciliary proteins followed by pulmonary radioaerosol mucociliary clearance study.

The number of gene mutations that are being identified in PCD patients has been rapidly increasing over the years. So far, at least 30 mutations have been reported and 85% of these are loss-of-function variants, while 15% are conservative missense mutations. The most prevalent mutations are *DNAH5* (15%–21%), *DNAI1* (2%–9%), *DNAAF1* (*LRRC50*) (4%–5%), *CCDC39* (2%–10%), *CCDC40* (2%–8%), *DNAH11* (6%) and *LRRC6* (3%). It is important to note that ciliary ultrastructural evaluation with transmission electron microscopy can be normal in up to 30% of patients, and the diagnosis in these patients may rest on genetic testing.

In addition to defects in ciliary ultrastructure, a new subgroup that has been recently identified includes mutations that are responsible for reduced number of cilia per cell. Normal respiratory epithelial cells have at least 200 cilia per cell. Many of these patients may have symptoms that are similar to classic PCD, and the mutations reported so far include cyclin O (*CCNO*) and the gene for multiciliate differentiation and DNA synthesis-associated cell cycle protein (*MCIDAS*).

Despite increased recognition of mutations associated with PCD, there is poor correlation between the genotypes and their associated clinical phenotypes. A better understanding of proteins that are involved in various stages of ciliary assembly, structure and function, and their regulation by different genes will provide more insights into this complex, heterogeneous disorder.

CHAPTER 82

Chest Pain and Shortness of Breath in a 15-Year-Old Boy

Presentation

A 15-year-old boy who has well-controlled, mild, intermittent asthma presents to the emergency department with a 5-hour history of chest pain and shortness of breath. He denies fever, wheezing, vomiting, cough, rhinorrhea, or recent trauma. A recent ankle injury has precluded excessive physical exertion, but he has been well otherwise. He denies the use of illicit drugs.

Physical examination reveals a well-developed Caucasian boy in no distress. His temperature is 98.6°F (37°C), heart rate is 72 beats/min, and respiratory rate is 18 breaths/min. The room air oxygen saturation is 98%. His lungs are clear, breath sounds are symmetric, and all other findings are normal.

Chest radiograph shows a pneumomediastinum without associated pneumothorax; computed tomography of the chest confirms the pneumomediastinum but yields no other findings. The patient is admitted to the observation unit for supplemental oxygen and pain control.

An additional piece of history leads to a procedure that reveals the source of the problem.

- **What is your differential diagnosis at this point?**
- **Are there any elements of history or physical examination that would help you?**
- **What additional diagnostic studies would you like performed?**

Discussion

Soon after admission, the patient began to complain of pain with swallowing. Additional questioning revealed that he had been eating mussels immediately prior to the onset of his symptoms and that the pain had begun suddenly during the meal.

He denied vomiting following eating, but he did consume a significant number of mussels in a short time. Because of this additional information, esophagography was obtained. Extravasation of contrast at the lower cervical junction indicated esophageal rupture.

The patient was managed nonsurgically with broad-spectrum antibiotics and nothing by mouth. On hospital day 4, he was free of all symptoms. Repeat esophagography revealed no abnormality. He was discharged from the hospital on a liquid diet and oral antibiotics. At follow-up 2 months later, he was completely well.

The Condition

Pneumomediastinum is defined as the escape of air into the mediastinal tissues. Pneumomediastinum occurs primarily in older children and adolescents and more often in boys than in girls. The most common cause is alveolar rupture, which allows air to travel along tissue planes into the mediastinum. Spontaneous pneumomediastinum (SPM) refers to cases that are not related to trauma or medical procedures. Most pediatric cases of SPM are due to asthma and respiratory infections, although some occur following the Valsalva maneuver or forceful vomiting. Pneumomediastinum due to inhalation drug use has been reported in recent years.

Patients who experience pneumomediastinum present most commonly with chest pain, shortness of breath, and subcutaneous emphysema. The presence of crepitations over the precordium is known as Hamman sign and is strongly suggestive of the diagnosis. The crepitus is heard best during systole and may obscure the heart sounds. Diagnosis is made with chest radiography in 98% of cases. Lateral views are associated with higher yields. Chest computed tomography scans yield the diagnosis when the radiograph appears normal.

Complications of pneumomediastinum are rare, including pneumopericardium and pneumothorax, and generally resolve without any intervention. Severe respiratory distress, stridor, and tamponade almost never occur. When these more serious complications do occur, they are usually seen in patients who are receiving mechanical ventilation or in those who have severe underlying disease.

Treatment is supportive and includes bed rest, analgesics, and avoidance of the Valsalva maneuver. The patient may be treated on an outpatient basis if the underlying cause is identified and controlled. Follow-up is recommended within 24 to 48 hours. Oxygen therapy is often instituted in hospitalized patients in an effort to speed reabsorption of the pneumomediastinum, although no conclusive evidence indicates that oxygen is beneficial. Repeat radiographs are not necessary unless the patient deteriorates clinically.

When managing pneumomediastinum, the primary condition to consider other than SPM is esophageal perforation. In cases in which an underlying cause for a pneumomediastinum is not identified or in which the history is suggestive, additional evaluation may be warranted to rule out esophageal perforation.

The Underlying Cause

Esophageal perforation is a rare but serious cause of pneumomediastinum in the pediatric population. Perforation results most often from foreign body ingestion, trauma, or a medical procedure. Rarely, it may occur after forceful vomiting associated with either binge drinking or eating, known as Boerhaave syndrome. Described first in 1724 by Hermann Boerhaave, the esophageal perforation in this syndrome results from increased intra-abdominal pressure transmitted to the esophagus against the closed glottis. Complications of an esophageal perforation include mediastinitis, emphysema, and pneumothorax. Mediastinitis can be fatal.

Signs and symptoms of esophageal perforation can include chest pain, abdominal pain, subcutaneous emphysema, neck pain, dyspnea, and sore throat. Patients in whom diagnosis and treatment are delayed may exhibit respiratory distress or signs of shock.

Radiologic evaluation generally begins with plain radiographs of the chest and soft tissue of the neck, followed by esophagography. Plain radiographs often appear normal, but suggestive findings include subcutaneous emphysema, pneumomediastinum, and mediastinal widening. Although esophagography with barium-containing contrast has the highest sensitivity for identifying an esophageal perforation, extravasation of barium into the mediastinum may lead to a fibrosing mediastinitis. Some experts, therefore, recommend beginning with esophagography that employs water-soluble contrast. If that study is not diagnostic, barium-containing contrast is used.

Treatment of esophageal perforation generally requires coordination with a surgical team, although most children and adolescents do not require operative intervention. Medical management usually consists of the cessation of oral intake, broad-spectrum antibiotics, and parenteral nutrition.

Lessons for the Physician

Esophageal perforation is a rare but serious condition that may present initially with pneumomediastinum. A thorough history must be obtained, focusing particularly on the circumstances surrounding the onset of symptoms. In cases in which no underlying cause of pneumomediastinum can be identified, esophagography may be warranted.

Brian Kit, MD, and Betina Franceschini, MD, Children's National Medical Center, Washington, DC, and Anne Arundel Medical Center, Annapolis, MD

CHAPTER 83

Hemoptysis of 1½ Years Duration in a 15-Year-Old Girl

Presentation

A 15-year-old girl presents with a 1½-year history of intermittent hemoptysis. The hemoptysis was initially infrequent and was associated with cough and upper respiratory tract symptoms. Over time, the hemoptysis has started to occur in 3-day episodes every 2 weeks with no associated symptoms. She has normal menses and denies epistaxis, black or tarry stools, and easy bleeding. She denies chronic cough, changes in stool patterns, fevers, night sweats, and weight loss.

Her past medical history is notable only for gastroesophageal reflux disease diagnosed at age 10 years, which was treated with ranitidine and has since resolved. She is not on medications currently. Her family history is notable for an uncle with ulcerative colitis and an aunt with hypothyroidism. She is an avid field hockey player but has had no history of traumatic injuries.

On examination, she is near the 50th percentile for height, weight, and body mass index. Her vital signs are appropriate for age. She is well appearing with completely normal physical examination findings. Stool guaiac is negative.

Her complete blood cell count shows microcytic anemia. Coagulation studies are normal. A tuberculin test has no induration at 48 hours. Sweat chloride test, anti-neutrophil cytoplasmic antibody, and anti-glomerular basement membrane antibody tests are negative.

A chest radiograph is unremarkable. There are no obvious nasopharyngeal lesions on direct laryngoscopy, and an echocardiogram is unremarkable. Computed tomography of the chest with angiography demonstrates ground-glass opacities suggestive of hemosiderosis or hemorrhage (Figure 83.1). Bronchoscopy confirms hemosiderosis (Figure 83.2), evidence of an old hemorrhage. Additional evaluation leads to diagnosis.

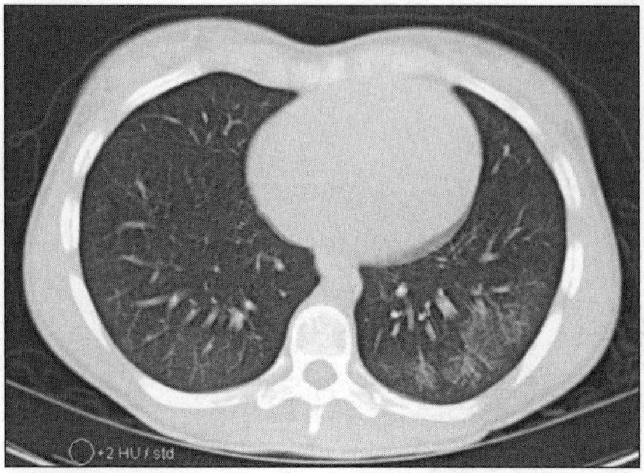

Figure 83.1. Chest computed tomography with angiography demonstrates ground-glass opacities, suggestive of hemosiderosis versus hemorrhage.

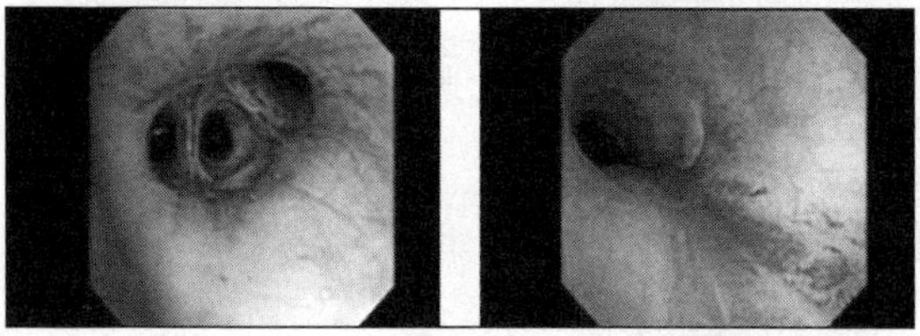

Figure 83.2. Bronchoscopy images from left lower lobe and bronchus intermedius (left to right) confirm hemosiderosis, evidence of old hemorrhage.

- **What is your differential diagnosis at this point?**
- **Are there any elements of history or physical examination that would help you?**
- **What additional diagnostic studies would you like performed?**

Discussion

The additional blood test showed elevated tissue transglutaminase IgA antibodies, suggestive of celiac disease. A duodenal biopsy was performed and showed abundant intraepithelial lymphocytes, villous blunting, and crypt hyperplasia, confirming the diagnosis. The girl's pulmonary hemosiderosis was thus consistent with Lane-Hamilton syndrome (LHS), a rare extraintestinal manifestation of celiac disease.

Differential Diagnosis

The differential diagnosis for hemoptysis is extensive, ranging from relatively common to quite rare conditions. Possible etiologies include infection, bronchiectasis, nonpulmonary bleeding, trauma, coagulopathy, cardiac disease, pulmonary tumor, vascular anomaly, autoimmune disease, and pulmonary-renal syndromes. The chronicity of this patient's symptoms, her age, and the lack of associated extrapulmonary symptoms narrowed the differential diagnosis. Her extensive workup did not support any of the above etiologies, resulting in a working diagnosis of idiopathic pulmonary hemosiderosis (IPH).

Idiopathic pulmonary hemosiderosis is a rare condition seen most commonly in children and adolescents and is characterized by recurrent hemoptysis of unknown etiology, iron deficiency anemia, and pulmonary infiltrates on imaging. The diagnosis is usually made by bronchoscopy and bronchoalveolar lavage after ruling out more common etiologies of hemoptysis. Idiopathic pulmonary hemosiderosis has been associated with celiac disease in rare cases, leading to this patient being screened for celiac disease by measuring serum transglutaminase IgA antibodies.

The Condition

Lane-Hamilton syndrome is a rare condition, defined as the association of celiac disease and IPH. First described in 1971, LHS has since been reported in approximately 35 cases in the literature. Twenty-two of these patients were children younger than 18 years. Interestingly, only half of them presented with gastrointestinal symptoms in addition to recurrent hemoptysis.

Over the last 2 decades, celiac disease is increasingly diagnosed among patients with a wide spectrum of gastrointestinal and extraintestinal manifestations. With the availability of highly sensitive and specific serologic testing, the incidence of celiac disease has increased to 1 in 120 to 300 persons in Europe and North America. Celiac disease results from an inappropriate T-cell mediated immune response against ingested gluten in genetically predisposed persons expressing antibodies against an autoantigen, tissue transglutaminase.

Idiopathic pulmonary hemosiderosis and celiac disease are both hypothesized to be immunologically mediated, but the common link between the 2 entities is not clearly understood. Several hypotheses regarding the pathogenic basis of LHS exist. Although the gut is the main route of exposure to food allergens, other sites of contact may exist. It has been proposed that in the case of gastroesophageal reflux, microinhalation may expose the lung mucosa to gluten, thus precipitating this disorder in genetically susceptible individuals. Another theory suggests that immune complexes against food allergens are deposited on the basal membrane of alveolar capillary cells. An alternative explanation implicates the cross-reactivity of antireticular antibodies with antigens on the basal membrane of alveoli. Finally, a specific strain of adenovirus has been proposed as another pathogenic mechanism.

While it is commonly suggested that LHS represents the overlap of 2 separate disease processes, IPH and celiac disease, others have suggested that LHS should be considered as a single disease entity.

Treatment and Prognosis

The patient described was started on a gluten-free diet and her hemoptysis resolved. She had recurrence of hemoptysis when she was unintentionally reexposed to gluten, but once again achieved symptomatic control when her gluten-free diet was resumed.

In LHS cases reported in the literature, pulmonary symptoms responded to a gluten-free diet in 14 out of 22 (63.6%) children. A gluten-free diet appears to control both gastrointestinal and respiratory symptoms in patients with LHS. For those who do not respond to a gluten-free diet, immunosuppressive therapy may be necessary. The typical first-line immunosuppressive treatment for IPH is systemic steroids. Additional treatment options include hydroxychloroquine, cytotoxic agents, or a combination of one of these medications with systemic steroids.

Lane-Hamilton syndrome results in significant morbidity and mortality. Recurrent alveolar hemorrhage may result in progressive pulmonary fibrosis if left untreated. The possibility of a favorable outcome with gluten-free diet alone, as illustrated in this case, highlights the importance of early recognition of LHS.

Lessons for the Physician

- Patients with idiopathic pulmonary hemosiderosis should be screened for celiac disease, even in the absence of gastrointestinal symptoms.
- Early recognition of Lane-Hamilton syndrome and initiation of treatment with a gluten-free diet may result in disease remission and may prevent progressive pulmonary disease.

Margot R. Nagan, MD; Marissa Hauptman, MD, MPH; and Scott E. Hadland, MD, MPH, Boston University School of Medicine, Department of Pediatrics, MA; Boston Children's Hospital, Department of Medicine, MA; and Harvard Medical School, Department of Pediatrics, Boston, MA

Amit Grover, MBBCh BAO, Boston Children's Hospital, Department of Medicine, MA, and Harvard Medical School, Department of Pediatrics, Boston, MA

Part 14

Obstetrics and Gynecology

CHAPTER 84

Newborn Girl With a Mass Protruding From Her Introitus

Presentation

A neonatal girl has a mass protruding from her introitus. She was born at an estimated gestational age of 39 weeks to a mother who is 26 years of age and gravida 6 (term 2, preterm 1, abortion 2) and had received prenatal care. The mother's blood type is O+, she is rubella immune and hepatitis B surface antigen negative, and she has had a negative serologic test for syphilis. Prenatal screening showed a decreased alpha fetoprotein value. The neonate was delivered vaginally and had Apgar scores of 9 at both 1 and 5 minutes.

On genitourinary examination, the neonate has normal labia majora and minora. A cauliflowerlike tissue mass measuring 1.5 × 2 cm appears to arise from the anterior wall of the vagina and protrudes when the neonate cries. No other malformations are noted. A catheter can be inserted into the urethra without any difficulty or evidence of obstruction, and the neonate urinates normally. Abdominal ultrasonography yields normal findings.

- **What is your differential diagnosis at this point?**
- **Are there any elements of history or physical examination that would help you?**
- **What additional diagnostic studies would you like performed?**

Discussion

Interlabial masses in a neonate or young girl cause concern for parents and physicians. Evaluation of the relationship of the urethral opening to the mass and the quality of the mass are keys to proper diagnosis.

Mucocolpos is the accumulation of fluid due to congenital vaginal obstruction and distention of the vagina. The most common cause of obstruction is an imperforate hymen. Less commonly, a transverse vaginal septum can cause obstruction but is less likely to be apparent in the neonate. Mucocolpos appears as a bulging, thin membrane at the introitus. The mass appears pearly gray because of the transparency of the hymen. The urethral meatus is cephalad to the mass, and an infant feeding tube or saline-moistened calcium alginate swab cannot be passed into the vagina. Treatment consists of an elliptical incision in the membrane and tacking back of the edges to prevent refusion of the hymen.

Urethral prolapse occurs most commonly in 5- to 8-year-old prepubertal girls (youngest reported patient, 5 days of age) and usually involves circumferential eversion of a portion of the distal urethral mucosa through the external meatus. The mass is smooth, bright red, or cyanotic and completely encircles the urethral meatus. The mucosa of the prolapsed urethra is friable, resulting in vaginal bleeding or hematuria. The vaginal opening is posterior to the mass. The prolapse usually resolves with symptomatic treatment, including sitz baths and application of topical estrogen cream. Tissue necrosis is rare and may require excision of the necrotic prolapsed urethral mucosa. For unclear reasons, urethral prolapse is more common in African American girls.

Prolapsed ectopic ureterocele is a congenital anomaly and appears as a smooth cystic dilation of the terminal ureter that sometimes obscures the urethral meatus and is round and red or purplish. Most ureteroceles remain fixed, but they may protrude into or through the urethra during voiding. They can be associated with a duplicated collecting system and may lead to urinary obstruction.

Rhabdomyosarcoma of the vagina (sarcoma botryoides) is the most common malignant tumor of the lower genitourinary tract in neonatal and infant girls. The peak incidence is in the first 2 years after birth, with 90% occurring before age 5 years. This tumor typically presents as grapelike clusters of pearly gray tissue protruding through the introitus or as vaginal bleeding.

Paraurethral cyst is a less common, epithelial-lined mass that arises from embryonic remnants of the urogenital duct, müllerian structures, or mesonephric duct. Such cysts can displace the urethral meatus laterally. The vaginal opening should be visible midline and posterior to the mass. In the neonate, the cysts may resolve spontaneously. Most paraurethral cysts involute spontaneously and do not require surgical excision. Before surgery is undertaken, a careful evaluation of the urinary and genital tracts is important to avoid misdiagnosing a congenital anomaly.

Gartner duct cysts can rarely present in the neonatal period or infancy as a smooth cyst emanating from the vagina.

Diagnosis

An interlabial mass can often be diagnosed definitively by history and physical examination findings. The color and location of the mass should be noted and surrounding structure evaluated.

Both prolapsed urethra and ureterocele appear smooth and red or cyanotic. Ureterocele is a congenital anomaly, and prolapsed urethra occurs in the older child. Mucocolpos appears pearly gray because of transparency of the hymen. Rhabdomyosarcoma presents as grapelike, pearly gray clusters. An infant feeding tube, urethral catheter, or saline-moistened calcium alginate swab is useful for evaluating the anatomy of the lower genital tract. The route of urine flow is also important, with paraurethral cyst displacement of the meatus causing an eccentric urinary stream. In this case, an infant feeding tube placed in the urethra showed no urinary retention and demonstrated the relation of the mass to the urethra and vagina.

Abdominal ultrasonography, abdominal computed tomography, or magnetic resonance imaging can be used for evaluation of abdominal masses or genitourinary tract abnormality. Biopsy should be performed on any vaginal mass, especially if rhabdomyosarcoma is in the differential diagnosis.

In this patient, excisional biopsy and frozen section were performed on the fifth day after birth. The excised mass measured 3 × 1 × 0.3 cm. Subsequent histopathologic analysis revealed that it was a fibroepithelial polyp arising from the vagina. The vaginal polyp was excised fully from the anterior vaginal wall without any complications.

The Condition

Vaginal polyp (fibroepithelial polyp) is a rare interlabial mass (Figure 84.1) in infants and the young child; such polyps are also uncommon in older children and adults. This mucosal polypoid lesion has a connective tissue core covered by benign squamous epithelium. Recurrence after excision is uncommon, although recurrence after incomplete excision has been reported.

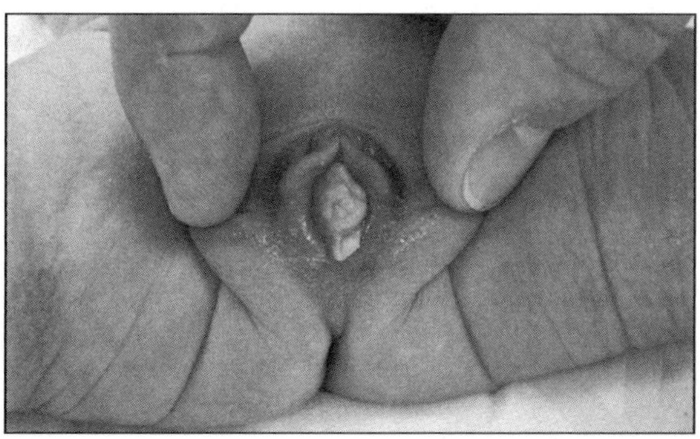

Figure 84.1. Vaginal fibroepithelial polyp in a neonatal girl.

Lessons for the Physician

Careful examination of the genitalia of the neonate can reinforce for the physician the range of normal genitalia and increase the likelihood of identifying anomalies and other abnormalities. Familiarity with the differential diagnosis of interlabial masses is necessary to determine the need for radiologic evaluation and referral to a pediatric gynecologist, surgeon, or urologist.

Reham El Gammal, MD; Christina Fernandez, MD; and Shahab Abdessalam, MD, Nebraska Medical Center, Omaha, NE

CHAPTER 85

Episodic Lower Abdominal Pain in an 11-Year-Old Girl

Presentation

An 11-year-old girl presents to the emergency department with a 1-day history of severe abdominal pain. The patient characterizes the pain as episodic, cramping, and localized to the suprapubic area and right lower quadrant. The episodes occur approximately every 2 to 4 weeks, during which she experiences pain several times a day for 3 to 5 days. The pain self-resolves, and she is pain-free between episodes. There are no alleviating or exacerbating factors. She reports associated nausea but no vomiting, diarrhea, constipation, or fever. The patient denies menarche.

On presentation, she is tachycardic with a heart rate of 124 beats/min. Other vital signs are normal. Her height is 167 cm (>95th percentile), and weight is 59.3 kg (95th percentile). She appears to be in significant pain; she is lying on her side in a fetal position. There is diffuse abdominal tenderness, which is most notable over the suprapubic region, with no rebound or guarding. The abdominal examination findings are otherwise normal, with normal bowel sounds and no distention, masses, or organomegaly. Genitourinary examination findings are consistent with a Sexual Maturity Rating of 2. The hymenal ring is open and intact without notches or tears. The breast Sexual Maturity Rating is 3.

Results of initial laboratory evaluation are as follows: white blood cell count, 1,500/mcL (1.5×10^9/L); hemoglobin, 12 g/dL (120 g/L); and platelet count, 256×10^3/mcL (256×10^9/L). The urinalysis result is positive for trace ketones with 1 white blood cell, and no bacteria are seen on microscopic examination. A urine pregnancy test result is negative. Abdominal ultrasonography reveals a uterine mass. Additional evaluation and imaging studies reveal the diagnosis.

- **What is your differential diagnosis at this point?**
- **Are there any elements of history or physical examination that would help you?**
- **What additional diagnostic studies would you like performed?**

Discussion

The patient was treated with ketorolac and morphine as needed for pain control. Pelvic magnetic resonance imaging performed to further evaluate the uterine mass revealed a vaginal obstruction with hematocolpos with mild distention of the uterus (Figure 85.1). The cervix and ovaries were normal. Pelvic examination with the patient under general anesthesia revealed a transverse vaginal septum. She underwent surgical resection of the septum and evacuation of retained blood. Intraoperative vaginal ultrasonography confirmed complete evacuation of hematocolpos. Her pain resolved postoperatively.

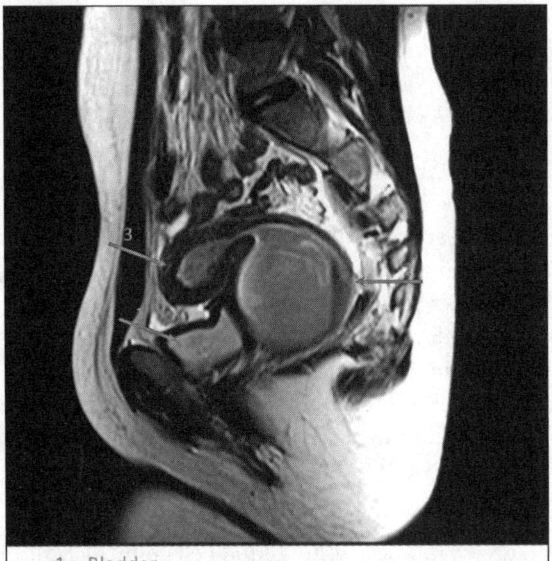

Figure 85.1. Pelvic magnetic resonance imaging reveals a distended vagina with layering of blood and a mildly distended uterus and bladder.

Differential Diagnosis

The differential diagnosis of abdominal pain in a girl of this age is vast but can be narrowed by classifying the pain as acute, chronic, or recurrent. The major organ systems to consider are the gastrointestinal, urologic, and gynecologic. This girl was experiencing recurrent abdominal pain; as such, the differential diagnosis included constipation, peptic ulcer disease, urinary tract infection, dysmenorrhea, and ruptured ovarian cyst. Less common diagnoses would include inflammatory bowel disease, cyclic vomiting syndrome, kidney stones, heavy metal poisoning, ovarian torsion, and imperforate hymen with hematocolpos. The possibility of a functional abdominal pain disorder should be considered when an organic origin of pain is not detected on thorough evaluation. Certainly, many children with organic abdominal pain may also have a component of functional pain, which makes diagnosis and management more challenging.

The Condition

Embryologically, the vagina is formed from 2 evaginations that originate from the urogenital sinus and müllerian duct. A transverse vaginal septum results from failure of fusion or canalization of these evaginations. These septae may be located at various levels in the vagina. Approximately 46% are found in the upper portion of the vagina; 35% to 40%, in the middle portion; and 15% to 20%, in the lower portion. Most septae are generally less than 1 cm in thickness and have fenestrations and therefore do not cause a complete obstruction.

A girl born with a vaginal septum will have normal-appearing external female genitalia. Younger children may present with mucocolpos, whereas adolescents commonly present with hematocolpos. Ascending infection is also possible through a perforation or fenestration, leading to pyohematocolpos. Occasionally, a mass may be palpated on abdominal or rectal examination, which may lead to symptoms secondary to a mass effect on the urinary system, such as urinary retention or hydronephrosis.

Hematocolpos is a condition in which the vagina becomes distended with blood because of accumulation of menstrual products. Hematometra is a related condition that refers to a distended uterus filled with blood caused by large accumulation of menstrual products. The most common causes of hematocolpos and hematometra are imperforate hymen, vaginal agenesis (1:5,000), and complete transverse vaginal septum (1:30,000–1:80,000). Vaginal agenesis is also known as müllerian aplasia or Mayer-Rokitansky-Küster-Hauser syndrome and refers to congenital absence of the vagina with variable cervical and uterine development. Symptoms secondary to hematocolpos or hematometra generally present at the time of menarche and include periodic lower abdominal pain and primary amenorrhea.

Approximately 25% to 50% of females with uterine or vaginal anomalies will have an associated urologic anomaly, such as unilateral renal agenesis, horseshoe kidney, or abnormalities of the collecting system. Skeletal anomalies of the spine, ribs, and extremities are also associated with uterine or vaginal anomalies in 10% to 15% of cases.

Diagnosis

Definitive diagnosis is usually made by ultrasonography or pelvic magnetic resonance imaging. Imaging is required to define the level and thickness of the septum. It is also important to differentiate between a high septum and a congenital absence of the cervix and to delineate any additional genitourinary abnormalities.

Management

Once the diagnosis is confirmed, the septum should be surgically excised with end-to-end anastomosis of vaginal mucosa. Endometriosis is a known complication of hematocolpos and often requires continued follow-up with a gynecologist. Although not completely understood, the endometriosis is presumed to be related to retrograde menstruation and implantation of endometrial cells.

As stated earlier, uterine and vaginal anomalies have been associated with other congenital anomalies and therefore may require additional evaluation.

Lessons for the Physician

- The differential diagnosis of abdominal pain is vast; however, a genitourinary cause of abdominal pain in children, particularly in young girls with recurrent or cyclic symptoms, should be considered.
- Girls with a vaginal septum will have normal-appearing external genitalia and often present with hematocolpos or pelvic mass.
- Vaginal septum is diagnosed with imaging studies, such as abdominal or pelvic ultrasonography or magnetic resonance imaging.
- Surgical resection is the primary treatment for vaginal septum.
- Congenital anomalies of the uterus and vagina may be associated with urologic or skeletal anomalies and require additional evaluation.

Lisa Didion, MD, and Ryan Nerland, MD, Blair E. Batson Children's Hospital, University of Mississippi Medical Center, Jackson, MS

Part 15

Ophthalmology

CHAPTER 86

18-Month-Old Girl With Esotropia of the Left Eye

Presentation

A healthy 18-month-old girl develops esotropia of her left eye 4 days after an episode of fever, constipation, and vomiting. There is no history of trauma, headaches, ataxia, medication ingestion, or travel abroad, and the family history is unremarkable.

Physical examination is difficult to perform because the child is uncooperative. She looks well and has no fever or signs of dehydration. Her left eye is deviated medially, and abduction of that eye seems to be reduced. The remaining physical findings, including neurologic and funduscopic findings, are normal. Cranial computed tomography and magnetic resonance imaging do not show any abnormalities. The vomiting has subsided, and she has passed normal stools. *Clostridium botulinum* toxin is not detected in the stools.

The following day, she is seen by an ophthalmologist. There is no ptosis, and her left eye abducts fully when the right eye is covered. The eye findings are otherwise normal, with no significant refractive error present. One year later, the esotropia remains, and the child is otherwise asymptomatic.

- **What is your differential diagnosis at this point?**
- **Are there any elements of history or physical examination that would help you?**
- **What additional diagnostic studies would you like performed?**

Discussion

Full abduction of the left eye while the right eye was covered ruled out left lateral rectus (abducens or sixth nerve) palsy. The child was diagnosed as having an acute basic-acquired left esotropia without underlying refractive error or associated neurologic disease.

The Condition

The most common type of acquired esotropia is *accommodative esotropia,* a term indicating that the deviation of the eye is caused by uncorrected refractive errors. Because this child's esotropia was not accommodative, it falls into the category of *basic-acquired esotropia.* Basic-acquired esotropia is rare in children. As illustrated by this case, it does not have to be associated with an underlying disease. Rarely, acquired esotropia may be associated with a significant underlying condition, such as Arnold-Chiari malformation, or serious intracranial disease, such as brain tumor. Although basic-acquired esotropia may develop at any age after 6 months, it occurs most commonly between the ages of 2 and 5 years.

Clinical Picture

The onset of basic-acquired esotropia is usually dramatic, with the sudden development of a large angle of deviation along with diplopia. Two mechanisms for acute basic-acquired esotropia that is not caused by intracranial disease are described. In some cases, the esotropia occurs after periods of interruption of fusion, such as after occlusion therapy for amblyopia in patients who have had no previous eye deviation. Similarly, the esotropia can be due to amblyopia following posttraumatic or postinfectious lid swelling that has caused a prolonged decrease in vision. The second type, which has no obvious cause, is usually intermittent but may become permanent and may be associated with diplopia but not with neurologic problems.

Differential Diagnosis

Other causes of esotropia besides the accommodative variety associated with refractive errors include Duane syndrome and infantile esotropia, which by definition occurs before the age of 6 months. Orbital conditions, such as orbital fracture, orbital mass, or extraocular muscle entrapment, need to be excluded, as does intracranial disease.

A significant condition that can cause acute esotropia is paralytic strabismus due to extraocular muscle paralysis from malfunctioning of the sixth cranial nerve. In that disorder, the deviation varies according to the direction of gaze, being most pronounced in the field of action of the paralyzed extraocular muscle and increasing when fixation is with the paretic eye.

Acquired sixth nerve paralysis may be caused by intracranial disease (tumor, increased intracranial pressure, meningitis, aneurysm), postinfectious phenomena (viral illness, varicella, Lyme disease), ear infection that has extended to cause petrositis, damage from trauma, a demyelinating process, or ocular myasthenia gravis.

Diagnosis

A detailed ophthalmologic examination is mandatory for esotropia. Assessment of visual acuity and testing for refractive errors are important elements of the evaluation. The angle of deviation should be measured by evaluating the corneal light reflex in each eye or by performing the alternate cover test. Examination of the anterior segment to assess the cornea, anterior chamber, and lens as well as direct and indirect funduscopy are required.

Detailed assessment of extraocular movements is necessary to exclude paretic eye deviation. In nonparalytic strabismus, the ocular movements are full when the undeviating eye is covered and the angle of eye deviation remains the same whichever eye is used for fixation. A detailed neurologic examination may be necessary.

Computed tomography of the orbits can exclude a fracture, an orbital mass, and extraocular muscle entrapment. Ultrasonography may be required to exclude loss of globe integrity. Neuroimaging studies such as computed tomography or magnetic resonance imaging are indicated in the presence of atypical features, craniofacial anomalies, or neurologic signs.

Therapy

The treatment of esotropia depends on the cause. Any underlying disorder, such as refractive error, must be treated. The earlier an accommodative esotropia is detected, the better the chances are that amblyopia can be prevented or treated successfully. Amblyopia may require patching of the nonamblyopic eye or penalization of that eye with atropine (to make the image in the stronger eye blurry). Treatment of the esotropia may include eyeglasses to eliminate diplopia and to reestablish binocular vision. Eye muscle surgery may be necessary in some cases. Achievement of a better balance of the extraocular muscles by using botulinum toxin is indicated in some cases.

Lessons for the Physician

Esotropia can occur for no apparent reason and with no other associated disorder, but it also can be a manifestation of serious intracranial disease. It is a sign that must be taken seriously and evaluated thoroughly, starting with a complete history and meticulous physical examination.

Hassib Narchi, MD, Sandwell General Hospital, Lyndon, England

COMMENTARY BY DR AIMEE LUAT, PEDIATRIC NEUROLOGIST, CHILDREN'S HOSPITAL OF MICHIGAN

Acquired esotropia in childhood is recently referred to in the literature as acute acquired comitant esotropia. The condition is still considered rare. However, a recent population-based study suggested that the acute non-accommodative esotropia type may be more common than previously thought and an incidence of 1 in 287 live births was noted. Since 2004, a new classification system based on etiology was proposed by Buch and Vinding: occlusion-related, non-accommodative with minimal refractive error, accommodative, decompensated monofixation syndrome, neurologic, cyclic, and secondary acute aquired comitant esotropia due to various etiologies such as optic neuritis and ataxia telangiectasia. There is still no clear-cut guideline as to when to image infants and children with acute acquired esotropia, as literature continues to show that it can still be only obvious manifestation of neurologic diseases such as Chiari malformation and pilocytic cerebellar tumor. Buch and Vinding identified 4 risk factors for intracranial disease: larger esodeviation at distance, recurrence, neurologic signs and symptoms (papilledema, ataxia and headache), and older age at onset (>6 years), suggesting that the presence of these risk factors in children with acute acquired esotropia may be used as a guide in ordering neuroimaging modalities.

References

1. Buch H, Vinding T. Acute acquired comitant esotropia of childhood: a classification based on 48 children. *Acta Ophthalmol.* 2015;93(6):568–574
2. Kothari M. Clinical characteristics of spontaneous late-onset comitant acute nonaccommodative esotropia in children. *Indian J Ophthalmol.* 2007;55(2):117–120
3. Jacobs SM, Green-Simms A, Diehl NN, Mohney BG. Long-term follow-up of acquired nonaccommodative esotropia in a population-based cohort. *Ophthalmology.* 2011;118(6):1170–1174
4. Hentschel SJ, Yen KG, Lang FF. Chiari I malformation and acute acquired comitant esotropia: case report and review of the literature. *J Neurosurgery.* 2005;102(4 Suppl):407–412
5. Lee JM, Kim SH, Lee JI, Ryou JY, Kim SY. Acute comitant esotropia in a child with a cerebellar tumor. *Korean J Ophthalmol.* 2009;23(3):228–231

CHAPTER 87

Eye Swelling, Redness, Discharge, and Pain With Movement in a 13-Year-Old Boy

Presentation

A 13-year-old boy comes to clinic having a 3-day history of swelling and redness of his eyes with discharge as well as pain with eye movement for 1 day. Acute bacterial conjunctivitis had been diagnosed elsewhere and topical antibiotic eyedrops, prescribed.

Now he complains of inability to see with his right eye. In addition, he has had non-projectile vomiting for 1 week and loose stools for 2 days but no headache. He has had no fever, trauma, sick contacts, illicit drug use, polyuria, nocturia, or recent travel. He has gained 27.0 kg over the last 6 months despite normal activity. His grandparents have type 2 diabetes.

Physical examination reveals a cooperative, obese adolescent who has a temperature of 98.7°F (37.1°C), heart rate of 110 beats/min, respiratory rate of 20 breaths/min, and blood pressure of 161/85 mm Hg. There is slight ptosis of the right upper lid, with lower lid chemosis and bilateral subconjunctival hemorrhage, more prominent on the right. The corneae and lenses are clear, and pupils are equally reactive bilaterally. Horizontal extraocular muscle movement is limited due to pain, with vertical movements intact. The optic discs appear normal. Visual acuity is 20/200 in the right eye and 20/20 in the left.

His white blood cell count is 10×10^3/mcL ($1\ 0\times 10^9$/L), hemoglobin level is 13 g/dL 130 g/L), hematocrit is 39% (0.39), and platelet count is 424×10^3/mcL (424×10^9/L). Electrolyte levels are within reference range. A computed tomography (CT) scan of the orbit is ordered, and an ophthalmologist is consulted.

- **What is your differential diagnosis at this point?**
- **Are there any elements of history or physical examination that would help you?**
- **What additional diagnostic studies would you like performed?**

Discussion

Possible diagnoses in a patient who has ptosis, eye swelling, pain, and sudden loss of vision include orbital cellulitis, carcinoma (primary or metastatic), retrobulbar abscess or hematoma, sarcoidosis, lymphoid tumor, Graves disease, optic neuritis, eosinophilic granuloma, and syphilis. The absence of fever in this patient argued against an acute infection. A CT scan of the orbit showed preseptal soft-tissue stranding, with no focal abscess or hemorrhage. The orbital contents appeared intact and symmetric.

Dilated eye examination showed sharp disc margins with an attached and well-perfused retina. Orbital pseudotumor was diagnosed. The patient was given high-dose prednisone, and his vision improved in 3 days without sequelae. His repeat blood pressure after pain medications was 122/84 mm Hg. Evaluation for autoimmune diseases was negative, but testing to explain his excessive recent weight gain showed dysmetabolic syndrome with insulin resistance. He was started on a regular exercise program, metformin, and diet monitoring to help with weight reduction.

The Condition

Orbital pseudotumor, also known as orbital inflammatory pseudotumor, is a rare, idiopathic, inflammatory process within the orbit. Some ophthalmologists prefer the term *idiopathic orbital inflammatory syndrome.* The condition is diagnosed by exclusion and affects adults primarily, with a 6% to 17% prevalence in children and adolescents. Although usually unilateral in adults, orbital inflammatory pseudotumor is commonly bilateral in children. Because this disorder affects the vision, prompt diagnosis and referral to an ophthalmologist are crucial so treatment can be started immediately.

Patients present with a sudden onset of pain, eyelid edema, proptosis, and subconjunctival hemorrhage, which may be associated with vision loss, photophobia, diplopia, ptosis, and motility restriction. Other potential findings include headache, vomiting, and weight loss, which are not seen in the adult population. Additional associations in pediatric and adolescent patients include bilateral involvement, iritis, and a history of trauma preceding the inflammatory process.

Another child who presented with a 3-week history of headaches and vomiting and had normal head CT scan results was initially believed to have migraine. She failed to respond to therapy with acetaminophen and propranolol and subsequently developed photophobia, diplopia, and eyelid swelling over 2 weeks. Orbital pseudotumor was diagnosed, and she was treated successfully with systemic corticosteroids.

Pathogenesis

The cause of orbital pseudotumor is unknown. Several theories point to an immune-mediated mechanism causing inflammation, which compresses the orbital structures and results in a mass lesion effect. Infections and genetic and environmental factors have also been postulated. Histologic findings include a mixture of plasma cells, macrophages, eosinophils, mature lymphocytes, and polymorphonuclear cells. In some cases, increasing amounts of fibrovascular stroma are seen.

Diagnosis

Orbital pseudotumor is diagnosed clinically. However, because this condition presents with variable symptoms that may mimic other disorders such as orbital cellulitis or malignancy, orbital imaging is crucial. A CT scan is the preferred imaging technique in the emergency setting because of its ease of use. On a CT scan, orbital pseudotumor may demonstrate contrast enhancement and infiltration of orbital tissue, extraocular muscle enlargement, absence of contiguous paranasal sinus disease, and absence of bony erosion or distortion of orbital contents.

Some authors prefer magnetic resonance imaging to CT scan. Magnetic resonance imaging demonstrates hypointensity on T1-weighted images and isointensity or minimal hyperintensity on T2-weighted images.[1] The findings depend on the degree of fibrosis. For example, a lesser degree of signal intensity is seen with the sclerosis variety on T2-weighted images, but enhancement is generally increased after the introduction of gadolinium.[1]

Some physicians believe that evaluation of a patient who is suspected of having orbital pseudotumor should include complete blood cell count, absolute eosinophil count, electrolytes, erythrocyte sedimentation rate, anti–double-stranded DNA, antineutrophilic cytoplasmic antibodies, angiotensin-converting enzyme, rapid plasma reagin test, thyroid function studies, and serum electrophoresis.

Treatment

Oral systemic corticosteroids are the mainstay of treating orbital pseudotumor. Rapid response to steroids is also considered diagnostic. Prednisone 1 to 1.5 mg/kg/d (up to 100 mg/d) leads to resolution of pain and proptosis within 24 to 48 hours. Intravenous steroids should be reserved for patients who experience rapid progression of symptoms or vision loss.

Low-dose radiotherapy has been used when corticosteroids fail or are medically contraindicated as well as during recurrences of signs and symptoms when the patient is receiving corticosteroid therapy. Surgery has been used to decompress localized tumors. Biopsy may be useful in evaluating patients who have presumed orbital pseudotumor, but because of the potential risk to surrounding orbital structures, surgery is typically not indicated.

Reference

1. Weber AL, Romo LV, Sabates NR. Pseudotumor of the orbit: clinical, pathologic, and radiologic evaluation. *Radiol Clin North Am.* 1999;37(1):151–168, xi

Lessons for the Physician

Orbital pseudotumor is a rare, benign inflammatory disorder of the orbit. The diagnosis is made by exclusion in patients presenting with eye pain, ptosis, chemosis, and vision loss. Findings on computed tomography scan or magnetic resonance imaging of the orbit, normal serologic test results, and a rapid response to steroids establish the diagnosis. Because this disorder affects vision, it is crucial to diagnose promptly and refer to an ophthalmologist for immediate treatment.

Mia Pingul, MD; Lopa Shah, MD; and Scott Denton, MD, University of Nevada School of Medicine, Las Vegas, NV

CHAPTER 88

Abnormal Eyelashes in 17-Year-Old Boy Who Has Congenital Heart Disease

Presentation

A 17-year-old boy with congenital heart disease (CHD) presents with a fever and fatigue. His past medical history includes a ventricular septal defect (VSD) with aortic regurgitation and distichiasis (double set of eyelashes arising from the meibomian glands) (Figure 88.1). Despite closure of his VSD, he developed progressive aortic insufficiency requiring multiple surgeries. His eyelashes were removed at 7 years of age because of persistent conjunctival irritation due to the distichiasis. After his last cardiac surgical (Ross) procedure, he developed chronic progressive right-sided pitting edema below the knee to the midfoot, without evidence of thrombosis.

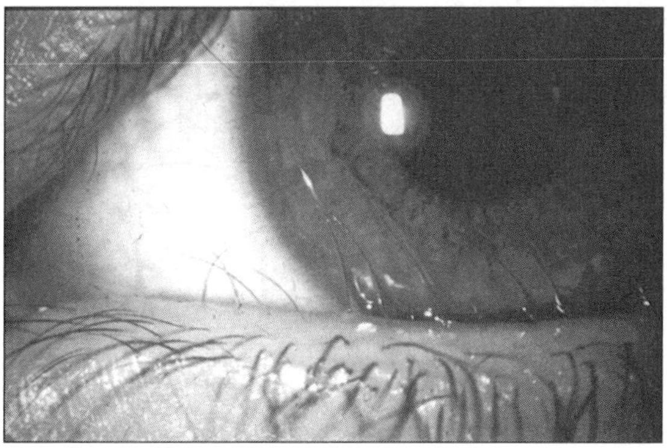

Figure 88.1. This patient has a double set of eyelashes (distichiasis). Photo courtesy of POSSUM-web 2009. Murdoch Childrens Research Institute.

Physical examination reveals a temperature of 98.6°F (37°C), heart rate of 90 beats/min, and blood pressure of 99/61 mm Hg. The right eye shows 2 aberrant eyelashes in the upper eyelid. His cardiovascular examination reveals a grade 2/6 systolic ejection murmur heard loudest at the pulmonic area. His right leg is edematous, cool, and nontender. The rest of the physical findings are normal.

His complete blood cell count is normal, and blood cultures are pending. An echocardiogram shows a successful valvular repair and no evidence of endocarditis. Consultation with a specialist provides the explanation for his CHD, distichiasis, and lymphedema.

- **What is your differential diagnosis at this point?**
- **Are there any elements of history or physical examination that would help you?**
- **What additional diagnostic studies would you like performed?**

Discussion

Entry of the features of CHD, distichiasis, and lymphedema into an online genetics database suggested a possible diagnosis of lymphedema-distichiasis syndrome. A clinical geneticist agreed with the diagnosis, and a mutation in the *FOXC2* gene confirmed lymphedema-distichiasis syndrome.

The Condition

Lymphedema-distichiasis syndrome classically presents with late-onset lymphedema (typically late childhood or puberty) and distichiasis. The lymphedema occurs exclusively in the lower extremities, is often asymmetric, and can be unilateral; the severity varies among patients, and boys usually present earlier than girls. Approximately 94% of affected individuals have distichiasis, which can cause photophobia, recurrent conjunctivitis, and corneal irritation. Congestive heart disease occurs in 7% of patients and may include VSD, atrial septal defect, patent ductus arteriosus, and tetralogy of Fallot. Other associated features of the syndrome include varicose veins, ptosis, cleft palate, spinal extradural cysts, and other ocular anomalies.

Diagnosis

This diagnosis is made clinically and confirmed by analysis of *FOXC2* gene, which reveals a mutation in about 95% of cases. There is clinical variability with no apparent genotype or phenotype correlation. Lymphedema-distichiasis syndrome is inherited in an autosomal dominant manner. There may be no known family history of distichiasis because relatives may not be aware of asymptomatic cases. Alternatively, the condition may be due to a new mutation, found in approximately 25% of affected patients.

Differential Diagnosis

Lymphedema should be considered as a cause of any peripheral edema that lacks pain or inflammation. Lymphedema can be difficult to differentiate from chronic venous insufficiency because both can have pitting edema (although lymphedema is typically not of the pitting type). Distinguishing features of lymphedema include a unilateral presentation, a squared-off appearance of the foot, and initial pitting edema progressing to nonpitting, brawny edema. In the later stages of lymphedema, the skin becomes hyperkeratotic, hyperpigmented, and papillomatous or verrucous. The Kaposi-Stemmer sign, in which an examiner is unable to pinch a fold of skin at the dorsal base of the second toe, is indicative of lymphedema.

Lymphedema is classified as either primary or secondary. In primary lymphedema, the dysfunction is caused by congenital hypoplasia or aplasia of the lymphatic vessels or by valvular incompetence, and the clinical changes may not become apparent until later in life. Primary lymphedema can be divided into 3 categories on the basis of age of onset of the edema. Congenital lymphedema (Milroy disease) manifests from birth to 1 year of age and is due to anaplastic lymphatic channels. The lower-extremity edema is bilateral, pitting, and nonpainful. Lymphedema praecox (Meige disease) manifests from age 1 to 35 years and is the most common form of primary lymphedema. This disorder is due to hypoplastic lymphatic channels. The edema is unilateral, more common in the distal extremity, and presents often at puberty. Lymphedema tarda manifests after age 35 years and is thought to be due to a defect in the lymphatic valves. Primary lymphedema is also associated with genetic syndromes, including Turner and Noonan syndromes, as well as with rarer disorders such as lymphedema-distichiasis syndrome.

In secondary lymphedema, there is blockage of the lymphatic system or disruption of the lymphatic drainage because of recurrent attacks of lymphangitis or infections with filariasis, malignancy, obesity, surgery, or trauma.

Management

Once the diagnosis of lymphedema-distichiasis is made, further evaluation is recommended to establish the extent of the disease. The following steps should be considered (the timing of which will depend on the initial presentation): referral to an ophthalmologist for slit-lamp examination, physical examination to identify a cardiac lesion or the complication of cellulitis, echocardiography, isotope lymphoscintigraphy to document the underlying abnormality of the lymphatic system, and referral to a geneticist for counseling.

The goal in managing primary lymphedema is to restore function and prevent deterioration. A multidisciplinary team is necessary for optimal management. Initial treatment includes the use of compression stockings, multilayer bandages, or pneumatic pumps; leg elevation; and skin care and debridement to prevent cellulitis, if needed. In cases of recurrent cellulitis or lymphangitis, long-term antibiotic therapy with penicillin or cephalosporins should be considered.

Some pharmacological therapies have proven to be effective in treating lymphedema, including benzopyrones, oral and topical retinoids, and topical emollients and keratolytics. Diuretics are not effective in treating lymphedema. Surgery is reserved for cases resistant to medical therapy. Ophthalmology referral is indicated for the management of the distichiasis, which can be conservative management with lubrication or more definitive surgical management.

This patient's lymphedema is currently well controlled, his distichiasis is asymptomatic after surgical repair, and his last echocardiography showed normal heart size and function.

Prognosis

Lower-extremity lymphedema can progress if uncontrolled and can be a disabling disease with functional, cosmetic, and psychological consequences. The severity of the edema is variable in lymphedema-distichiasis syndrome. A multidisciplinary team approach, in combination with patient education and compliance, can improve outcome. Prognosis depends also on associated comorbidities.

Lessons for the Physician

- A high level of suspicion for a genetic syndrome is required in the presence of a rare anomaly.
- The presence of 2 major anomalies significantly increases the likelihood of an underlying genetic condition. Especially with respect to the many rare diseases that manifest phenotypic variability, it is important to have a low threshold for considering genetic syndrome.
- Physicians should also be familiar with Web-based databases and regional clinical genetics resources.

Shalea Piteau, MD; Michael Storr, MD; and Jennifer MacKenzie, MD, Kingston General Hospital, Kingston, Canada

CHAPTER 89

18-Year-Old Girl With Pain, Redness, and Photophobia in Left Eye for 1 Week

Presentation

An 18-year-old African American girl has had pain, redness, and photophobia in her left eye for 1 week. For the last 3 days, she has also experienced blurred vision and floaters in her left eye. Today she has noted worsening vision in that eye. She has no concerns about her right eye. She denies any trauma to the left eye, headache, vomiting, or other neurologic symptoms, and she has been healthy otherwise. She is sexually active and has a history of *Chlamydia* infection that was treated 2 months ago.

On physical examination, the girl is alert and oriented. Her initial eye examination reveals bilaterally dilated pupils, possibly iatrogenic from an emergency department visit 2 days earlier. She has 20/60 vision in the left eye, which is injected and tender with palpation of the globe. On detailed examination by the ophthalmologist, the left eye has increased intraocular pressure, and keratic precipitates (accumulation of inflammatory cells on the cornea) are seen in the anterior chamber. Funduscopic examination of the same eye shows choroiditis, vitreous hemorrhage, and yellow patches in the periphery of the retina. The right eye vision, intraocular pressure, and funduscopic findings are normal. All other physical findings are normal. A series of blood tests and aqueous humor sampling leads to the cause of her eye condition.

- **What is your differential diagnosis at this point?**
- **Are there any elements of history or physical examination that would help you?**
- **What additional diagnostic studies would you like performed?**

Discussion

The clinical presentation was consistent with acute retinal necrosis (ARN) with panuveitis of the left eye. The girl was tested for antibodies against herpes simplex virus (HSV), *Toxoplasma,* varicella-zoster virus (VZV), cytomegalovirus (CMV), and Epstein-Barr virus (EBV). She had IgG and IgM antibodies against HSV-1. Subsequently, an aqueous humor sample was positive for HSV-1 by polymerase chain reaction testing. She was treated with intravenous acyclovir for 14 days and continued on oral acyclovir for a total of 12 weeks. She underwent laser photocoagulation of the left eye after 2 weeks to prevent retinal detachment. On 3-month follow-up, she had a residual visual deficit in her left eye (20/40) but no involvement of the right eye.

The Condition

Acute retinal necrosis was described initially by Urayama and colleagues in Japan in 1971. It is a fulminant type of necrotizing retinitis caused by members of the herpesvirus family and is characterized by anterior and posterior uveitis (panuveitis), vitreitis, diffuse retinal vasculitis, and late-onset retinal detachment. In the United States, ARN accounted for 5.5% cases of uveitis over a 10-year period. It usually affects healthy people ages 20 to 50 years but can affect younger children as well.

Multiple members of the herpes virus family have been implicated as the causative agents, including VZV, which accounts for most cases, HSV-1, HSV-2, and, rarely, CMV and EBV. The pathogenesis of ARN remains to be elucidated. Both primary infection, probably through involvement of the anterior segment of the eye (conjunctivitis and keratitis), and latent viral reactivation have been reported. There have been reports of predisposition to this disease in association with specific human white blood cell antigens, suggesting an immune basis for the condition. Affected patients present with red eye, periorbital pain, floaters, and hazy, decreased vision. The hallmark finding is yellow patches in the periphery of the retina, with keratic precipitates suggestive of anterior uveitis. In 67% of cases, the condition is unilateral, and in 33% of cases, it becomes bilateral, which can happen months after involvement of one eye.

Acute retinal necrosis is diagnosed clinically, but laboratory testing can help establish the cause. The evaluation includes viral titers for HSV, VZV, EBV, and CMV. Culturing of aqueous or vitreous specimens is useful. Polymerase chain reaction analysis of a fluid sample is highly sensitive, specific, and rapid and requires only a small sample.

The goal of medical treatment is rapid recovery and prevention of involvement of the contralateral eye. Prompt initiation of intravenous antiviral medication is the major therapeutic measure. Oral steroids are administered to reduce inflammation. There is no proven efficacy of antithrombotic agents. Retinal detachment is a common complication that can be prevented by prophylactic laser photocoagulation. If retinal detachment occurs, surgery such as vitrectomy or scleral buckle surgery might be needed.

Currently, there is no consensus on long-term oral antiviral prophylactic therapy. Close follow-up is needed to watch for reactivation, involvement of the other eye, and retinal detachment. The disease carries a poor visual prognosis, especially in the presence of complications such as retinal detachment, anterior ischemic optic neuropathy, or central retinal artery occlusion.

Differential Diagnosis

Although retinitis is rare in children and young adults, it can occur in various guises and have different causes. Cytomegalovirus retinitis is a common form of necrotizing retinitis, generally occurring in immunocompromised individuals. The course is chronic and associated with minimal vitreous inflammation. The lesions are distributed near retinal vessels. Hemorrhage is more common than in ARN. Diagnosis is essential because CMV does not respond to acyclovir.

Toxoplasma chorioretinitis caused by the protozoa *Toxoplasma gondii* is characterized by a diffuse multifocal retinitis and vitreitis that has a more fulminant presentation and more inflammation than does ARN. The peripheral retina is less involved. Polymerase chain reaction analysis of a vitreous sample helps in diagnosis.

Ocular syphilis caused by *Treponema pallidum* can present with diffuse patchy retinitis and vasculitis. A history of previous syphilis infection should be determined. The rapid plasma reagin test and the fluorescent treponemal antibody test help in diagnosis.

Behçet disease is a multisystem inflammatory syndrome characterized by recurrent oral ulcers, genital ulcers, and ocular inflammation. Patients who have this condition can also have arthritis, intestinal ulcers, and neuropsychiatric symptoms. Retinal vasculitis, with hemorrhages, is present. Affected patients respond to corticosteroids, cyclosporine, and colchicine.

Sarcoidosis can involve the eyes in 25% of cases. Findings include retinal periphlebitis that has an appearance described as "candle wax drippings," a finding considered as pathognomonic of sarcoidosis. The treatment consists of steroids, azathioprine, and cyclophosphamide.

The Agent

Herpes simplex virus is a ubiquitous virus whose involvement in chronic and repetitive infections is well known. It is a double-stranded DNA virus. The 2 serotypes are HSV-1, which usually involves the face and skin above the waist, and HSV-2, which usually infects genitalia and skin below the waist. Herpes simplex virus may be transmitted from both symptomatic and asymptomatic individuals. Infections with HSV result from direct contact with infected secretions. The clinical manifestations vary with age and immune status of the host.

Neonatal disease is usually from HSV-2 and can have 3 presentations, including skin, eye, and mucous membrane infection; central nervous system infection; and disseminated disease. Older children and adults usually have mucocutaneous disease, which includes herpes labialis, gingivostomatitis, eczema herpeticum, herpetic whitlow, and genital herpes. Herpes simplex virus can also cause encephalitis that is associated with significant neurologic sequelae.

Eye manifestations of HSV infection include blepharitis, conjunctivitis, epithelial keratitis, corneal ulceration, stromal keratitis, episcleritis, uveitis, and ARN. After active infection, the HSV lies dormant within the trigeminal ganglion or the cornea and may reactivate to produce many varieties of ocular herpetic disease. Ocular involvement may be caused by direct infection of the cornea or conjunctiva or through HSV-induced immune reactions that can affect any ocular structure. The exact pathophysiology for ocular inflammation still is not known.

Lessons for the Physician

Acute retinal necrosis should be suspected and treated as early as possible. Therapy consists of prolonged antiviral treatment combined with anti-inflammatory agents. In spite of treatment, the condition carries a poor prognosis, with chances for eventual involvement of the other eye, making it important to monitor the health of the other eye closely. The initiation of prophylactic laser therapy to prevent retinal detachment has improved the outcome for this condition.

Bhawana Arora, MD, and Sauraby Goel, MD, Children's Hospital of Michigan, Detroit, MI

Part 16

Orthopedics

CHAPTER 90

Bowlegs in a 2-Year-Old Girl

Presentation

A healthy 2-year-old girl presents to the clinic for evaluation of bowlegs. She was born at term and had a birthweight of 3.03 kg. Her development has been normal, and she eats a regular diet. However, the bowing of her legs has increased progressively since she started walking at 1 year of age. There is no parental consanguinity, and the family history has no findings of note.

Physical examination reveals an obese child who walks with a waddling gait. Her weight is 22 kg (above the 95th percentile), and height is 88 cm (50th percentile). Her body mass index is 28 kg/m^2 (>95th percentile). She has exaggerated bowing of both legs (Figures 90.1 and 90.2) and acanthosis nigricans on her neck. The findings on the rest of the physical examination are normal.

Laboratory studies demonstrate a serum 25-hydroxyvitamin D of 25 ng/mL (63 nmol/L) (reference range, 13 to 40 ng/mL [32–100 nmol/L]), 1,25-dihydroxyvitamin D of 36 pg/mL (93.6 pmol/L) (reference range, 16–56 pg/mL [41.6–145.6 pmol/L]), parathyroid hormone of 27 pg/mL (2.8 ng/L) (reference range, 15–65 pg/mL [1.6–6.8 ng/L]), and phosphorus of 5.9 mg/dL (1.9 mmol/L) (reference range, 3.3–6.6 mg/dL [1.1–2.1 mmol/L]). Results of a complete blood cell count and a comprehensive electrolyte panel, including calcium and alkaline phosphatase, as well as urinary phosphorus and calcium excretions, are within reference range. A lipid panel shows a borderline high cholesterol concentration of 181 mg/dL (4.7 mmol/L). Radiographs of the wrist appear normal. Lower extremity radiographs reveal the diagnosis.

- **What is your differential diagnosis at this point?**
- **Are there any elements of history or physical examination that would help you?**
- **What additional diagnostic studies would you like performed?**

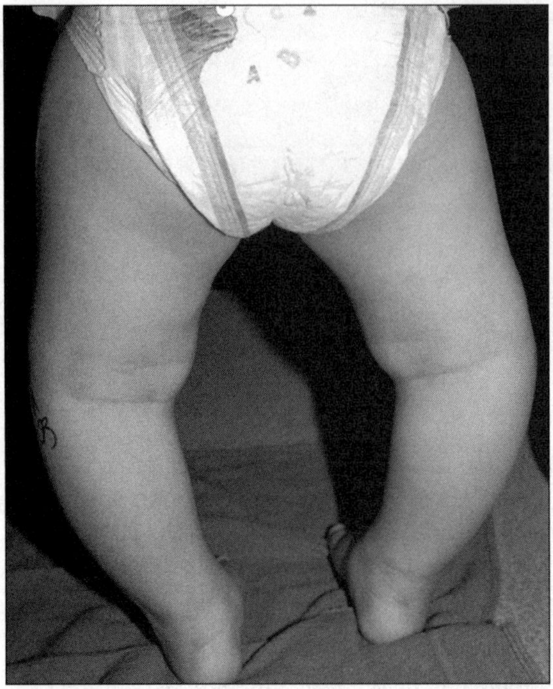

Figure 90.1. Clinical appearance of the legs from a posterior view.

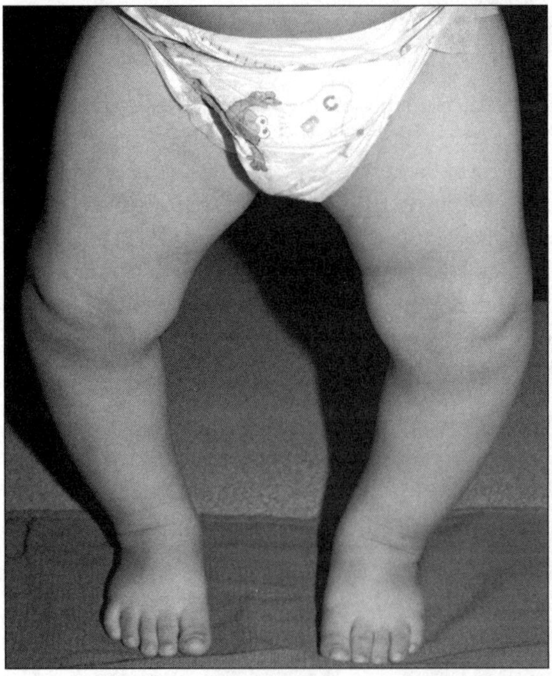

Figure 90.2. Clinical appearance of the legs from an anterior view.

Discussion

Radiographs of the knees showed bilateral changes of infantile Blount disease, also called "infantile tibia vara." Characteristic radiographic findings in Blount disease are irregular medial tibial metaphyses, beaking of medial tibial metaphyses, and wedging of the medial portion of the epiphyses (Figures 90.3 and 90.4). The child was referred to pediatric orthopedics. Because of the severity of her disease, she ultimately underwent a surgical intervention and continues to be monitored closely for recurrence of any deformity.

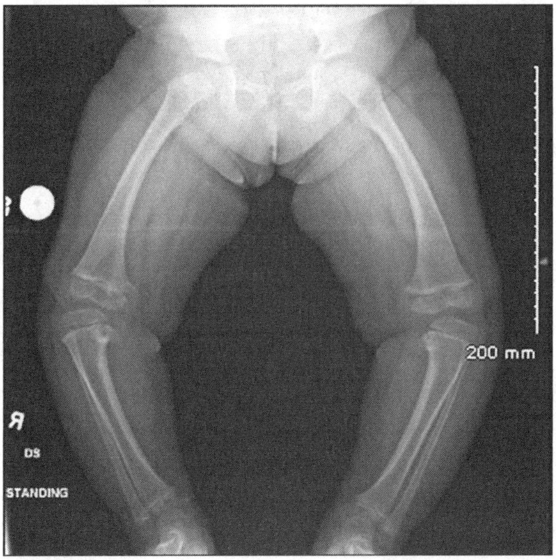

Figure 90.3. Full-length standing anteroposterior radiograph showing irregular medial tibial metaphyses and medially sloped and irregularly ossified epiphyses.

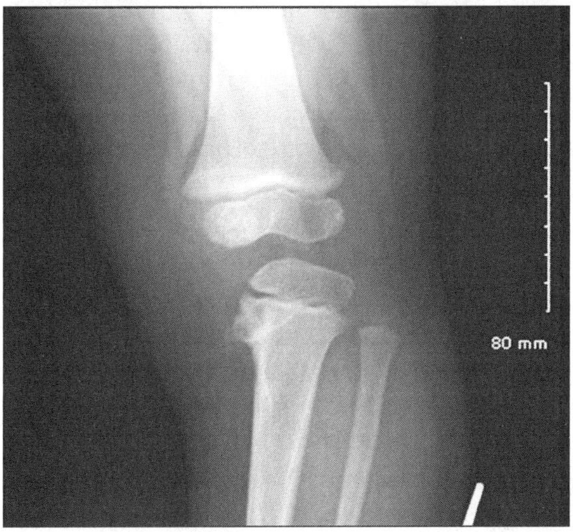

Figure 90.4. Prominent "beaking" of the medial tibial metaphysis, with lucent cartilage islands within the beak.

The Condition

Blount disease is a developmental disorder of unknown cause that affects the medial aspect of the proximal tibial physis, resulting in bowleg. The mechanism of bowing is believed to be an abnormal compression of the medial tibial growth plate, resulting in partial growth inhibition of the tibia and relative overgrowth of the fibula. The changes in infants and children who have infantile Blount disease are believed to result from increased weight in the presence of physiologic varus. The deformity is bilateral in 80% of cases and has been associated with early walking.

Although infantile Blount disease is a rare disorder, it is an important cause of pathologic bowlegs in the 1- to 3-year-old age group, especially in the context of the increasing incidence of obesity in younger children. A recent study identified body mass index more than 22 kg/m^2 as a risk factor for the development of infantile Blount disease.[1] A less aggressive type of Blount disease occurs in overweight adolescents, in whom the deformity is usually unilateral.

Diagnosis

Lower extremity bowing is a normal physiologic process that is bilateral, symmetric, and nonprogressive, resolving by age 2 years in most children. Pathologic bowing should be considered in any child who has persistent bowing after that time or who demonstrates progressive deformity at any age. Clinical and radiographic evaluations are necessary to differentiate physiologic bowing from infantile Blount disease and to identify other pathologic causes of bowing. Laboratory evaluation may be used to help rule out underlying bone diseases.

The gait and the overall appearance of the legs must be observed carefully because children who have Blount disease often demonstrate a lateral thrusting of the knee when walking. The child should be evaluated in the supine position with the lower extremities aligned and gently rotated so the kneecaps point straight up. Deformity related to normal physiologic bowing typically corrects with this maneuver. Relative proportion of the upper and lower extremities and the torso, as well as leg lengths, should be assessed. Dermatologic examination also may prove helpful in detecting disorders such as neurofibromatosis 1 (NF-1).

A single anteroposterior view hip-to-ankle radiograph that includes both legs (see Figure 90.3) should be performed in the standing position, although supine positioning may be used if the child is uncooperative. For supine positioning, the child's legs should be positioned with the kneecaps pointing toward the ceiling. The degree of proximal tibial deformity is measured via the metaphyseal-diaphyseal angle and predicts disease progression in the absence of the characteristic changes of more severe Blount disease. A metaphyseal-diaphyseal angle of more than 16 degrees suggests early Blount disease; less than 10 degrees suggests a physiologic varus.[2]

Laboratory evaluation of a child who has early or severe bowing may include measuring serum 1,25-dihydroxyvitamin D, 25-hydroxyvitamin D, intact parathyroid hormone, alkaline phosphatase, calcium, and phosphorus as well as urinary phosphorus excretion. These laboratory values are normal in Blount disease. Hence, diagnosis of infantile Blount disease is on the basis of the characteristic radiographic changes and progressive deformity.

Differential Diagnosis for Bowlegs

Other causes of pathologic bowing include metabolic bone diseases such as rickets, various genetic disorders, and congenital leg deformities. Physeal injury from trauma, infection, or tumor can also cause bowing deformity of the lower extremity.

Children who have rickets due to vitamin D deficiency frequently present with bowlegs but have additional skeletal findings such as thickening of the wrists, rachitic rosary, and frontal bossing. Radiographs show evidence of widening and fraying of the metaphyses. A family history of bowlegs and significant short stature is concerning for hereditary hypophosphatemic rickets. A mild form of hypophosphatasia may also present with leg bowing and short stature. In contrast to rickets, the serum alkaline phosphatase activity is low.

Bowed tubular bones can be a manifestation of multiple genetic disorders, which include skeletal dysplasias such as achondroplasia, pseudoachondroplasia, camptomelic dysplasia, and diastrophic dysplasia. These entities can be differentiated by assessment that uses full skeletal surveys and, in certain conditions such as achondroplasia, DNA testing. Because anterolateral tibial bowing is one of the skeletal manifestations of NF-1, patients must have a full evaluation for the presence of other criteria diagnostic of NF-1.

Some forms of osteogenesis imperfecta may also lead to lower extremity deformities in the form of bowing and can be investigated by obtaining a thorough family history, physical examination, history of fractures, and evidence of osteopenia in skeletal radiographs. Finally, infants of diabetic mothers can present with lower extremity anomalies.

Treatment

Treatment for Blount disease depends on the age of the child and the degree of deformity. Bracing is an option for children younger than 3 years who have minimal deformity. Bracing puts valgus stress on the knee and decreases the stress on the medial physis, potentially allowing for recovery of medial physeal growth. Surgical intervention is reserved for severe bowing, for children older than 3 years, or when bracing fails to improve the deformity. Operative options include osteotomy, hemiepiphysiodesis, and physeal stapling.

References

1. Scott AC, Kelly CH, Sullivan E. Body mass index as a prognostic factor in development of infantile Blount disease. *J Pediatr Orthop.* 2007;27(8):921–925
2. Feldman MD, Schoenecker PL. Use of metaphyseal-diaphyseal angle in the evaluation of bowed legs. *J Bone Joint Surg Am.* 1993;75(11):1602–1609

Lessons for the Physician

- Most bowlegs in the 1- to 3-year-old age group are physiologically normal and resolve over time.
- True pathologic variants require early recognition and referral to a subspecialist for additional management.

Mikla Derlet, MD, Department of Pediatrics, UC Davis School of Medicine, Sacramento, CA

CHAPTER 91

Intermittent Groin Pain in a 5-Year-Old Boy

Presentation

A 5-year-old previously healthy boy presents to the emergency department (ED) with a 2-week history of intermittent left groin pain, usually occurring later in the day. Pain is not related to eating, movement, urination, or stooling. There is no report of trauma or precipitating event. He screams and refuses to stand up during pain episodes, which occur suddenly and last approximately 1 to 2 hours at a time. He otherwise has normal gait and activity when pain-free. He does not wake up at night in pain. No recent illnesses or fevers are reported. Review of systems and his examination findings are unremarkable.

Two days prior, he was evaluated in the ED for the same issue and had normal urinalysis and urine culture and scrotal ultrasonogram results. The consulting urologist did not suspect a urologic process. He was discharged home with pain medication. Today, he returns to the ED because of the intense pain. The patient is admitted for further evaluation and pain management.

Complete blood cell count, C-reactive protein level, urinalysis results, and plain radiographs of the hips are unremarkable. Computed tomography of the abdomen and pelvis reveals a trace amount of nonspecific free fluid in the pelvis. His pain appears to be alleviated with ibuprofen and bed rest. The following day, he has another episode of intense groin pain after returning from the playroom. Physical examination at this time demonstrates only point tenderness on palpation over his symphysis pubis area. No swelling, erythema, or increased warmth was noted in that area. An additional imaging study reveals the diagnosis.

- **What is your differential diagnosis at this point?**
- **Are there any elements of history or physical examination that would help you?**
- **What additional diagnostic studies would you like performed?**

Discussion

Magnetic resonance imaging (MRI) of the pelvis revealed increased signal intensity of the symphysis pubis and the bilateral obturator externus muscles (Figure 91.1). There was no evidence of ischiopubic synchondrosis, associated or remote stress fracture, or enhancement after contrast administration to indicate infection in this case. These findings are consistent with posttraumatic osteitis pubis (PTOP) and myositis. After discussion of the MRI findings with his primary care physician and mother, both recalled a recent outpatient visit at which he reported being forced into a lateral split by his older brother in an attempt to teach him karate. This event occurred immediately before the onset of his pain. The boy was discharged home with instructions for limited physical activity. He was prescribed over-the-counter nonsteroidal analgesia for use. Several weeks after his hospital discharge, a follow-up telephone call to his parents revealed that he had recovered from the condition and had not had further pain episodes.

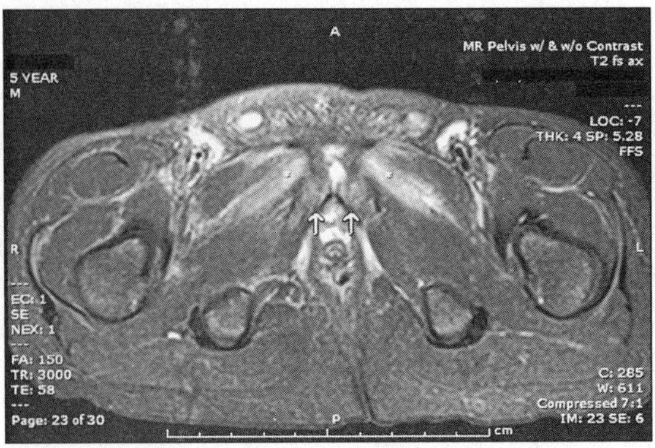

Figure 91.1. Axial fat-saturated T2 image through the symphysis pubis demonstrates symmetric increased signal intensity of the anterior aspect of the ischial bones (arrows) and symmetric increased signal intensity of the anterior aspects of the obturator externus muscles (asterisks).

Differential Diagnosis

Sources of groin area pain include kidney stones, musculoskeletal disorders, and, in boys, scrotal and testicular disorders. If testicular torsion or trauma is suspected, boys should be evaluated immediately. Musculoskeletal causes include transient synovitis, septic arthritis, osteomyelitis, malignancy, fracture, Legg-Calvé-Perthes disease, slipped capital femoral epiphysis, myositis, muscle strain, and PTOP.

The Condition

Posttraumatic osteitis pubis is a common cause of pain in the pelvis among athletes. However, this condition is rare in children. More common causes of groin pain would include ischiopubic synchondrosis, osteomyelitis, stress fracture, and scrotal disease. Magnetic resonance imaging is the most sensitive study for PTOP, and the diagnosis is one of exclusion. The symmetric occurrence of the bone marrow edema and associated myositis is the key. Other findings that may be seen on pelvic MRI include periarticular swelling, subchondral edema, or fluid at the symphysis pubis area. Additional causes of pubalgia, such as scrotal disease and anteroinferior abdominal wall insufficiency, are better confirmed with dynamic ultrasonography. Imaging must be integrated with clinical findings to exclude infection as a cause.

Although it is more common in adults, this condition can occur in children and should be considered in those with intermittent intense groin pain and, in boys, without apparent scrotal involvement. Typically, children with PTOP experience pain over the symphysis pubis area with possible radiation to the groin, thigh, or abdomen. Onset may be abrupt or insidious. Pain episodes may be precipitated by activities such as running, kicking, walking, and climbing. Although laboratory studies are not usually needed for PTOP, studies such as a complete blood cell count might be useful in ruling out other potential causes of groin pain.

Treatment

Rest and avoidance of vigorous physical activity typically result in resolution of PTOP in approximately 2 weeks to 3 months. In addition, nonsteroidal anti-inflammatory drugs and corticosteroids are helpful in alleviating the pain and reducing the inflammation of PTOP. Physical therapy, especially in athletes, is beneficial in the rehabilitation. Surgical intervention could be considered for athletes with severe PTOP in whom medical management fails.

Lessons for Physician

- Physicians should consider posttraumatic osteitis pubis as a cause of acute groin pain in children and athletes who are involved in exertional physical activities that involve the lower extremities.
- Rest and avoidance of vigorous physical activity along with analgesia is the recommended treatment for posttraumatic osteitis pubis.

Katherine Quinones, DO, and John C. Luk, MD, UT Southwestern Austin, Austin, TX

Lori L. Barr, MD, Austin Radiological Association, Austin, TX

Jay Shapiro, MD, Dell Children's Medical Center of Central Texas, Austin, TX

CHAPTER 92

Swelling Behind the Knee in a 15-Year-Old Boy

Magnetic Resonance Imaging Presentation

A 15-year-old boy presents to the pediatric clinic with a 3-week history of a mass behind his right knee. He found it incidentally while bathing and experiences no pain or discomfort in his right knee during sports activities. He denies a history of preceding trauma. His medical history, including personal history and family history, are negative for inflammatory arthritis and malignant tumor.

Physical examination reveals an adolescent boy with an ovoid, nontender, mobile mass with a cystic feeling in the posteromedial aspect of the right knee (Figure 92.1). The mass is approximately 9.8 × 3 × 2 cm, firm, and noncompressible. The swelling becomes prominent on extension of the knee. The swelling is also brilliant with transillumination. The rest of the examination findings are within reference range. A radiologic test confirms the physical finding.

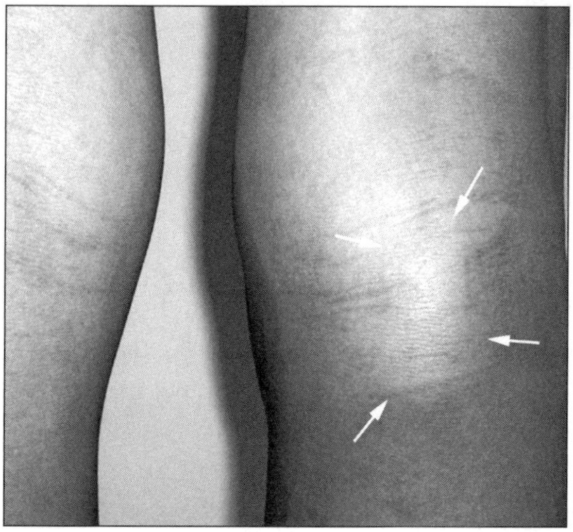

Figure 92.1. Clinical photograph showing a popliteal cyst in the posteromedial aspect of the right knee (white arrows).

- **What is your differential diagnosis at this point?**
- **Are there any elements of history or physical examination that would help you?**
- **What additional diagnostic studies would you like performed?**

Discussion

A radiograph of the knee did not reveal any abnormality. However, ultrasonography demonstrated a well-circumscribed hypoechoic cystic swelling in the posteromedial aspect of the right knee without joint effusion (Figures 92.2 and 92.3). A popliteal cyst was diagnosed in view of the benign nature of this cystic swelling.

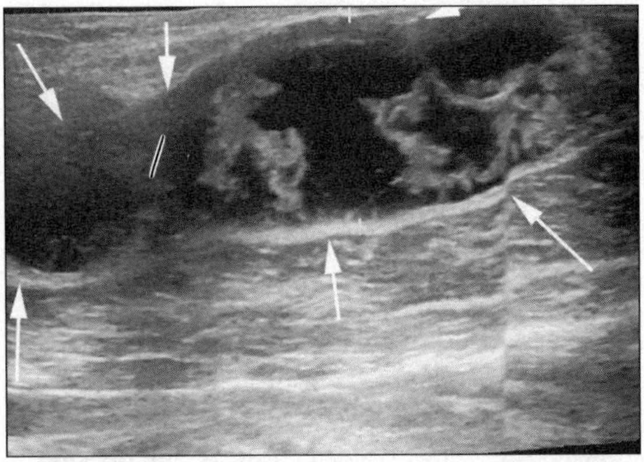

Figure 92.2. Ultrasonogram of the right knee (posterior sagittal view) showing the hypoechoic cystic mass (white arrows) with internal debris.

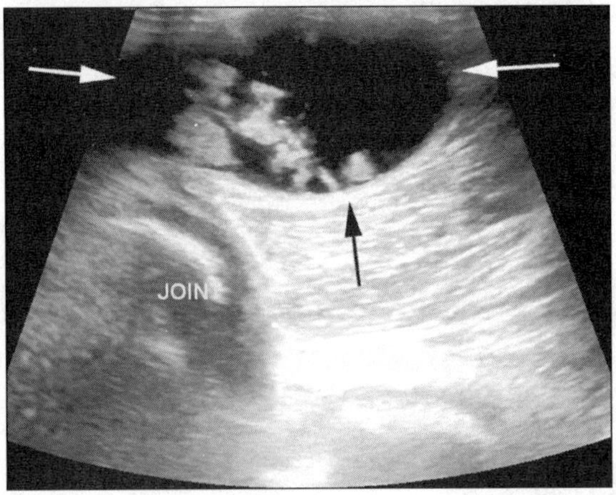

Figure 92.3. Ultrasonogram (posterior transverse view) showing the relationship of the popliteal cyst (black and white arrows) with the knee joint.

The Condition

A popliteal cyst is a synovial fluid–filled mass located in the popliteal fossa. It is commonly seen in both adults and children, although only approximately one-third of popliteal cysts are reported in children. Popliteal cysts are also referred to as Baker cysts, named after William Morrant Baker, who described it in 1877.

Popliteal cysts in children are mostly idiopathic. The occurrence in boys outnumbers the occurrence in girls in a ratio of 2:1, and most cases occur unilaterally. The patients are often asymptomatic, and most cases are detected incidentally by the patient, parent, or physician as a painless mass behind the knee. In one study, the prevalence of asymptomatic popliteal cysts in children detected by ultrasonography was reported as 2.4%. The mass gradually increases in size and may be fairly large when the patient first notices it. Physical examination reveals a firm cystic mass located in the medial aspect of the popliteal fossa, usually distal to the popliteal crease. It also becomes prominent on extension of the knee joint. Positive transillumination is a useful bedside diagnostic test. Secondary popliteal cysts are commonly encountered in children with underlying joint disorders that cause knee effusions, such as juvenile idiopathic arthritis, septic arthritis, psoriatic arthritis, meniscal tears, hemophilia, pigmented villonodular synovitis, or unstable osteochondritis dissecans.

The common mean age of presentation of idiopathic popliteal cysts is 6 years, with a range of 2 to 14 years. The most common site of origin is the bursa of the gastrocnemius and semimembranosus muscles. Another common site of origin is herniation of the synovium through the posterior joint capsule of the knee. In adults, popliteal cysts are usually secondary to osteoarthritis, meniscal tears, and inflammatory joint conditions. Unlike in adults, the presence of underlying intra-articular disease is rare in children. However, children with knee pain or joint swelling should undergo evaluation for an underlying cause, such as septic arthritis, Lyme disease (for patients living in, or visiting, endemic areas in the last year), inflammatory arthritis, or structural injury. Normal debris inside the cyst can be seen as echogenic internal signals on ultrasonography (see Figure 92.2). In a recent study in children, the presence of these echogenic internal signals was frequently encountered in patients with arthritis and further investigation with magnetic resonance imaging (MRI) was recommended.

Differential Diagnosis

Soft-tissue tumors, such as lipoma, xanthoma, hemangioma, fibrosarcoma, synovial cell sarcoma, and tumors of the tendon sheath, should be included in the differential diagnosis. In older children and adults, a ruptured popliteal cyst may mimic deep venous thrombosis or thrombophlebitis. Knee radiographs should be obtained to evaluate bony lesions, such as osteochondromas, osteochondritis dissecans, and malignant bone tumors. The diagnosis of a popliteal cyst is confirmed by ultrasonography, which differentiates a solid mass from a hypoechoic cystic lesion. Aspiration of the cyst in children is seldom required for diagnosis. In some instances, MRI may be required if the ultrasonogram is equivocal in delineating cystic mass from solid tumors. The presence of a solid mass warrants urgent referral to a specialist for further evaluation, possible biopsy, and appropriate treatment (including excision, chemotherapy, radiotherapy, or a combination of the three). Magnetic resonance imaging is also recommended for further evaluation if there is clinical suspicion for underlying joint conditions due to persistent knee pain, joint swelling, or systemic symptoms.

Management

Most authors report a spontaneous resolution of idiopathic popliteal cysts within a period of 20 months. Hence, conservative management by watchful waiting is strongly recommended in children. On the contrary, in adults, treatment is directed toward intra-articular disease and recurrence of popliteal cyst is common. Rupture of the cyst, hemorrhage, infection, or malignant transformation can occur rarely in children, so new or increased pain should warrant immediate evaluation. Surgical treatment is indicated in children only in the presence of symptoms (pain or increasing size that limits motion).

Our patient is older than the typical patient with idiopathic popliteal cysts, and ultrasonography also revealed echogenic internal signals. Hence, we recommended further evaluation with MRI for the presence of underlying joint diseases. However, the patient's family decided to wait because he is mostly asymptomatic. He participates in basketball without any pain or discomfort and is under follow-up.

Lessons for the Physician

- Baker cysts or popliteal cysts are common in children.
- Popliteal cysts are mostly asymptomatic and incidentally found as painless masses behind the knee.
- In children, most cases are idiopathic and resolve spontaneously, so surgical excision is not required.
- Ultrasonography confirms the cystic nature of the swelling, which is also helpful in the evaluation of the characteristics of the swelling and also reveals the presence or absence of the joint effusion.
- On the basis of clinical or radiologic suspicion, magnetic resonance imaging is recommended for further evaluation of underlying joint disorders in secondary popliteal cysts.

Senthilkumar Sankararaman, MD; Kamakshya Patra, MD; and Wanda Wells, MD, Louisiana State University Health Sciences Center, Shreveport, LA

Part 17

Surgery

CHAPTER 93

An 11-Month-Old With Nausea, Vomiting, and an Abdominal Mass (Visual Diagnosis)

Presentation

An 11-month-old girl presents to the emergency department (ED) with 12 episodes of nonbilious, nonbloody vomiting and decreased activity for the past 24 hours. Her medical history and family history are notable. She was born at term via an uncomplicated, induced vaginal delivery. There is a paternal history of diabetes. The patient's half sister, who has phenylketonuria, was ill with nausea without vomiting 2 days before the patient's presentation. Yesterday the patient was seen in the ED for nausea and 5 bouts of vomiting. She was discharged after receiving one dose of ondansetron and could tolerate clear liquids by mouth. She now returns to the ED for continued vomiting.

On physical examination the patient's temperature is 100.2°F (37.9°C), heart rate is 114 beats/min, respiratory rate is 30 breaths/min, blood pressure is 105/65 mm Hg, and oxygen saturation is 98% on room air. She is comfortable and sleeping but awakens when physically examined. Mucous membranes are slightly dry, and her posterior oropharynx is erythematous. Cardiac auscultation reveals normal S_1 and S_2 without a murmur. She has good peripheral perfusion and normal capillary refill. Her lungs are clear to auscultation. She has no abdominal scars, and bowel sounds are normal. Her abdomen is soft and nontender, and no masses are palpable. The spleen and liver are not enlarged. Abdominal radiography reveals a normal bowel gas pattern.

The patient is admitted for intravenous hydration. Despite treatment with ondansetron, frequent vomiting persists. During her second hospital night, she has several large bowel movements that contain blood and mucus. Her father notices a visible mass in her abdomen (Figure 93.1). Laboratory evaluation reveals that her stool sample is negative for *Shiga*-like toxin and rotavirus. An abdominal radiograph is

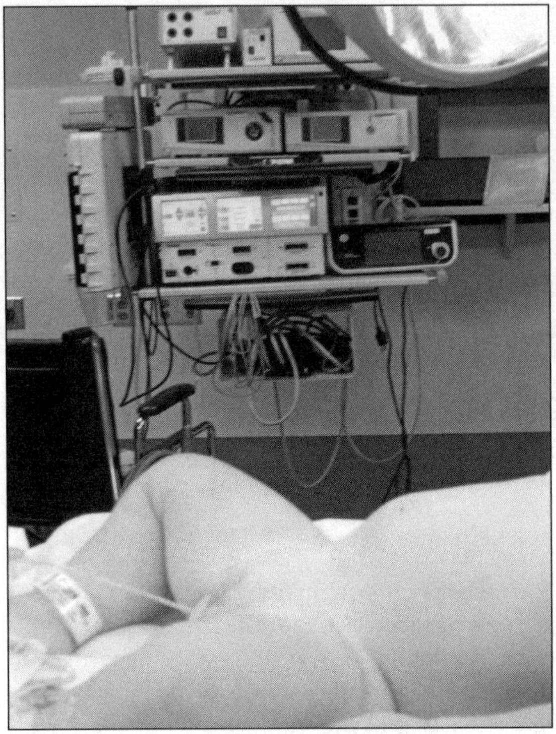

Figure 93.1. Abdominal bulge due to underlying mass.

suggestive of underlying disease (Figure 93.2). On the basis of the radiographic findings, a water-soluble contrast enema is performed (Figure 93.3) that confirms the suspected underlying diagnosis.

- **What is your differential diagnosis at this point?**
- **Are there any elements of history or physical examination that would help you?**
- **What additional diagnostic studies would you like performed?**

Diagnosis

Intussusception

The patient's history of bloody stools, a palpable abdominal mass, and the soft tissue opacification on abdominal radiography are highly suggestive of ileocecal intussusception. Subsequent contrast enema revealed a large intussusception that involves the ileum, cecum, and ascending and transverse colon.

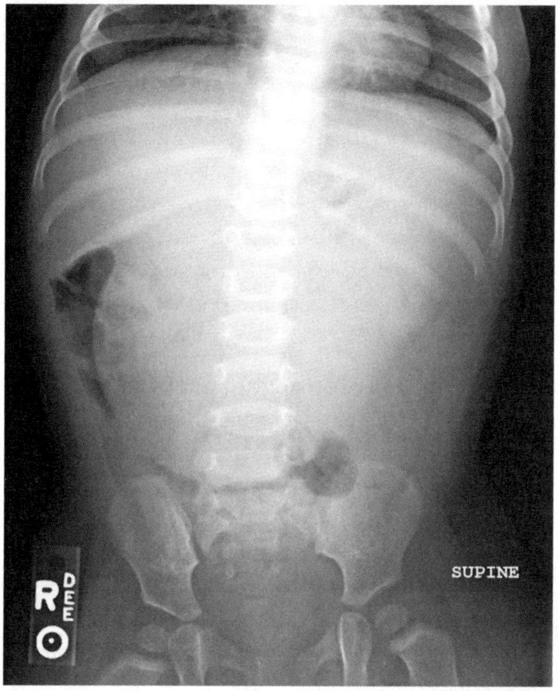

Figure 93.2. Abdominal radiograph showing paucity of air in bowel and a curvilinear mass within the course of the colon.

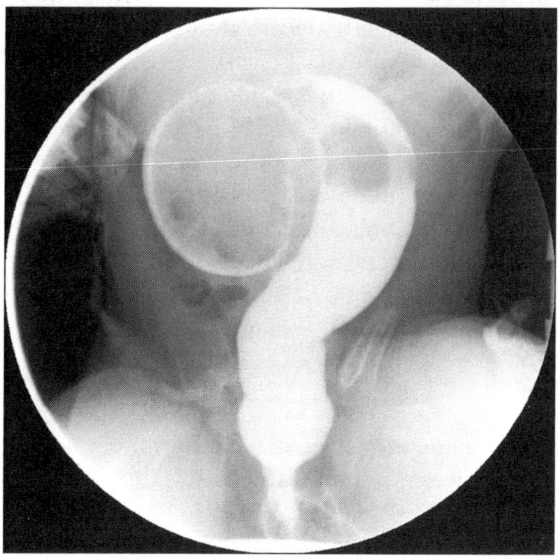

Figure 93.3. Water-soluble contrast enema reveals an intra-intestinal mass.

Discussion

Intussusception occurs when a portion of the proximal segment of the bowel (the intussusceptum) invaginates into a distal bowel segment (the intussuscipiens). Without treatment, bowel obstruction, necrosis, perforation, and death can ensue. Fortunately, most intussusceptions can be reduced by contrast enema. However, some patients require surgical intervention with manual reduction or excision of the affected portion of the bowel. Longer duration of intussusception is associated with increased morbidity and mortality. Thus, prompt recognition and treatment are imperative. Diagnosis is contingent on clinical suspicion and confirmation by abdominal ultrasonography or contrast enema.

Intussusception is the most common cause of bowel obstruction in infants and children between ages 6 and 36 months. Infants between ages 4 and 7 months are most commonly affected. Intussusception rarely occurs in children younger than 2 months, and 70% of cases occur in the first year of life. Most cases are idiopathic, but some, particularly those occurring in children outside the reference age range, form around pathologic lead points, such as a Meckel diverticulum, intestinal polyp, or edema caused by Henoch-Schönlein purpura. Males develop intussusception at roughly twice the rate of females. The incidence is estimated to be 18 to 56 per 100,000 live births, and there is evidence in the United States and abroad that the incidence is decreasing overall.

Infants and children with intussusception present with a variety of signs and symptoms. Vomiting, abdominal pain, bloody stool, and lethargy are among the most common. Unfortunately, these symptoms are nonspecific and carry a vast differential diagnosis. The classic currant jelly stool is generally a late finding that occurs when the bowel wall undergoes significant vascular injury and blood mixes with mucoid material to produce this characteristic appearance. Either gross or occult blood in the stool is present in more than half of children with confirmed intussusception. The classic triad of abdominal pain, vomiting, and bloody stool is observed in less than 50% of affected individuals and should not be relied on for diagnosis. However, this triad is highly predictive of intussusception. To date, no reliable individual discriminating factors have been identified, and the diagnosis of intussusception continues to rely on a high degree of clinical suspicion and confirmatory imaging studies.

Abdominal radiography, ultrasonography, and contrast enema are the 3 most common imaging modalities used in the evaluation of a child with possible intussusception. Abdominal radiography is occasionally indicative of intussusception, but the sensitivity of radiography is too low (29%–50%) to safely exclude the diagnosis. When intussusception is suspected, it must be definitely ruled out with either ultrasonography or contrast enema. The sensitivity and specificity of both studies approach 100%. However, ultrasonography is the preferred initial test because it is not invasive and does not expose the patient to ionizing radiation. If intussusception is found on ultrasonography, stable patients should proceed to contrast enema under ultrasonic or fluoroscopic guidance for initial therapy. Unstable patients and those with evidence of bowel rupture should have emergent surgical consultation.

Differential Diagnosis

The differential diagnosis depends on the presenting symptoms. Gastrointestinal bleeding and abdominal pain in children can be caused by Henoch-Schönlein purpura, hemolytic uremic syndrome, and allergic colitis. Vomiting and abdominal pain have an equally broad differential diagnosis, including infectious gastroenteritis and malrotation with volvulus. From a surgical standpoint, the presence of hematochezia, a palpable abdominal mass, and a curvilinear mass within the course of the colon with a paucity of air in the bowel on abdominal radiography suggests segmental bowel obstruction from either volvulus or a persistent omphalomesenteric duct besides an intussusception.

Management

Contrast enema continues to be the diagnostic criterion standard and first-line therapy for an intussusception. A total of 46% to 80% of intussusceptions can be reduced with enema. Traditionally, a liquid enema was performed under fluoroscopic guidance; however, the current trend is toward air enemas under ultrasonic guidance, which do not use ionizing radiation. The efficacy of the 2 treatments is similar, and the choice of technique primarily depends on the experience of the attending radiologist.

Before any planned contrast enema, intravenous access should be obtained, the infant or child should be fully fluid resuscitated, and a pediatric surgeon should be notified. Many physicians will also administer a dose of intravenous antibiotics. When contrast enema reduces intussusception, the child should be closely monitored because 10% of patients will experience intussusception again. Primary surgical treatment is indicated for unstable patients and those with signs of bowel perforation. Surgical treatment is also necessary when contrast enema fails to reduce the intussusception. Most pediatric surgeons approach uncomplicated, irreducible intussusception with laparoscopic reduction. If necessary, manual reduction of the intussusception is often successful; however, bowel excision may also be necessary. A delay in definitive diagnosis may lead to greater bowel ischemia and greater likelihood of resection.

Patient Course

Unfortunately, the patient's intussusception could not be reduced by contrast enema. The patient was taken to the operating room for an exploratory laparotomy and manual reduction of the intussusception. During the exploratory laparotomy, the patient was found to have necrotic ileum within the intussuscipiens (Figure 93.4). A right hemicolectomy with primary anastomosis was performed. Two days later the patient had abdominal distention with free air seen on abdominal radiography. She returned to the operating room, where an anastomotic leak was repaired. After 3 weeks in the pediatric intensive care unit, she was discharged home in good condition.

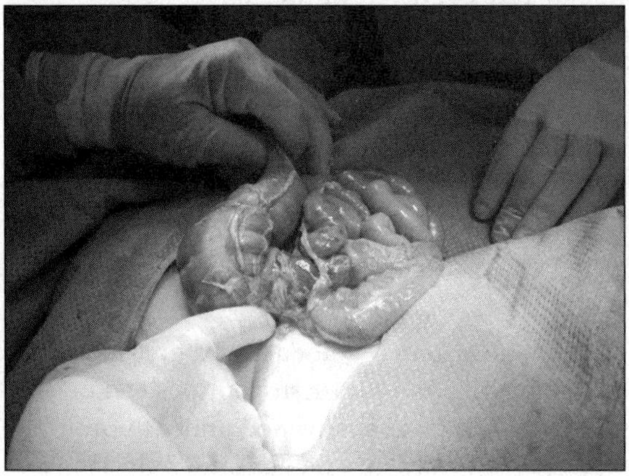

Figure 93.4. Necrotic ileum within the intussuscepted colon.

Summary

- Infants and children with intussusception can present with a wide variety of symptoms, including vomiting, fever, lethargy, and abdominal pain. The classic triad of abdominal pain, hematochezia, and palpable abdominal mass is seen in a few patients.
- Early diagnosis of intussusception depends on a high level of clinical suspicion in any child with nonspecific abdominal findings followed by appropriate radiographic or ultrasonographic evaluation and confirmation with a contrast enema.
- Abdominal radiography, although an appropriate component of the initial workup for gastrointestinal symptoms, lacks the sensitivity to reliably exclude the presence of intussusception.
- Because ultrasonography is a safe, sensitive, and specific test for the diagnosis of intussusceptions, it should be performed early whenever there is clinical suspicion of intussusception.
- Contrast enema is the criterion standard for diagnosis and first-line treatment of intussusception. There is an increasing trend for pneumatic reduction of intussusception compared with hydrostatic reduction. Intravenous line placement, fluid resuscitation, and notification of the pediatric surgeon should be completed before contrast enema.

Laura A. Whittington, DO; David C. Stevens, MD; and Sarah A. Jones, MD, Department of Pediatrics, University of South Dakota Sanford School of Medicine, Sioux Falls, SD

Julie M. Mayo, DO, Department of Pediatrics, University of South Dakota Sanford School of Medicine, Sioux Falls, SD, and Pediatric Hospital Service/Sanford Children's Hospital, Sioux Falls, SD

CHAPTER 94

Intermittent Swelling and Bleeding From the Gums in a 3-Year-Old Girl

Presentation

A 3-year-old girl presents to the emergency department with a history of intermittent swelling and bleeding from her gums for the past 2 months. She has no history of bleeding from any other site. Yesterday she had one episode of hematemesis and appeared pale. There is no fever, cough, runny nose, dental caries, or trauma to the face. Past medical history and family history, including bleeding disorders, are negative. She is not taking any medications.

On examination, her temperature is 98.6°F (37.0°C), heart rate is 132 beats/min, respiratory rate is 26 breaths/min, and blood pressure is 113/52 mm Hg. She appears pale and anxious. A swelling is apparent on her left-sided lower gum, with active bleeding near the second molar tooth and mild swelling of her left cheek. There is associated painless left-sided submandibular lymphadenopathy. The rest of the physical examination findings are normal.

Laboratory investigations reveal hemoglobin of 4.2 g/dL (42 g/L), white blood cell count of 14.2 × 10^3/mcL (14.2 × 10^9/L), platelet count of 249 × 10^3/mcL (249 × 10^9/L), mean corpuscular volume of 62 mcm^3 (62 fL), red blood cell distribution width of 18%, and reticulocyte count of 2%. Serum iron concentration is 13 mcg/dL (2.3 mcmol/L), ferritin is less than 2 ng/mL (4.5 pmol/L), and total iron binding capacity is 571 mcg/dL (102.2 mcmol/L). She receives a packed red blood cell transfusion because of severe anemia. Computed tomography scan of the mandible reveals a lucent, lytic lesion in the left-sided mandible with adjacent soft-tissue involvement (Figure 94.1).

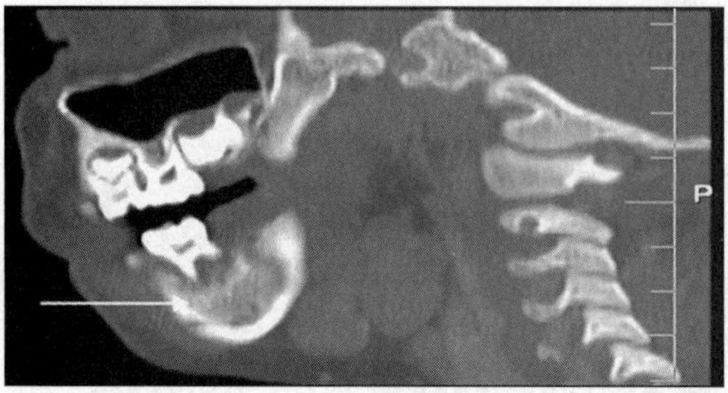

Figure 94.1. Computed tomography scan showing a lucent, lytic lesion on the left side of mandible (arrow), with displacement of tooth and soft-tissue extension.

- **What is your differential diagnosis at this point?**
- **Are there any elements of history or physical examination that would help you?**
- **What additional diagnostic studies would you like performed?**

Discussion

Magnetic resonance imaging revealed an expansive bony lesion in the left-sided mandible with patchy enhancement and cortical breakthrough. Magnetic resonance angiography did not show any feeding vessels. The child was taken to the operating room for evaluation and biopsy. In the operating room, a pulsating mass was felt at the base of the tooth, and aspiration yielded frank blood. The biopsy was aborted and the child underwent arteriography, which revealed a left-sided posterior mandibular arteriovenous malformation (AVM) with the nidus supplied by the distal facial artery branches and by hypertrophied inferior alveolar artery branches. Transcatheter embolization of the facial artery branches was performed, and the parents were advised of the need for a second embolization of the hypertrophied inferior alveolar artery a few months later. The girl was discharged from the hospital receiving iron supplementation and with instructions for follow up with oral maxillofacial and interventional radiology.

The Condition

Vascular malformations are caused by disturbances in angiogenesis and result in the persistence of arteriovenous anastomoses, which are formed during embryonic life. They may be arterial, venous, capillary, lymphatic, or mixed. Vascular malformations of arterial or arteriovenous origin are termed *high-flow vascular malformations* and are the causes of massive hemorrhages. They can occur in any organ in the body, in order of frequency: head and face, upper and lower extremities, trunk, and internal organs. Half of all intraosseous AVMs occur in the maxillofacial region and seldom in the mandible. Such lesions can go unrecognized for years. Arteriovenous malformations are usually present as developmental anomalies from birth and grow in size with physical growth. The peak incidence of presentation of intraosseous vascular lesions is at puberty, with equal frequency in boys and girls. Spontaneous involution has not been described.

Clinical Symptoms

Patients usually present with soft-tissue swelling, local pain, teeth mobility, discoloration of overlying skin and oral mucosal surfaces, paraesthesia and facial asymmetry, local pulsation, periodontal bleeding, or spontaneous bleeding from the tooth. Intraosseous AVMs near the alveolar bone often present with pericoronal bleeding, mobile teeth, and occlusal anomalies. Gingival bleeding seems to be a symptom common in most documented cases. The recurrent bleeding can lead to severe anemia, as seen in our patient. Instances of massive hemorrhage, even exsanguinations, have been documented following the extraction of teeth associated with such AVMs.

Diagnosis

Plain radiography does not reveal any pathognomonic features for these lesions. Arteriovenous malformations may appear as honeycomb radiolucencies or have a soap bubble appearance, and the differential diagnosis includes the conditions mentioned in Box 94.1. Root resorption may be seen on a plain radiograph, creating an appearance of a tooth floating in the adjacent alveolar osseous erosion. An incision biopsy can help in making a definitive diagnosis of the lesions, which mimic AVM on radiography. A computed tomography scan and magnetic resonance image can show the shape, extent, and boundaries of lytic lesion and the involvement of major vessels in intraosseous AVM. Superselective angiography can provide crucial information on the feeder arteries, draining veins, flow rate, and collateral flows of the AVM. Such examinations can be of great help for definitive diagnosis.

Box 94.1. Differential Diagnosis of Lesions Appearing as Honeycomb Radiolucencies or Soap Bubble

- Follicular cyst
- Aneurysmal cyst
- Ameloblastomas
- Ameloblastic fibromas
- Odontogenic keratocysts
- Giant cell granulomas
- Malignant primary or metastatic tumors

Management

Management of AVMs in the maxillofacial area is typically complex and requires a multidisciplinary team approach. In the case of intraosseous AVMs of the mandible, a combination of embolization and surgery is recommended. Endovascular embolization therapy alone can cure mandibular and maxillary vascular malformations that have limited soft-tissue involvement without the functional limitation and cosmetic deformities incurred with surgical resections. For larger AVMs that have soft-tissue involvement, an embolization procedure controls the acute hemorrhage but does not eliminate the risk of a recurrence due to the presence of a collateral circulation. Resection of the mandibular fragment containing the lesion is needed for complete healing. In some cases, curettage of the resected fragment with immediate reimplantation has been tried, which reduces the morbidity associated with the procedure and the difficulty of reconstruction. Lesional curettage without resection preserves bone support, but the excision is often inadequate. Rarely, in extensive vascular malformations, total eradication of the vascular malformation may become difficult.

Lessons for the Physician

- Arteriovenous malformations of the mandible may lead to fatal hemorrhages, especially during routine dental procedures.
- Any child presenting with gingival bleeding or swelling should be suspected of having this condition.
- Aggressive management with embolization to stop the bleeding and a close follow-up evaluation and possible surgical management should be considered.

Bhawana Arora, MD, and Usha Sethuraman, MD, Children's Hospital of Michigan, Detroit, MI

CHAPTER 95

Sharp, Right-Sided Abdominal Pain in an 8-Year-Old Boy

Presentation

An 8-year-old boy who has asthma presents to the emergency department with the acute onset of sharp, right-sided abdominal pain. His pain is 10/10 on the pain scale. He denies fever, nausea, vomiting, diarrhea, or trauma to the abdomen. His last bowel movement was yesterday. He admits to some pain with urination. He remains hungry despite the pain. He has no known sick contacts.

Physical examination reveals an uncomfortable child, crying with pain. His temperature is 98.6°F (37.0°C), heart rate is 85 beats/min, blood pressure is 118/71 mm Hg, respiratory rate is 20 breaths/min, and oxygen saturation is 99% on room air. He weighs 40 kg, which is at the 95th percentile for his age. He has hypoactive bowel sounds, a mildly distended abdomen, and right lower quadrant abdominal tenderness. He also has voluntary guarding but no rebound tenderness. The Rovsing and obturator signs are negative.

His laboratory results are as follows: white blood cell count, 8.1×10^3/mcL (8.1×10^9/L) (63% neutrophils, 21% lymphocytes, 9% monocytes, 6% eosinophils); hemoglobin, 11.7 g/dL (117 g/L); hematocrit, 35% (0.35); and platelet count, 268×10^3/mcL (268×10^9/L). His serum electrolyte concentrations are normal, and urinalysis shows clear yellow urine with negative white blood cell esterase and nitrite tests, 1 white blood cell per high-power field, and 1 red blood cell per high-power field. An imaging study reveals the diagnosis.

- **What is your differential diagnosis at this point?**
- **Are there any elements of history or physical examination that would help you?**
- **What additional diagnostic studies would you like performed?**

Discussion

A computed tomography scan of the abdomen and pelvis revealed a hazy density in the anterior mesenteric fat of the right lower quadrant, suggesting inflammation (Figure 95.1). The appendix was normal in caliber and showed air throughout. There was mild thickening of the terminal ileum, but the cecum and ascending colon appeared normal. There was a moderate amount of free fluid collected in the pelvis. These findings are characteristic of omental infarction.

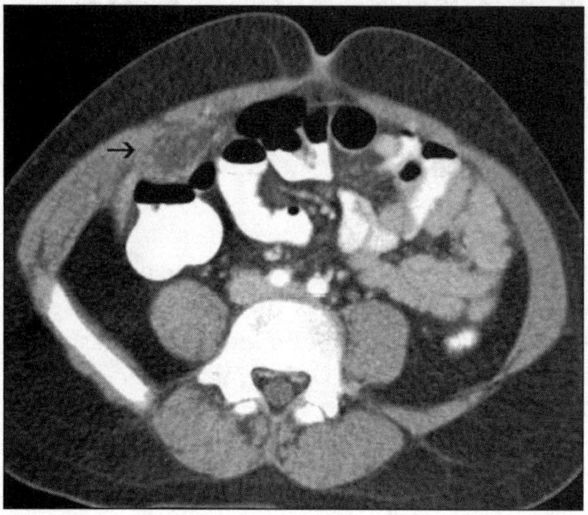

Figure 95.1. Computed tomography scan showing an area of focal mesenteric inflammation immediately inferior to the liver edge, suggesting omental infarction.

The Condition

Omental infarction results when the omentum twists around a pivotal point and compromises venous return. The distal omentum becomes congested and edematous. Hemorrhagic extravasation results in the characteristic serosanguineous free fluid in the peritoneal cavity. As the torsion progresses, arterial occlusion leads to necrosis of the omentum.

There are both primary and secondary forms of omental infarction. The primary form has no associated intra-abdominal pathology. Predisposing factors include anatomic variations of the omentum, such as accessory omentum, bifid omentum, irregular accumulations of omental fat in obese patients, and a narrowed omental pedicle. In addition, there may be an embryonic variant of blood supply to the omentum that makes it susceptible to kinking and twisting. Precipitating factors are those that cause displacement of the omentum, such as trauma, exercise, and hyperperistalsis. Secondary omental infarction is more common and is associated with such abdominal diseases as cysts, tumors, and hernial sacs.

The incidence of torsion is higher on the right side of the omentum due to its greater size and mobility. Therefore, omental infarction typically presents with right-sided abdominal pain and localized peritoneal signs. Frequently, fever and gastrointestinal complaints (such as nausea, vomiting, and diarrhea) are absent. Leukocytosis is an inconsistent finding. The diagnosis should be suspected in obese children.

Diagnosis

The diagnosis of omental infarction is confirmed with imaging studies. Ultrasonography usually shows a focal area of increased echogenicity in the omentum between the umbilicus and right side of the colon, corresponding to the point of maximal tenderness. The omental mass is typically nonmobile and fixed to the right side of the colon. However, the diagnosis is based primarily on computed tomography scan findings of a heterogenous soft-tissue mass within an area of omental fat located between the anterior abdominal wall and the transverse or ascending colon. There are surrounding inflammatory changes and, rarely, reactive bowel wall changes leading to bowel wall thickening adjacent to the area of omental infarction.

Management

The treatment of omental infarction remains controversial. Operative management, either open or laparoscopic, is the traditional approach and is aimed at preventing the development of local abscess and adhesions due to the presence of necrotic tissue in the abdomen. However, case reports of a nonoperative approach to treatment that consists of prophylactic antibiotics and analgesics indicate that omental infarction can be self-limited without significant sequelae.

This patient was admitted to the hospital for nonoperative management, focusing on pain control. He remained afebrile throughout his hospital stay, and his pain gradually improved over the next 48 hours. A repeat white blood cell count the day after admission was 7.0×10^3/mcL (7.0×10^9/L). He had no complications and was discharged from the hospital 2 days after admission.

Lessons for the Physician

- The differential diagnosis of acute, right-sided abdominal pain in children includes appendicitis, cholecystitis, pyelonephritis, nephrolithiasis, and ovarian torsion.
- Omental infarction is an important diagnosis to consider, yet it is often overlooked because traditionally it has been considered rare in the pediatric population. However, an increasing number of cases of omental infarction have been diagnosed with more frequent use of computed tomography scans and the increasing incidence of childhood obesity.
- Although omental infarction is often diagnosed during surgery for presumed appendicitis, a conservative approach is possible if the diagnosis can be made preoperatively.

Gia Bradley, MD, and Hoover Adger Jr, MD, MPH, The Johns Hopkins School of Medicine, Baltimore, MD

CHAPTER 96

Severe Right Lower Quadrant Colicky Pain and Mild Right-Sided Flank Pain in an 8-Year-Old Girl

Presentation

An 8-year-old girl presents with the acute onset of severe right lower quadrant colicky pain and mild right-sided flank pain associated with nausea and vomiting. She has no fever, dysuria, or diarrhea. Yesterday she had a similar but milder episode that lasted for a few hours and resolved spontaneously. At the age of 2 years, she underwent an uneventful bilateral inguinal hernia repair.

On physical examination, the girl is in severe pain. Her temperature is 97.6°F (36.4°C), pulse is 93 beats/min, blood pressure is 100/62 mm Hg, and respirations are 22 breaths/min. Her abdomen is soft and nondistended. Bowel sounds are normal. There is mild right lower quadrant tenderness to deep palpation without any peritoneal signs. Neither costovertebral tenderness nor palpable masses are present.

Normal values are found on a complete blood cell count and measurements of serum electrolytes, glucose, and urea nitrogen. Urinalysis reveals 5 to 10 red blood cells per high-power field.

One additional test helps determine the cause of her illness.

- **What is your differential diagnosis at this point?**
- **Are there any elements of history or physical examination that would help you?**
- **What additional diagnostic studies would you like performed?**

Discussion

Computed tomography of the abdomen showed ovarian enlargement, small peripheral follicles, and some intraperitoneal fluid. These findings were consistent with the diagnosis of ovarian torsion. At surgery, the right ovary and fallopian tube were found to be twisted and infarcted. A large, hemorrhagic follicular cyst occupied the right ovary.

Abdominal pain is the most common chief concern of patients seen in pediatric emergency departments. The causative condition is often obscure, with an unconfirmed or uncertain diagnosis reported in more than 40% of patients.

Ovarian torsion is a well-known yet poorly recognized clinical entity that can involve the fallopian tube, ovary, and ancillary structures. It is the fifth most common gynecologic emergency, with a reported incidence of 3% in one series of acute gynecologic complaints. However, the diagnosis of ovarian torsion is often missed. The diagnosis is delayed in most affected patients because of failure to consider this condition, which can have nonspecific clinical findings.

Pathophysiology

Adnexal torsion is typically associated with a mass such as a cyst, which is most likely, or a benign or malignant tumor. Functional ovarian cysts in children usually develop following hormonal stimulation that occurs during 2 peak periods: the first year of life and around the time of menarche. Even cysts that occur normally with ovulation may cause ovarian enlargement and predispose to torsion, as can large hemorrhagic cysts. It is believed that the increase in the weight and the size of the ovary may alter the anatomy of the fallopian tube and cause twisting.

Adnexal torsion presents as severe sudden pain due to twisting of the ovary, the fallopian tube, or a paratubal cyst. The most common form of torsion involves the ovary and the distal aspect of the fallopian tube, wherein the ovary rotates on its pedicle and compromises the blood supply. Torsion of the ovary initially interferes with the venous and lymphatic circulation. If unrelieved, torsion of the ovary progresses rapidly to occlusion of the arterial circulation, which may be irreversible and lead to necrosis. Because necrosis can lead to loss of fertility, infection, sepsis, and death, torsion is considered a surgical emergency.

Clinical Features

The symptoms and signs associated with ovarian torsion are variable, often nonspecific, and can be misleading. The classic history in ovarian torsion is the abrupt onset of colicky pain in a lower quadrant, with radiation to the flank or groin that mimics renal colic. The pain associated with torsion is acute, severe, and unilateral. Most patients have nausea, vomiting, and lower quadrant pain, but these findings are associated with many other abdominal causes of pain and are not specific for ovarian torsion. Objective findings also are variable and rarely impressive in patients experiencing ovarian torsion. This paucity of objective findings may suggest the need to consider ovarian torsion. Patients who have ovarian torsion generally present without fever and have a normal white blood cell count and differential, although some may have an elevated white blood cell count or low-grade fever. The patient may describe a prior history of similar episodes.

The ability to diagnose adnexal torsion depends on the physician's consideration of the condition in the differential diagnosis, which is especially important when a patient has an ovarian mass. It is important to remember that even if the patient is pregnant, ovarian torsion may still occur. Ovarian torsion has been reported in patients who underwent untwisting of the ischemic adnexa when they were 6 to 20 weeks pregnant. It also is very important in pregnant patients to differentiate torsion from an ectopic pregnancy, which can present as severe abrupt pain and an adnexal mass.

Differential Diagnosis

The first priority in evaluating a child who has abdominal pain is to determine if he or she requires immediate surgical intervention. Besides ovarian torsion, the differential diagnosis of acute lower abdominal pain in a girl must include acute appendicitis, ectopic pregnancy, intussusception, intestinal obstruction, and ruptured ovarian cyst. Significant pain can also be caused by kidney stones, pelvic inflammatory disease, constipation, gastroenteritis, mittelschmerz, and urinary tract infection.

Ovarian torsion should be considered in patients who have moderate to severe unilateral adnexal pain and tenderness. In addition, an adnexal mass is often palpable. A history of prior torsion is important. Patients may present with recurrent episodes of pain over several months, which may be caused by incomplete torsions that resolve. It is important to realize that prepubertal girls can experience torsion of the ovary; the physician should not discount this condition in a young girl who has a compatible clinical picture.

Gastroenteritis is the most common cause of abdominal pain not requiring surgery; appendicitis is the most common cause for which surgery is necessary. Acute appendicitis is the condition misdiagnosed most frequently in patients who have adnexal torsion. In many cases, torsion is indistinguishable from acute appendicitis on clinical grounds. Initially, patients who have appendicitis often report poorly defined, constant pain in the periumbilical region. As the disease progresses, the pain shifts from the periumbilical region to the right lower quadrant. Anorexia, nausea, vomiting, and fever often follow the pain. The differentiation of appendicitis from adnexal torsion often requires imaging studies.

It is difficult to diagnose ectopic pregnancy accurately by history and physical examination alone. Abdominal pain associated with amenorrhea is the most common presenting complaint. Diagnostic accuracy has improved with the combination of serum quantitative chorionic gonadotropin assays and transvaginal ultrasonography.

Laboratory Testing

General laboratory studies are usually not helpful in diagnosing ovarian torsion, but they may help diagnose other conditions. A pregnancy test must be performed in the emergency department on all female patients of reproductive age who have abdominal pain, regardless of their sexual or menstrual history, which may be unreliable. In a variety of situations, it is essential that physicians consider adolescent girls pregnant until they have been tested. Ectopic pregnancy is a fatal condition without intervention and is the leading cause of death in the first trimester of pregnancy. A pregnant patient having abdominal pain must be considered to have an ectopic pregnancy until proven otherwise.

This patient had microscopic hematuria, which has been noted in several case reports of adnexal torsion. The hematuria may be related to the retroperitoneal inflammation associated with torsion, similar to what occurs in cases of retroperitoneal appendicitis.

Ultrasonography is the primary modality used to diagnose torsion and reveals the affected ovary, usually as a uniformly echogenic mass. Sonographic findings consistent with torsion include a solid, cystic, or complex pelvic mass with or without a fluid collection in the pouch of Douglas. A more specific finding is the demonstration of multiple follicles (8–12 mm in size) in the cortical portions of a unilaterally enlarged ovary. This finding is attributed to the transudation of fluid into the follicles as part of the congestion of the ovary that results from circulatory impairment. Sonographic identification of a normal ovary in its normal position may help exclude the diagnosis of torsion. Because most cases of torsion are due to large ovarian cysts or masses, the finding of a normal-size ovary makes adnexal torsion unlikely.

Doppler ultrasonography commonly is used to evaluate suspected adnexal torsion. When torsion is present, the lack of blood flow on Doppler examination probably indicates that an ovary is beyond salvage.

Computed tomography often reveals a complex ovarian mass and can demonstrate or exclude other abdominal and pelvic disease, such as appendicitis. However, the definitive diagnosis and management of torsion require laparotomy.

Management

Prompt diagnosis is important both to establish the diagnosis and to increase the rate of salvage of the ovary. An ovarian salvage rate of less than 10% has been reported. The interval between the onset of symptoms and the necrosis of adnexal structures is not known, but in the case of testicular torsion, irreversible changes may occur after only 4 hours. Early surgical intervention is required in both entities to preserve fertility.

Treatment of ovarian torsion mandates early surgical exploration and may require unilateral salpingo-oophorectomy. When the diagnosis remains unclear, laparoscopy can assist in making the diagnosis. Laparoscopy is often performed when an adnexal mass is not demonstrated on physical examination or on imaging studies and the diagnosis is unclear. Salpingo-oophorectomy may be necessary if there is evidence of necrotic tissue and was the treatment of choice for all torsions in the past; however, multiple studies support the concept of untwisting nonnecrotic adnexa if possible. When unilateral torsion is diagnosed, oophoropexy (plication) of the contralateral adnexa may be indicated.

Lessons for the Physician

Ovarian torsion is a cause of acute abdominal pain that requires prompt surgical intervention and should always be considered in the differential diagnosis of a girl who has acute abdominal pain. Considering torsion is especially relevant when evaluating patients who are being observed for the possibility of appendicitis. Early diagnosis of adnexal torsion is imperative to preserve fertility. Time is critical when ovarian torsion is present. A high level of clinical suspicion and expeditious imaging may decrease the surgical delay and improve the likelihood of ovarian salvage.

Muhammad Waseem, MD; Sandhya Ganti, MD; and Joel Gernsheimer, MD, Lincoln Hospital, Bronx, NY

CHAPTER 97

11-Year-Old Boy With Pain in the Left Lower Quadrant of His Abdomen, Radiating to His Back

Presentation

An 11-year-old boy comes to the emergency department in the evening complaining of pain in the left lower quadrant (LLQ) of his abdomen that has been present all day, is worsening, and now radiates to his back. The pain is sharp and stabbing and is aggravated by walking and stretching but not by deep breathing. Positioning and rest do not relieve the pain. He has had one soft stool today and denies vomiting, fever, dysuria, cough, and trauma.

On physical examination, the boy is afebrile and has a pulse of 102 beats/min, respiratory rate of 20 breaths/min, and blood pressure of 116/68 mm Hg. There is tenderness on deep palpation in the LLQ as well as rebound tenderness. No psoas or obturator signs are detected, and bowel sounds are normal. Rectal examination does not cause abdominal pain, and the stool is negative for occult blood. No back or scrotal tenderness is present. The remainder of the physical findings are normal.

His white blood cell count is 8.1×10^3/mcL (8.1×10^9/L), amylase level is 54 U/L, and blood glucose level is 92 mg/dL (5.1 mmol/L). Electrolyte and liver function levels are normal. Urinalysis is negative for nitrites and white blood cell esterase and shows 3 to 5 white blood cells and 1 to 3 red blood cells per high-power field. Abdominal radiography documents a normal gas pattern and a moderate amount of fecal matter.

The patent is admitted and given intravenous fluids. He awakens when the LLQ is palpated. Abdominal ultrasonography shows normal findings. Further imaging leads to a diagnosis.

- **What is your differential diagnosis at this point?**
- **Are there any elements of history or physical examination that would help you?**
- **What additional diagnostic studies would you like performed?**

Discussion

Computed tomography of the abdomen and pelvis with oral and rectal contrast showed a localized infiltration of blood or edema fluid into the fat between the colon and the abdominal wall muscle in the LLQ, just below the level of the iliac crest. The findings were consistent with epiploic appendagitis (EA).

The family and patient were educated and reassured about this condition. The boy was discharged from the hospital to follow up with his pediatrician in 1 week. The abdominal pain resolved in 1 month with no complications.

The Condition

The epiploic appendages are located along the colon and are outpouchings comprised of both fat and blood vessels. They run along the serosal surface, from the cecum to the rectosigmoid junction, and vary in thickness and length. Among their functions are carrying out local defense against infection (similar to the omentum), storing fat, and acting as a cushion against peristalsis or as a reservoir for blood when there is contraction. Epiploic appendagitis is caused by an ischemic event that is believed to result from either torsion of the epiploic appendage or spontaneous venous thrombosis.

A similar condition, segmental omental infarction (OI), is hypothesized to also be caused by vascular compromise, either from increased abdominal pressure or postprandial vascular congestion. The susceptibility to infarction is high because the blood supply of the omentum is prone to injury. It is embryonic in nature, can be supplied by 1 or 2 arteries, and is drained by 1 vein.

Torsion of an appendage is the most common cause of EA. Keeping in mind that EA and OI are diagnoses of exclusion, the incidence is more common in males and is not associated with any particular ethnic group, lifestyle, or genetic pattern. The adult literature states that the condition is more common in the fourth and fifth decades of life. Pediatric data suggest that the structure of fat in children younger than 2 years might be protective, although patients as young as 2 years have experienced EA.

Differential Diagnosis

There are several approaches to developing a differential diagnosis for abdominal pain. When the history and physical findings suggest a specific location for the pain, an anatomic approach can be useful. In this case, the physician must consider systems in the LLQ, including gastrointestinal, genitourinary, and musculoskeletal. Had the patient been female, a gynecologic disorder would have to be considered.

The gastrointestinal structure in the LLQ is colon. The most common cause of pain in this area is constipation, which can present with a wide spectrum of discomfort patterns. Inflammatory bowel disease, as well as inflammation of an appendix located to the left of the midline, must be considered. Less common are internal hernias.

Genitourinary pathology includes kidney stones, which classically produce a severe, colicky pain that is felt in the flank. Musculoskeletal injuries consist of abdominal wall strains and tears that present as more superficial pain. Disorders affecting females include diseases of the ovary or fallopian tube, such as torsion, pelvic inflammatory disease, tubo-ovarian abscess, and ruptured ovarian cyst. Pain localizing to the right lower quadrant produces a similar list of possibilities, although appendicitis is much more likely.

Making the Diagnosis

Distinguishing between EA and OI is impossible clinically. Both may present similarly with a gradual onset. Most often, the patient does not appear ill, is afebrile, does not complain of nausea and vomiting, and has normal bowel movements and an unchanged appetite. The pain can range from dull to sharp and can be colicky or constant. It is usually localized, and palpation can elicit rebound tenderness. Epiploic appendagitis is more common on the left side. The pain may begin after an increase in intra-abdominal pressure, such as caused by coughing, deep inhalation, or stretching.

Laboratory results are usually unremarkable and should prompt the physician to consider this diagnosis by exclusion. Computed tomography and ultrasonography can help confirm the diagnosis. The lesion of EA is generally small and prone to developing a thickened rim of visceral peritoneum, which is referred to as the "ring sign." The lesion resulting from OI is larger and has a greater mass effect on the adjacent bowel wall. It lacks the ring sign.

If the clinical findings and results of imaging convince the physician that EA or OI is likely and disorders requiring surgery are excluded, a conservative approach is appropriate. There may be situations in which laparotomy may be necessary to resolve the diagnostic dilemma.

Treatment

Surgical ligation is the treatment when the diagnosis results from exploratory laparotomy. Nonsteroidal anti-inflammatory drugs are the mainstay of therapy, along with education and support, when the condition is diagnosed without surgery. Potential sequelae include obstruction, intussusception, abscess formation, fever, anorexia, and obstipation.

Lessons for the Physician

A patient who presents with abdominal pain forces the physician to construct a long differential list of conditions. A comprehensive history and thorough physical examination help narrow the diagnostic possibilities and should focus any further diagnostic testing. Imaging can assist in making the diagnosis, especially when a specific process is suspected. When a patient is found to have epiploic appendagitis or omental infarction (which are diagnoses made by exclusion with corroboration by imaging), pain relief, education, and encouragement constitute appropriate therapy.

Francesco Mulè, MD, Jacobi Medical Center, Bronx, NY

Daniel Rauch, MD, Children's Hospital at Westchester Medical Center, Valhalla, NY

CHAPTER 98

Sudden, Sharp Left Upper Quadrant Abdominal Pain, Nausea, and Vomiting in an 11-Year-Old Girl

Presentation

An 11-year-old girl is admitted to the hospital because of sudden, sharp left upper quadrant (LUQ) abdominal pain, nausea, and vomiting. She has no history of chronic illness, recent acute illness, or trauma. Physical examination reveals normal blood pressure (110/80 mm Hg), mild tachycardia (95 beats/min), and moderate tachypnea (30 breaths/min). Abdominal examination documents a 10-cm tender, mobile mass in her left-sided flank with associated guarding.

Her hemoglobin level is 13.6 g/dL (136 g/L), white blood cell count is 17.2 × 10^3/mcL (17.2 × 10^9/L), and platelet count is 127 × 10^3/mcL (127 × 10^9/L). Blood electrolyte values and hepatic and pancreatic enzyme levels are within the reference range. Abdominal ultrasonography shows free peritoneal fluid in the LUQ as well as another finding, further delineated by abdominal computed tomography (CT), that reveals the cause of her pain.

- **What is your differential diagnosis at this point?**
- **Are there any elements of history or physical examination that would help you?**
- **What additional diagnostic studies would you like performed?**

Discussion

Imaging revealed a moderately enlarged spleen located in the left-sided flank that showed signs of infarction. A left-sided subcostal laparotomy was performed, the diagnosis of torsion of a wandering spleen was confirmed, and a total splenectomy was performed. The patient's postoperative course was uneventful, and she was discharged on postoperative day 6 after receiving vaccination for *Streptococcus pneumoniae* and *Haemophilus influenzae.* Oral penicillin V was prescribed for life. Eighteen months later, the patient is in good health.

The Symptom

The differential diagnosis of LUQ abdominal pain in children includes disorders of the spleen, stomach, colon, and kidneys. Splenic disorders are the most common and include congestion (primarily in hematologic diseases), rupture (posttraumatic or with hematologic conditions), and infarction (often related to sickle cell disease).

Upper digestive tract disorders such as gastroenteritis or mesenteric lymphadenitis (often accompanied by fever, vomiting, and viral symptoms) and ulcer (commonly causing pain related to eating patterns) may also cause LUQ abdominal pain. Colonic diseases, especially those affecting the splenic flexure, such as colitis (either inflammatory or infectious), which are often accompanied by diarrhea and bleeding, should be considered. Less commonly, constipation resulting from Hirschsprung disease causes LUQ pain.

Urologic disorders are a common cause of LUQ abdominal pain. Associated findings include fever, as with infection and some tumors, or hematuria (tumors). Obstruction of the collecting system can lead to hydronephrosis. Physical examination often discloses an abdominal or flank mass.

Although far less common, extra-abdominal causes of LUQ pain should not be ignored, including pericarditis and pneumonia.

The Condition

Wandering spleen (WS) is characterized by incomplete fixation of the spleen's ligaments. Torsion of a WS, a very rare disorder, occurring in only 0.2% of all cases of splenectomy, usually affects young adults and adults between 20 and 40 years of age. Only 33% of cases occur in children, as in this case. In adults, there is a female predominance of 2 to 4:1; in children, the ratio is nearly 1:1.

Wandering spleen, the second most frequent splenic malformation after accessory spleen (AS), may be acquired or congenital. The acquired form is usually due to hormonal changes in multiparous females, including slackening of the abdominal wall and laxity of the splenic ligaments. The congenital form is due to a failure of development of the dorsal mesogastrium by lack of fusion of the dorsal peritoneum. Consequently, splenic ligaments (phrenicosplenic, splenorenal, phrenicocolic, pancreaticosplenic, gastrosplenic, splenocolic) are missing or only partially formed.

Accessory spleen is a different entity and occurs far more frequently than WS. It is estimated that 10% to 30% of the population has an AS. Accessory spleen can be defined as a small globular mass of supernumerary splenic tissue. The most frequent location (around 20%) is the splenic hilum. Other sites include the vicinity of the tail of the pancreas and the gastrosplenic or splenorenal ligaments within the pancreatic tail, in the wall of the stomach or bowel, in the greater omentum or mesentery, or even in the pelvis and scrotum. Accessory spleens are usually about 1 cm in diameter.

An AS is an incidental finding of no clinical significance in most patients. Awareness of its presence is important in a patient who requires splenectomy because failure to remove it may result in persistence of the condition that created the need for splenectomy. An AS may be of clinical importance as a source of preservable splenic tissue in cases of a ruptured primary spleen.

Clinical Findings

Clinical presentations of WS can range from an asymptomatic, painless state in 60% of cases to acute or chronic abdominal pain in 40%. Physical findings often include a firm, painful, ovoid mass palpable in the LUQ associated with fullness and rebound tenderness.

Complications of WS, occurring in up to 60% of cases, include torsion, infarction, partial portal hypertension, hemorrhage, and thrombosis. Patients experiencing splenic torsion usually present with vomiting, fever, acute pain, and hypovolemic shock. If overlooked, torsion may lead to infarction, gangrene, abscess, pancreatic necrosis, or variceal hemorrhage. Wandering spleen can cause partial portal hypertension prior to splenic infarction by mechanical modification of the flux in the splenic vein. Over time, this mechanism can cause the development of esophageal varices, which can bleed, especially if torsion occurs. It is interesting that the detection of portal hypertension can lead to discovery of a WS and allow treatment before torsion occurs.

Diagnosis

Diagnosing torsion of a WS is difficult and usually requires imaging. Abdominal ultrasonography demonstrates the absence of a spleen in the left-sided upper abdomen and a hypoechoic abdominal mass. Later, due to infarction, a hyperechoic or heterogeneous mass may appear. Doppler ultrasonography shows torsion of the pedicle and absent blood flow.

Abdominal CT is the definitive diagnostic technique. The most diagnostically accurate finding is a circular, whorled structure that has alternating bands of radiolucency and radiodensity, representing the twisted splenic pedicle (Figure 98.1).

Generally, the spleen is located in an abnormal position and fails to enhance with the use of intravenous contrast material because of complete infarction (Figure 98.2). Occasionally, the enhancement may be heterogeneous or peripheral (subcapsular).

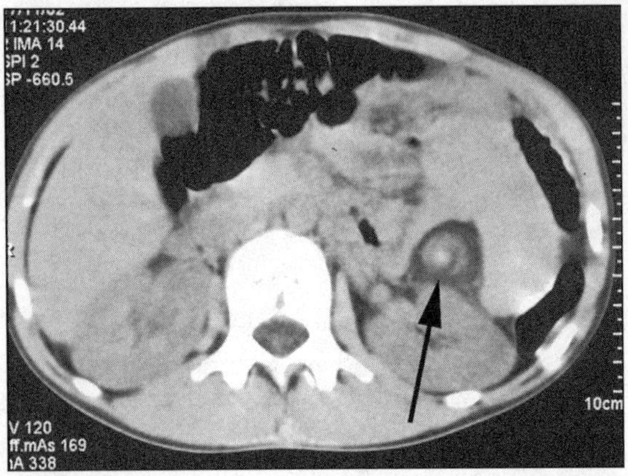

Figure 98.1. Computed tomography scan without contrast showing a twisted splenic pedicle with edema (black arrow) associated with a round filling defect area representing a fresh thrombus in a splenic vessel (hyperdense center).

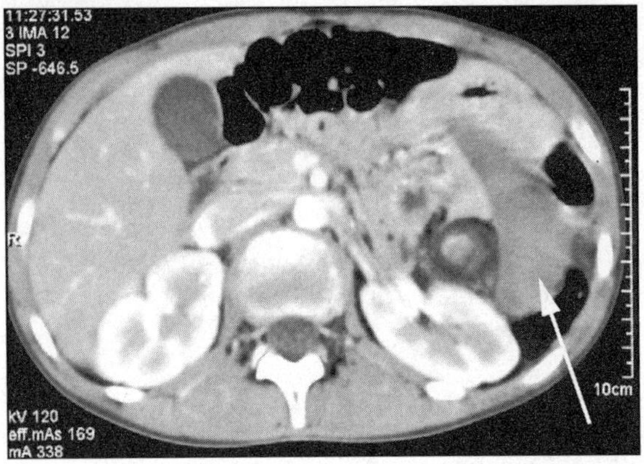

Figure 98.2. Computed tomography scan showing the absence of splenic contrast enhancement after injection (white arrow).

Treatment

The treatment of WS, if diagnosed before torsion, is splenopexy rather than splenectomy, to preserve splenic function. The spleen may be repositioned in the LUQ laparoscopically. If torsion and infarction have occurred, as in this case, either laparoscopic or open splenectomy is mandatory (Figure 98.3). In the rare cases in which the spleen is viable after detorsion, conservative treatment by splenopexy is appropriate. One surgical technique involves creating a pocket out of mesh, into which the spleen is placed. The mesh is sutured to the abdominal wall, preventing torsion.

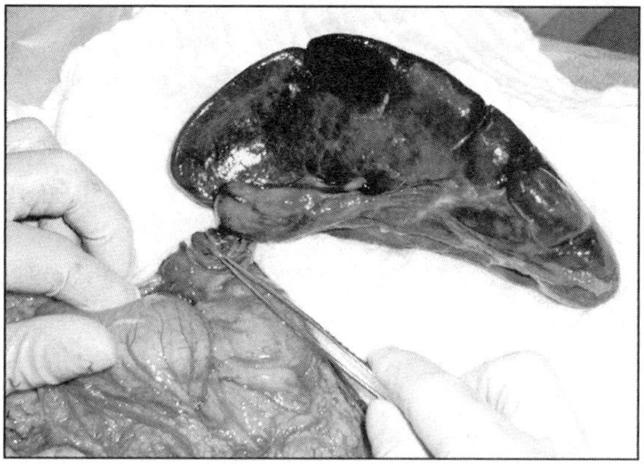

Figure 98.3. Operative view of the infarcted spleen showing the twisted pedicle.

Lessons for the Physician

Deficiencies in the function of splenic ligaments, either from a congenital condition or acquired because of hormonal effects, may lead to wandering spleen, a very rare entity occurring primarily in multiparous women and children. Wandering spleen predisposes to torsion, which may lead to serious complications such as infarction, abscess, variceal hemorrhage, or pancreatic necrosis. Splenectomy is the only treatment when infarction occurs.

Le ́on Maggiori, MD; Olivier Poujade, MD; Toufic Ata, MD; and Elie Chouillard, MD, Center Hospitalier Intercommunal, Poissy, France

Part 18

Urology

CHAPTER 99

Scrotal Swelling in a 7-Year-Old Boy

Presentation

A 7-year-old boy comes to the clinic because of scrotal swelling that he first noted 36 hours ago and disclosed to his mother today. He has been well and denies trauma, fever, nausea, vomiting, hematuria, or dysuria. He is taking no medications. His mother's brother had testicular cancer at 20 years of age.

Physical examination reveals a well-developed, friendly boy whose axillary temperature is 98.6°F (37.0°C), pulse is 90 beats/min, respirations are 20 breaths/min, blood pressure is 100/70 mm Hg, pulse oximetry saturation is 100%, height is 122 cm (50th percentile), and weight is 22.5 kg (50th percentile). Examination yields normal results, with the exception of the scrotal swelling. Inspection of the genitalia shows Sexual Maturity Rating 1 (prepubertal) sexual development. The testes are of normal size, shape, and position, with no palpable masses or obvious deformities. The scrotum is diffusely edematous over the left side and slightly tender to palpation. Transillumination of the scrotum appears normal, and there are no hernias. Laboratory evaluation reveals a normal urinalysis, complete blood cell count, and chemistry panel results. Further testing suggests a diagnosis.

- **What is your differential diagnosis at this point?**
- **Are there any elements of history or physical examination that would help you?**
- **What additional diagnostic studies would you like performed?**

Discussion

Differential Diagnosis

Acute swelling of the scrotum represents a potential emergency that requires prompt evaluation and management. The differential diagnosis is broad and encompasses both medical and surgical diseases. Often it is useful to classify conditions causing acute scrotal swelling as those associated with pain and those not associated with pain. Conditions causing painful scrotal swelling include testicular torsion, torsion of the appendix testis, orchitis, epididymitis, incarcerated hernia, Henoch-Schönlein purpura, and severe scrotal trauma. Conditions causing painless scrotal swelling include varicocele, hydrocele, testicular tumor, inguinal hernia, and acute idiopathic scrotal edema.

Testicular torsion presents with the abrupt onset of severe pain and swelling in the scrotum. It is associated with the so-called bell-clapper deformity, an anomaly in which a thin membrane called the tunica vaginalis completely surrounds the testis, epididymis, and the distal portion of the spermatic cord in such a way that the testis is allowed to rotate freely, leading to vascular compromise. Physical examination usually demonstrates unilateral swelling of the involved side of the scrotum and testis. Discoloration is a late finding. In addition, a high-riding testis, with the other testis demonstrating an abnormal, transverse lie, may suggest the diagnosis. The cremasteric reflex is notably absent, and lack of pain relief with gentle lifting of the affected testis (negative Prehn sign) is also suggestive. Results of urinalysis are normal. The diagnosis is made most often clinically, but color Doppler ultrasonography is frequently employed when the clinical picture is not clear. Treatment, which consists of surgical detorsion and fixation of the testis to the scrotal wall (orchiopexy), may lead to salvage of the affected gonad if initiated promptly. Torsion of the testis is considered a bilateral disorder, and the other testis is fixated to avoid future torsion.

Torsion of a testicular appendage, an embryonic remnant of the developing gonad, may also present with acute swelling and pain, although the pain is usually less severe than that of testicular torsion. This condition is probably the most common cause of acute scrotal pain and swelling in the preadolescent boy. Occasionally, a "blue dot" discoloration may be visible through the skin of the affected testis (positive "blue dot sign"). Urinalysis and color Doppler ultrasonography yield negative results. Treatment is conservative, although the diagnosis is often made on surgical exploration for a suspected testicular torsion.

An incarcerated inguinal hernia may also present with painful swelling of the scrotum and should be suspected in any child who has a history of intermittent groin swelling. Immediate surgical referral is indicated. Occasionally, severe scrotal trauma may result in scrotal swelling. Urgent evaluation by an urologist is necessary to evaluate for a testicular hematoma or rupture.

Epididymitis is rare in the preadolescent boy and usually associated with a urinary tract anomaly. Urinalysis typically demonstrates pyuria. Orchitis is also rare in the preadolescent boy and may be caused by coxsackievirus, mumps, or echovirus. When caused by the mumps virus, orchitis usually follows parotitis within 1 week, although it may occur in the absence of salivary gland involvement. Treatment is typically conservative, but the infection may result in testicular atrophy and decreased fertility.

Leukemic infiltration of the testis represents one of the most common sites of relapse following complete bone marrow remission and may present either with painful or painless scrotal and testicular enlargement. Rarely, Henoch-Schönlein purpura, a systemic vasculitic disease characterized by abdominal pain, nonthrombocytopenic purpura, arthralgia, gastrointestinal bleeding, and renal disease, will present with acute, painful scrotal swelling. Treatment is conservative.

A varicocele, a dilatation of the venous plexus of the spermatic cord, rarely occurs prior to puberty. A palpable mass classically described as a "bag of worms" can be felt, usually above the left testis. The mass is accentuated by the standing position and may cause mild to moderate discomfort. Referral to an urologist is indicated if discomfort persists or if there is a discrepancy in testicular volume, in which case the varicocele may be affecting testicular growth, with adverse effects on fertility. A hydrocele is caused by the accumulation of peritoneal fluid inside a patent process vaginalis. Although most hydroceles resolve spontaneously between the ages of 12 to 18 months, occasionally one will remain undetected and present later in life. Surgical correction is indicated in some cases, especially when the hydrocele remains in communication with the peritoneal cavity and is likely to be associated with a hernia.

Testicular cancer most commonly affects males during late puberty to young adulthood. It presents usually as a firm, enlarged, nontender testicular mass. The combination of surgery and chemotherapy has improved survival significantly.

Acute idiopathic scrotal edema is a relatively uncommon condition characterized by the rapid onset of significant scrotal edema. Erythema may be present, and the edema may extend to the skin adjacent to the scrotum, perineum, abdomen, or penis. The condition is usually unilateral and the skin, mildly tender, although the underlying testis is not tender. It is most common in prepubertal boys, but cases in older boys and adults have been reported. Normal findings on physical examination of the genitalia, with the exception of a thickened, edematous scrotal wall, as well as normal results of urinalysis and color Doppler ultrasonography help differentiate this disorder from other conditions causing acute scrotal swelling. The etiology of acute idiopathic scrotal edema is unknown, although it has been suggested to represent a form of angioneurotic edema. The condition resolves spontaneously, without sequelae, in 1 to 3 days.

Management

In this case, ultrasonography of the scrotum demonstrated diffuse scrotal wall edema with normal scrotal contents. The mother of the patient was reassured that a diagnosis of testicular cancer was extremely unlikely. Bed rest was prescribed, and the condition resolved spontaneously without further problems.

Derek S. Wheeler, MD, United States Naval Hospital, Guam

COMMENTARY BY DR YEGAPPAN LAKSHMANAN, PEDIATRIC UROLOGIST, CHILDREN'S HOSPITAL OF MICHIGAN

A short course of oral steroid may be considered if the scrotal swelling does not seem to be improving after a period of 24 to 48 hours of observation.

CHAPTER 100

Persistent Flank Pain and Voiding Dysfunction in an 11-Year-Old Boy

Presentation

An 11-year-old boy presents with a long history of left flank pain and enuresis and a new finding of left renal atrophy. The patient's left flank pain began at age 3 years during potty training. At age 4 years, he underwent computed tomography and renal ultrasonography (RUS), which revealed a thickened bladder and a smaller left kidney (left kidney, 7.1 cm; right kidney, 8.0 cm). Urinalysis results were normal. A pediatric urologist at another institution thought the pain was musculoskeletal.

The patient's pain continued, and he was reevaluated at age 10 years when he began experiencing penile pain concomitant to the flank pain. Subsequent RUS revealed a lack of left renal growth. Voiding cystourethrogram (VCUG) was nondiagnostic because the patient could not void at that time. A technetium-99m-mercaptoacetyltriglycine scan revealed reduced radiotracer uptake on the left, which was consistent with a minimally functioning left kidney (13%) but good clearance of tracer bilaterally demonstrating no evidence of obstruction.

Our pediatric urology team was subsequently consulted out of concern for infravesical obstruction from posterior urethral valves (PUVs), leading to secondary, left-sided, vesicoureteral reflux (VUR). Voiding cystourethrogram findings (Figure 100.1) are abnormal in that the patient's bladder capacity was 500 mL, greater than expected given his age, and he required 2 attempts to void to completion. No dilation of the posterior urethra, as typically seen with PUV, or VUR, was identified.

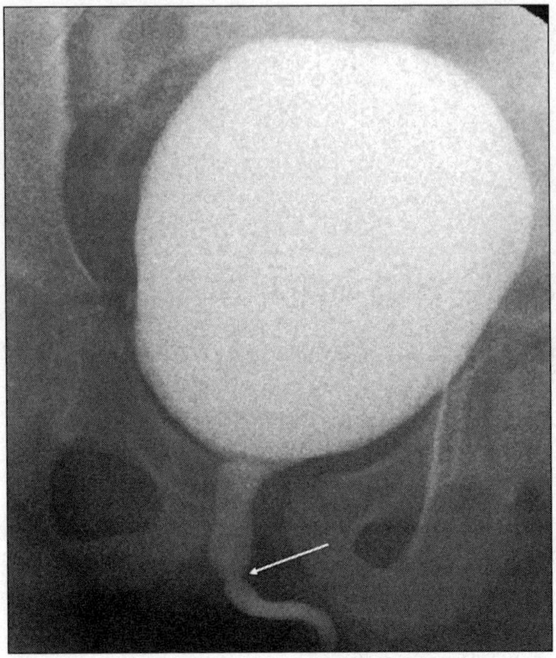

Figure 100.1. Voiding cystourethrogram shows elevated bladder capacity and normal urethra. Arrow indicates the sphincter.

Because of the patient's difficulty voiding and decline in renal function, the patient is taken to the operating room, where a cystourethroscopy is performed, revealing his diagnosis.

- **What is your differential diagnosis at this point?**
- **Are there any elements of history or physical examination that would help you?**
- **What additional diagnostic studies would you like performed?**

Discussion

On cystourethroscopy, a membranous structure was identified distal to the urethral sphincter, in the anterior urethra, consistent with anterior urethral valves (AUVs). This was resected endoscopically (Figure 100.2). The remainder of the urethra was without abnormality, and there was no evidence of PUVs. A Foley catheter was placed intraoperatively and left in place for 24 hours. Postoperatively, the patient has improved bladder emptying and is free of flank and penile pain. He continues to have occasional nocturnal enuresis.

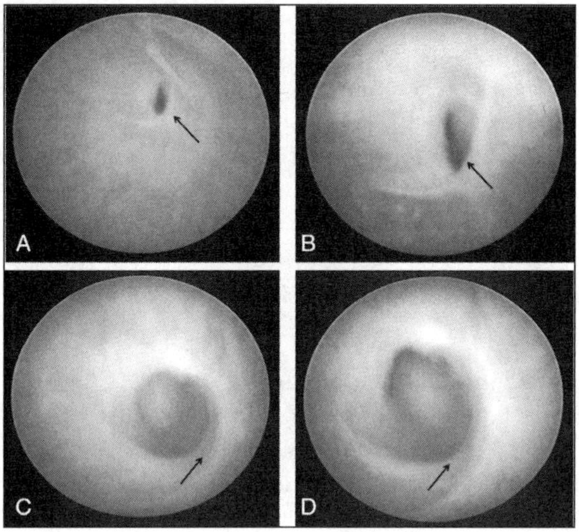

Figure 100.2. Endoscopic images revealing anterior urethral valves (arrow).

The Condition

Anterior urethral valves are a rare cause of urinary obstruction in boys, being 10 times less frequent than PUVs. They may occur at any portion of the anterior urethra, which begins at the level of the urogenital diaphragm and extends distally, with approximately 40% occurring in the bulbous urethra; 30%, at the penoscrotal junction; and 30%, in the penile urethra. They are frequently associated with urethral diverticula. Given their rarity, the pathophysiology behind an AUV is not well understood, although embryologic developmental anomalies, including aborted urethral duplication, incomplete hypospadias, ruptured syringocele, or Cowper duct cyst remnants, have been suggested as causes.

The severity of the disease varies widely, and symptoms have been categorized into 4 classes, ranging from cases with only mild proximal urethral dilation (class I) to those with severe upper tract involvement (class IV). It has been suggested that 30% of patients have associated VUR. Milder cases may present at an older age with a multitude of urologic symptoms, including urinary tract infection, penile swelling, enuresis, and postvoid dribbling. Severe cases present with urinary retention, hydronephrosis, renal failure, and bladder rupture. It is estimated that nearly one-third of patients with AUVs will present in the neonatal period, whereas half of all patients with AUVs will present by age 2 years.

The Diagnosis

Because the severity symptoms in patients with AUVs vary greatly, a high index of suspicion is required in evaluating for AUVs. In patients with symptoms of obstructive uropathy, initial diagnostic tests include RUS and VCUG. Renal ultrasonography may reveal bladder anomalies, including poor emptying or thickened bladder wall, or renal abnormalities, such as hydronephrosis or poor renal growth. On VCUG, an area of narrowing is classically seen at the level of the AUV with dilation of the urethra noted proximal to that level. Associated urethral diverticulum may also be seen on VCUG. Voiding cystourethrogram may also detect associated bladder involvement (diverticula, trabeculation, or elevated bladder capacities) or upper tract involvement (VUR). As with our patient, however, VCUG results may appear normal in patients with AUVs; it has been suggested that the presence of a catheter during VCUG can prevent full appreciation of anomalies of the anterior urethra.

If the VCUG result is negative but the index of suspicion remains high, VCUG may be performed again, or retrograde studies may be performed. Retrograde urethrogram may detect valves missed on VCUG, although the retrograde flow can compress the valves, giving the appearance of a normal urethra. Urodynamics may demonstrate decreased urinary flow consistent with obstruction. As in our case, endoscopic evaluation via cystourethroscopy may detect AUVs that have been missed on previous diagnostic studies.

Treatment

On initial diagnosis of AUVs, bladder drainage is a priority to prevent further damage to the bladder and upper tracts. Urinary catheters may be placed as a temporizing maneuver, although patients with AUVs require urologic intervention for definitive management of their disease.

Most patients with mild disease may be fully treated, as our patient was, with endoscopic resection. In patients with associated urethral diverticula, open repair with diverticulectomy may be required. Furthermore, these patients may undergo open resection of valves at the time of diverticulectomy, or they may warrant a formal urethroplasty, depending on the severity of the AUVs. In patients with severe disease with bladder pressures not adequately relieved by catheterization, vesicostomy may temporize the patient until he/she has grown enough for urethroplasty. Rarely, some patients with severe disease may not experience adequate relief of upper tract pressure despite adequate bladder drainage. Upper tract drainage via ureterostomy has been described.

Lessons for the Physician

- As with posterior urethral valves, urinary obstruction from anterior urethral valves (AUVs) may lead to bladder dysfunction and upper tract damage.
- Given the possibility of serious sequelae, AUVs are an important diagnosis to consider in children with common urologic symptoms, including difficulty voiding, weak stream, urinary tract infections, and enuresis.
- Endoscopic valve ablation can improve bladder function and symptoms in patients with AUVs.
- Urologic consultation is warranted in patients in whom conservative treatment, such as bladder and bowel treatment, behavioral therapy, and medication, fails.

Janae Preece, MD, Division of Urology, University of Maryland, Baltimore, MD

Kristina D. Suson, MD, Division of Pediatric Urology, The Johns Hopkins Hospital, Baltimore, MD, and Department of Urology, Children's Hospital of Michigan, Detroit, MI

Ming-Hsien Wang, MD, Division of Pediatric Urology, The Johns Hopkins Hospital, Baltimore, MD

Index

Page numbers with a *b* denote a box; an *f*, figure; and a *t*, table.

B

C

D

E

F

G

H

I

J

K

L

M

O

P

Q

R

S

T

W

X